THE

Vitamin Cure

THE
Vitamin Cure

Clinically Proven Remedies to Prevent and Treat
75 Chronic Diseases and Conditions

MONTE LAI, PhD

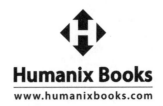

Humanix Books
www.humanixbooks.com

Humanix Books

The Vitamin Cure
Copyright © 2018 by Ching-San Lai
All rights reserved

Humanix Books, P.O. Box 20989, West Palm Beach, FL 33416, USA
www.humanixbooks.com | info@humanixbooks.com

Library of Congress Cataloguing-in-Publication data is available upon request.

Interior Design: Scribe, Inc.

Humanix Books is a division of Humanix Publishing, LLC. Its trademark, consisting of the word "Humanix," is registered in the Patent and Trademark Office and in other countries.

Disclaimer: The information presented in this book is not specific medical advice for any individual and should not substitute medical advice from a health professional. If you have (or think you may have) a medical problem, speak to your doctor or a health professional immediately about your risk and possible treatments. Do not engage in any care of treatment without consulting a medical professional.

ISBN: 9781630060954 (Trade Paper)
ISBN: 9781630060961 (E-book)

Printed in the United States of America
10 9 8 7 6 5 4 3 2 1

In memory of
Lawrence H. Piette

ACKNOWLEDGMENTS

This book is a culmination of over forty years of my academic and industrial work in which I engaged with an aim to find ways to improve health and wellbeing of the public. My interest in antioxidant vitamins dates back four decades when I was pursuing my Ph.D. degree in biophysics in late professor Lawrence H Piette's lab in Honolulu, Hawaii. Professor Piette who was the pioneer in the field of free radicals in biology and medicine was my mentor and inspiration in science. This book is dedicated to him.

I would like to thank all the people who provided their time and valuable advices when I worked in the pharmaceutical industry in San Diego. It is not possible to mention them all here, Timothy R. Billiar, M.D., Mike Ziegler, M.D, Marv Rosenthal, Ph.D., Chung Y. Hsu, M.D, Ph.D., George Gill, M.D, Fu-Tong Liu, M.D, Ph.D., Ferid Murad, M.D., Ph.D., the late Mitchell Fink, M.D and the late Leonard Arthur Herzenberg, Ph.D.

I also would like to express my appreciation to Ron Epstein, Ph.D. and Larry Wade for reading a part of the manuscript. This book would not be possible without relentless support and love of my son Shawn and my dear friend Hena Hsu. I wholeheartedly appreciate their enthusiasm and encouragement throughout the course of this work.

Poison is in everything, and nothing is without poison. The dosage makes it either a poison or a remedy.

Paracelsus (1493–1541)
Father of Toxicology

CONTENTS

Part Four: Prevention and Treatment

**Part Five: Summary of Recommended Daily Doses
of Vitamins and Essential Elements for Prevention
and Treatment of 75 Diseases and Conditions..............483**

INTRODUCTION

In the 1970s, Linus Pauling, a two-time Nobel laureate, recommended large doses of vitamin C to prevent and cure cancers. He himself was taking 8 g of vitamin C daily, and he was fit and healthy well into his 70s. Pauling's claim received tremendous media attention; he was frequently in the news. During that time, I was a graduate student pursuing my PhD in biophysics in Honolulu, Hawai'i. Pauling's media exposure was of particular interest to me because my dissertation investigated free radicals and antioxidants. High-dose vitamin C produces hydrogen peroxide, which kills cancer cells in the body. Recently, the National Institutes of Health (NIH) recommended intravenous high-dose vitamin C injections as a form of cancer therapy for treating certain advanced stages of cancer. Owing to my own research work, I had already become aware of the ways in which antioxidants like vitamin C and vitamin E work to scavenge harmful free radicals (molecules with unpaired electrons) in the body.

I continued my research work in the field of free radicals in biology and medicine after I joined the Medical College of Wisconsin in Milwaukee as a faculty member, devoting my research to nitric oxide, a gaseous free radical that is crucial for countless aspects of human health, ranging from the heart to the reproductive organs. In 1995, while taking a sabbatical leave, I decided to resign from my position as a full professor of biophysics at the medical school and serve as president and CEO of a new pharmaceutical company, focusing on the design and development of new drugs, in San Diego. Over the past two decades, I have acquired extensive knowledge in the pharmaceutical field by being at the forefront of the research on the pros and cons of therapeutic drugs in treating diseases and conditions.

Diseases and conditions can be divided into categories of *acute* and *chronic*. Modern medicine has done much in the field of acute conditions—such as trauma, infections, burns, bone fractures, or migraine attacks—but it has had limited success in treating chronic diseases like Alzheimer's, Parkinson's, or diabetes, among others. Therapeutic drugs for chronic diseases are largely designed to treat symptoms rather than causes.

Take type 2 diabetes as an example: Most diabetes drugs can lower blood glucose. But high blood glucose is a symptom, not a cause, of type 2 diabetes. Compare this to how a fever is a symptom rather than the cause of an infection—bacteria or viruses are the causes. Antipyretic agents that prevent or reduce fever, such as naproxen or acetaminophen, may control the fever, but they cannot eradicate the pathogen that causes the infection—the agents treat only the feverish symptom, not the causative pathogen. Likewise, diabetes drugs treat only the symptom of high blood glucose, not the cause of type 2 diabetes.

At present, the root causes of most chronic diseases are still elusive. Both genetic and environmental factors are known to play pivotal roles in etiologies of chronic diseases. Chronic diseases are often related to gene mutations. A single gene mutation rarely causes chronic disease; although people who carry a hereditary mutated gene may be at an elevated risk, it does not mean that they will inevitably suffer from the disease. Environmental factors are known to affect epigenetics (how our genes interact with the environment) as well as trigger the expression of predisposed hereditary genes. A nutrient-deficient diet and an unhealthy lifestyle are by far the two most important environmental factors associated with the causes of a host of chronic diseases. Conversely, a nutrient-rich diet and a healthy lifestyle can stave off chronic diseases.

You may have browsed through the internet or read a newspaper and found an article claiming that vitamins are effective in treating diseases. Yet several months later, you may have seen another news report make the opposite claim, suggesting that vitamins are not only useless but also possibly harmful to health. You might not know what to believe anymore. I am certain many people feel this way. Nowadays, information is readily available on the internet. With just a few keystrokes, you can find ample health-related data about vitamins and essential elements. Nevertheless, it is difficult to sort through all the available findings to build a reliable knowledge base that will improve your health and that of your loved ones. The aim of this book is to provide you with easily accessible, evidence-based knowledge about vitamins and essential elements for the prevention and treatment of chronic diseases.

Before you dive into the contents of the book, you need to know how clinical data are generated. First, several kinds of clinical studies exist. Let us start with the simplest one. A doctor prescribes vitamins to treat a patient suffering from a disease, and after taking vitamins for a few months, the patient recovers from the illness. The doctor publishes his findings in a scientific journal. This is called a "case study." If the doctor prescribes vitamins to a group of patients rather than a single patient and publishes his findings in a scientific journal, that is called an "observational study." On the other hand, if the same doctor publishes the findings of a study in which he divides his patients into two groups, in which one group receives vitamins and the other group receives a placebo, and neither the doctor nor the patients know who is taking vitamins and who is taking the placebo, that is called a "randomized controlled trial."

Many doctors and scientists worldwide are conducting clinical studies to test the effectiveness of vitamins for preventing or treating chronic diseases. For example, in the past 10 years, at least eight clinical studies have been published on the use of vitamin D for the prevention of osteoporosis. Although their topics and design might have been similar, these eight clinical studies produced different results and conclusions due to factors like patient selection, dosage, environment, and the like. Can vitamin D prevent osteoporosis? Of those eight clinical studies, which one should you believe?

Fortunately, a statistical method known as meta-analysis has been widely used to assess the efficacy of pharmaceutical agents in treating diseases. In the case of the abovementioned example, a meta-analysis would combine all the clinical data obtained from those eight clinical studies, excluding the data deemed to be biased, and analyze the remainder of the combined data to reach a statistical conclusion on whether vitamin D can or cannot prevent osteoporosis. Meta-analysis is currently the most reliable method for assessing the efficacy of vitamins or essential elements in preventing or treating chronic diseases. All the information on how vitamins and essential elements prevent and treat chronic diseases in this book is based solely on meta-analyses published in peer-reviewed scientific journals, not any single clinical study report.

This book contains five parts. Part 1 contains a brief history of the discovery of each of the 13 essential vitamins—namely, vitamin A, vitamin B1, vitamin B2, vitamin B3, vitamin B5, vitamin B6, vitamin B7, vitamin B9, vitamin B12, vitamin C, vitamin D, vitamin E, and vitamin K. Part 2 covers essential elements, including the five essential elements—calcium, potassium, sodium, magnesium, and phosphorus—as well as the eight essential trace elements, which are iron, zinc, manganese, copper, molybdenum, iodine, chromium, and selenium. Both parts 1 and 2 also present meta-analytic evidence of the efficacy of each vitamin/essential element in the prevention and treatment of diseases, its recommended daily allowance, and best food sources of it. Part 3 provides important secrets for staying healthy. These include an explanation of how sugar makes you fat, why patients with autoimmune diseases should not eat meat, and how exercise benefits the brain. Part 4 provides meta-analytic evidence of which vitamins and essential elements should be taken to prevent and/or treat 75 chronic diseases and conditions, including lung cancer, breast cancer, colorectal cancer, prostate cancer, endometrial cancer, blood cancer, bladder cancer, glioma, diabetes, stroke, heart disease, cataracts, hypertension, Alzheimer's disease, osteoporosis, arthritis, hepatitis C, fatty liver disease, Parkinson's disease, sleep apnea, and others. Part 5 summarizes the clinically proven remedies for preventing and treating the 75 chronic diseases and conditions presented in part 4.

For the purpose of easy reference, all vitamins, essential elements, secrets for staying healthy, and diseases in this book have been assigned a specific chapter number: vitamins are numbered from 1 to 13, essential elements from 14 to 27, secrets for staying healthy from 28 to 36, and diseases from 37 to 111. For example, vitamin A is 1, calcium is 14, and Alzheimer's disease is 37.

Author's disclaimer: The book provides readers with relevant health information about vitamins and essential elements, but it does not intend to be a substitute for any medical advice given to readers by health-care professionals. Efficacies of vitamins and essential elements in preventing or treating diseases may vary greatly among individuals. Recommendations from the book should not replace any nutrient-balanced diets or prescribed medications.

PART ONE

Vitamins

Vitamins are essential nutrients that the body does not make; therefore, they have to be obtained from foods. Some vitamins are derived from animal-based foods, while others are from plant-based foods. Only by consuming nutrient-balanced foods can one obtain sufficient amounts of all 13 vitamins—vitamin A, vitamin B1, vitamin B2, vitamin B3, vitamin B5, vitamin B6, vitamin B7, vitamin B9, vitamin B12, vitamin C, vitamin D, vitamin E, and vitamin K—to maintain good health. These 13 vitamins are distributed to various organs and tissues, and each one is involved in a multitude of essential physiological functions in the body. *Vitamin* literally means "being vital for life."

1

VITAMIN A (RETINOL)

Vitamin A is also known as the anti–dry eye vitamin. In 2000 BCE, physicians in ancient Egypt and Greece already knew that beef liver could cure night blindness. Of course, they had no way of knowing that this was because beef liver contains high amounts of vitamin A. In 1913, Lafayette Mendel and Thomas Osborne were able to isolate a "lipid-soluble" substance from chicken eggs and fish liver and called it vitamin A. In 1930, the chemical structure of vitamin A was identified as retinol.

Vitamin A enhances vision, allowing us to differentiate people from objects in our surroundings in dim light. In the eye, vitamin A binds to opsin, a photosensitive protein, to form rhodopsin. The photosensitivity of rhodopsin essentially establishes our eyesight and vision.

Vitamin A is also called the "anti-infective vitamin." The body's first-line defense against infections involves the skin, respiratory tract, digestive tract, and urinary tract. Vitamin A activates immune cells in these tissues.

Since our bodies cannot make vitamin A, it has to be obtained from foods. Preformed vitamin A and provitamin A are two kinds of vitamin A found in foods. Vitamin A from animal-based foods, such as beef liver, is preformed vitamin A, which the body uses promptly. Plants, such as carrots, contain carotenes. Carotenes are made up of provitamin A, which must be converted to vitamin A in the digestive tract before our bodies can utilize them.

What Are the Symptoms of Vitamin A Deficiency?

- *Xerophthalmia.* Xerophthalmia, or abnormal dryness of the conjunctive cornea of the eye, is the most common symptom in vitamin A–deficient children. Symptoms related to vitamin A deficiency in adults include night blindness and diminished adaptability of eyesight under dim light or at nighttime. In severe cases, patients might be afraid of driving or being outdoors alone at night because of their weakened vision.

- *Eye disease and blindness.* Severe vitamin A deficiency can cause blindness. Pregnant women deficient in vitamin A have an elevated risk of giving birth to babies with dry eye syndrome and even blindness. Globally, about half a million children suffer from blindness related to vitamin A deficiency; it is the most preventable cause of blindness in children. Hippocrates, the celebrated physician of Greek antiquity, told his patients who had eye diseases to eat cooked beef liver, which is rich in vitamin A.

- *Infectious diseases.* Infectious diseases can consume and deplete vitamin A stored in the liver, causing vitamin A deficiency. Measles infections depleting vitamin A can also lead to dry eye syndrome and xerophthalmia or even blindness in children.

- *Thyroid malfunction.* The thyroid gland produces thyroid hormones T3 and T4. T3 is the active form of the thyroid hormone, and vitamin A enhances the conversion of T4 to T3. Vitamin A deficiency can hinder this conversion and cause thyroid malfunction.

What Are the Causes of Vitamin A Deficiency?

- *Lipid malabsorption.* Lipids, or fats, facilitate the absorption of lipid-soluble vitamin A in the intestines, so lipid malabsorption can reduce the absorption of vitamin A, resulting in vitamin A deficiency. Lipid malabsorption is often caused by a blockage of pancreatic or gallbladder juice secretion, Crohn's disease, celiac disease, or inflammatory bowel disease.

Prevention and Treatment of Diseases

- *Prevention.* Meta-analysis confirms that vitamin A can prevent lung cancer (82), bladder cancer (44), stomach cancer (107), glioma (70), cervical cancer (50), asthma (38), and cataracts (49).
- *Treatment.* High doses of vitamin A can be used as an adjuvant therapy for treating blood cancers (45).

Which Food Items Are Vitamin A Rich?

Beef liver and fish liver oil contain high amounts of vitamin A. Milk and eggs are also excellent sources of vitamin A. Vegetables and fruits contain high levels of carotenoids.

This list of food items that are rich in vitamin A and beta-carotene is adapted from information provided by the USDA.

FOODS	PORTION	VITAMIN A CONTENT, IU	% DAILY REFERENCE VALUE
Beef liver (cooked)	1 slice (68 g)	21,566	431
Sweet potato (cooked)	½ cup	19,218	384
Pumpkin (cooked)	½ cup	19,065	381
Carrots (raw)	½ cup	10,692	214

continued

FOODS	PORTION	VITAMIN A CONTENT, IU	% DAILY REFERENCE VALUE
Spinach (cooked)	½ cup	9,433	214
Cantaloupe	½	9,334	187
Mango	1	3,636	73
Broccoli (cooked)	½ cup	1,207	24
Milk	1 cup	395	8
Eggs	1	270	5

Daily reference value of vitamin A is 5,000 IU according to the 2013 FDA food-labeling guidelines.

How to Calculate the Dosage of Vitamin A

International Units (IU) are commonly used to quantify vitamin A in food items and supplements.

- 1 IU of vitamin A is equal to 0.3 mcg of retinol
- 1 IU of beta-carotene is equal to 0.15 mcg of retinol
- 1 IU of beta-carotene in food is equal to 0.025 mcg of retinol

What Are the Recommended Dietary Allowances for Vitamin A?

1–3 years	1,000 IU
4–8 years	1,333 IU
9–13 years	2,000 IU
14 years and older	3,000 IU (men); 2,333 IU (women)

The upper daily intake limit of vitamin A is 10,000 IU.

Vitamin A Supplements

- *Dosage.* The common dosage for vitamin A supplements ranges from 5,000 to 25,000 IU. Vitamin A supplements can be taken either daily or weekly. The recommended dose is 3,000 IU daily or 20,000 IU weekly.
- *Types.* Vitamin A supplements are mainly composed of retinol, retinyl acetate, and retinyl palmitate. Their weight-to-unit conversion factors are as follows:
  - ○ 0.3 mcg of retinol is equal to 1 IU of vitamin A
  - ○ 0.344 mcg of retinyl acetate is equal to 1 IU of vitamin A
  - ○ 0.55 mcg of retinyl palmitate is equal to 1 IU of vitamin A
- *Fish liver oil.* Fish liver oil contains vitamin A, vitamin D, and omega-3 fatty acids, including EPA (eicosapentaenoic acid) and DHA (docosahexaenoic acid). There are two types of fish liver oil supplements: regular and fermented. Fermented fish liver oil supplements are more expensive compared to regular fish liver oil supplements. The fermentation process enhances the contents and purity of vitamin A, vitamin D, and the omega-3 fatty acids. The vitamin A in fish liver oil is a natural retinyl palmitate, which is the same as synthetic retinyl palmitate.
- *Melanoma.* Vitamin A can prevent melanoma. Clinical studies have shown that taking a dose of 4,000 IU of vitamin A daily for six months reduced the risk of melanoma by 40%. The protective effect was more profound in women than in men.
- *Wrinkles.* Vitamin A reduces wrinkles, making older skin look younger. Topical vitamin A at a dose of 0.4% applied three times weekly was effective in reducing wrinkles within weeks.

Safety Issues

- *Overdose.* Long-term consumption of high doses of vitamin A may cause hypervitaminosis A. Symptoms include blurred vision, lack of appetite, dry skin, and muscle weakness. High doses of vitamin A can cause liver damage as well as osteoporosis.

- *Pregnant women.* During pregnancy, women should take no more than 25,000 IU of vitamin A supplement daily to avoid hypervitaminosis A, which can lead to birth defects in infants.
- *Recommended daily dose.* Vitamin A is lipid-soluble and, once absorbed, will be retained in the body for a long time. It is recommended that you take no more than 10,000 IU of vitamin A per day.

What Types of Drugs May Interact with Vitamin A?

- Alcohol can exacerbate liver damage caused by high doses of vitamin A. Drinking alcoholic beverages with beef liver slices as a side dish is prevalent in some Asian cultures, which can lead to vitamin A toxicity. Furthermore, cholesterol-lowering drugs that hinder lipid absorption may also diminish vitamin A absorption.
- Long-term consumption of high doses of vitamin A can decrease vitamin K absorption, leading to vitamin K deficiency. Vitamin A enhances the drug action of warfarin. People who take warfarin to treat and prevent blood clots together with high-dose vitamin A should consult with health-care professionals.

2

VITAMIN B1 (THIAMINE)

Thiamine was the first B vitamin discovered; therefore, it was named vitamin B1. Vitamin B1 deficiency leads to beriberi disease. In 2600 BCE, ancient Chinese writings recorded the prevalence of beriberi disease in China. Dutch physicians in the 19th century noted that chickens fed only polished rice developed paralysis. Certain important nutrients seemed to be missing from polished rice. In the early 20th century, Casimir Funk isolated a water-soluble antineuritic substance from bran, the hard outer layer of cereal grain, and demonstrated that it could treat beriberi disease. He named the antineuritic substance "vitamine." *Vita* in Latin means "life," so a "vitamine" is required for life and was originally thought to be an amine.

Vitamin B1 obtained from foods is stored mostly in bones and muscles and the brain, heart, liver, kidneys, and other organs. Vitamin B1 participates in the conversion of carbohydrates and lipids into energy, and it is required for the synthesis of thiamine pyrophosphate, or TPP, a cofactor that is essential for a multitude of enzymes involved in energy production in the cell. Without TPP, the body would be unable to produce energy, leading to paralysis.

Which Diseases Are Associated with Vitamin B1 Deficiency?

Vitamin B1 deficiency can cause beriberi disease and Wernicke-Korsakoff syndrome. In addition, TPP deficiency may lead to neuro-degenerative diseases as well as hereditary metabolic malfunction.

- *Beriberi disease.* The two major types of beriberi are wet beriberi and dry beriberi. Wet beriberi affects heart and blood circulation, while dry beriberi damages the nervous system. In extreme cases, it can cause paralysis. Symptoms of beriberi also include dementia, waddling, and foot edema.
- *Wernicke-Korsakoff syndrome.* Vitamin B1 deficiency can exacerbate Wernicke-Korsakoff syndrome, an alcohol-induced nerve-damaging disease. Symptoms include memory loss, jerky eyeball movements, disorientation, and a staggering gait. Alcohol abstinence may reverse the course of the disease. Untreated, it can lead to psychosis and even death.

What Are the Causes of Vitamin B1 Deficiency?

- Major causes of vitamin B1 deficiency are insufficient intake from foods, malabsorption, transport malfunction, increased demand, or excessive loss. Diseases and conditions that elevate the risk of vitamin B1 deficiency include alcoholism, AIDS, digestive tract disease, liver disease, and severe vomiting. People who are on hunger strike or suffer from anorexia are prone to vitamin B1 deficiency.

Prevention and Treatment of Diseases

- *Treatment.* Meta-analysis confirms that vitamin B1 can treat heart failure (74). Vitamin B1 may also be effective in Alzheimer's disease (37), glaucoma (69), and cataracts (49).
- *Prevention.* Vitamin B1 may prevent cataracts (49) and type 2 diabetes (60).

Which Food Items Are Vitamin B1 Rich?

Vitamin B1–rich foods include beef, nuts, milk, oats, oranges, pork, eggs, and legumes. Vitamin B1–fortified foods include rice, spaghetti, breakfast cereals, bread, and flour. The recommended dietary allowance of vitamin B1 is only 1.5 mg, an amount readily obtainable from foods. However, vitamin B1 is water soluble; therefore, it cannot be stored in the body and needs to be replenished daily via food.

This list of vitamin B1–rich food items is adapted from information provided by the USDA.

FOOD	PORTION	VITAMIN B1 CONTENT, MG	% DAILY REFERENCE VALUE
Pork	3 ounces	0.81	54
Green beans	½ cup	0.21	14
Brown rice	1 cup	0.19	13
Walnuts	1 ounce	0.19	13
Hyacinth beans	½ cup	0.17	7
Oranges	1	0.11	7
Cantaloupes	½	0.11	7
Milk	1 cup	0.10	7
Bread	1 slice	0.10	7
Eggs	1	0.03	2

Daily reference value of vitamin B1 is 1.5 mg according to the 2013 FDA food-labeling guidelines.

What Are the Recommended Dietary Allowances for Vitamin B1?

1–3 years	0.5 mg
4–8 years	0.6 mg
9–13 years	0.9 mg
14–18 years	1.2 mg (boys); 1.0 mg (girls)
19 years and older	1.2 mg (men); 1.1 mg (women)

There is currently no upper intake limit for vitamin B1.

Vitamin B1 Supplements

- *Dosage.* The most common dosage for vitamin B1 supplements is 100 mg. Vitamin B1 is relatively safe, and so far, there is no known toxicity.
- *Types.* Vitamin B1 supplements are made of benfotiamine, thiamine hydrochloride, and thiamine mononitrate. Among them, benfotiamine has the best absorption rate in the intestines.
- *Diabetes.* Randomized controlled trials have shown that benfotiamine was effective in mitigating symptoms and complications associated with both type 1 and type 2 diabetes, such as peripheral neuropathy and pain. The suggested daily dose of benfotiamine is 200 mg (50 mg four times per day) for three months.
- *Heart failure.* Vitamin B1 can treat heart failure (74). The recommended daily dose is 100 mg.
- *Stress.* Vitamin B1 is also known as the "antistress vitamin." It boosts immune functions and regulates mood, thus increasing resistance to stressful conditions.

What Types of Drugs May Interact with Vitamin B1?

- *Digoxin.* Digoxin is a drug commonly prescribed to treat heart disease. Digoxin may interfere with the absorption of vitamin B1 by cardiac cells.

- *Diuretics.* Diuretics reduce the blood level of vitamin B1, thus increasing the risk of vitamin B1 deficiency. People who take diuretic medications to reduce the amount of water in the body should consider taking vitamin B1 supplements at a daily dose of 100 mg.
- *Antibiotics.* Antibiotics hinder the absorption of vitamin B1 by the intestines, thus reducing the blood level of vitamin B1.

3

VITAMIN B2 (RIBOFLAVIN)

Vitamin B2 is also called riboflavin. Its discovery has a colorful history. In the late 19th century, scientists discovered a bright-yellow fluorescent substance in milk. At that time, no one knew anything about this fluorescent substance. In 1930, Otto Warburg and his associates isolated the same substance in yeasts. They showed that it could repair damaged cells. In later years, Warburg's group confirmed that the bright-yellow substance was riboflavin. Since it was the second vitamin B discovered, it was called vitamin B2.

Riboflavin by itself has no biological activity. It is involved in the synthesis of two important cofactors, FMN (flavin mononucleotide) and FAD (flavin adenine dinucleotide), which support the activities of many enzymes in the body. These enzymes participate in energy production, drug metabolism, and toxin degradation. FAD is also involved in the antioxidant enzymatic reaction that gets rid of free radicals, preventing them from causing cellular and DNA damage. Glutathione is often thought of as the mother of all antioxidants in the body. Glutathione deficiency is common in many chronic diseases, including Alzheimer's disease, heart disease, stroke, cancer, and diabetes. FAD boosts glutathione levels and enhances the body's antioxidant capacity. It is also required as a cofactor for the synthesis of new red blood cells. Riboflavin insufficiency can hamper iron absorption and cause anemia.

What Are the Symptoms of Vitamin B2 Deficiency?
- The major symptoms of vitamin B2 deficiency include throat pain, fatigue, skin inflammation and peeling, swollen and inflamed lips, new blood vessels growing in the corneas, anemia, endocrine malfunction, and neurodegeneration.

What Are the Causes of Vitamin B2 Deficiency?
- *Diseases.* People with congestive heart disease and alcoholism are at high risk of vitamin B2 deficiency. Conversion of riboflavin to cofactors FMN and FAD is blocked in patients with hypothyroid disease and adrenalin insufficiency.
- *Insufficient intake from foods.* Milk, eggs, and meat are the major food sources of vitamin B2. Researchers in Poland revealed that among people aged 20–25, about 33.7% of women and 25% of men were vitamin B2 deficient due to insufficient intake of vitamin B2 from foods.

Prevention and Treatment of Diseases
- *Prevention.* Vitamin B2 may prevent cataracts (49), cardiovascular disease (48), lung cancer (82), breast cancer (47), and colon cancer.
- *Treatment.* Vitamin B2 may help treat migraines (88), hypertension (78), and corneal disorders.

Which Food Items Are Vitamin B2 Rich?
Milk and dairy products are excellent sources of vitamin B2. Animals' internal organs (e.g., liver, kidneys, heart) as well as plant-based

foods—such as nuts, legumes, and dark-green leafy vegetables—are good sources of vitamin B2. Vitamin B2–fortified foods include bread, spaghetti, and breakfast cereal.

This list of vitamin B2–rich food items is adapted from information provided by the USDA.

FOOD	PORTION	VITAMIN B2 CONTENT, MG	% DAILY REFERENCE VALUE
Lamb	3 ounces	3.90	229
Beef liver	3 ounces	2.90	170
Yogurt	1 cup	0.57	34
Milk	1 cup	0.45	26
Almonds	1 ounce	0.32	19
Eggs	1	0.26	15
Mushrooms	½ cup	0.23	14
Spinach	½ cup	0.21	12
Chicken	3 ounces	0.16	9
Beef	3 ounces	0.15	9

Daily reference value of vitamin B2 is 1.7 mg according to the 2013 FDA food-labeling guidelines.

What Are the Recommended Dietary Allowances for Vitamin B2?

1–3 years	0.5 mg
4–8 years	0.6 mg
9–13 years	0.9 mg
14–18 years	1.2 mg (boys); 1.0 mg (girls)
19 years and older	1.2 mg (men); 1.1 mg (women)

There is currently no known toxicity of vitamin B2 and no upper intake limit for vitamin B2.

Vitamin B2 Supplements

- *Dosage.* The most common dosages of vitamin B2 supplements are 50–100 mg, which is much higher than the recommended dietary allowance of 1.2 mg. Nevertheless, vitamin B2 is relatively safe, even when taken at high doses. Various B vitamins seem to act in synchrony and exert complementary effects in the body. If you are a vegetarian and need to take vitamin B2, you may consider taking a vitamin B complex supplement. Vitamin B is bright-yellowish in color, so you should expect your urine to turn bright yellowish when taking a vitamin B2 supplement.

- *Hypertension.* The MTHFR gene encodes methylenetetrahydrofolate reductase, an enzyme that is critical for folate metabolism, and vitamin B2 is required as its cofactor. Globally, about 10% of people have MTHFR gene polymorphic variants, while 20% of the people in northern China and 32% of all Mexicans carry variants of this gene. Certain MTHFR gene variants cause congenital hypertension, a condition that cannot be controlled by antihypertensive drugs alone. Clinical studies have shown that a combination therapy consisting of antihypertensive drugs and vitamin B2 lowered systolic pressure by 9.2 mmHg and diastolic pressure by 6.0 mmHg in patients with congenital hypertension. The suggested vitamin B2 dose is 1.6 mg daily for 16 months.

- *Migraine.* Vitamin B2 may mitigate symptoms during a migraine attack. Randomized controlled trials have shown that taking vitamin B2 reduced the incidence of migraine attacks and pain by 50%. In this case, the suggested vitamin B2 dosage is 400 mg daily for three months.

What Types of Drugs May Interact with Vitamin B2?

- Anticonvulsant drugs that prevent seizures and Adriamycin (doxorubicin), used to treat breast cancer, reduce the blood level of vitamin B2.

4

VITAMIN B3 (NIACIN)

Vitamin B3 is also known as niacin. Vitamin B3 deficiency can cause pellagra, which comes from the Italian word for "rough skin." In the late 15th century, Christopher Columbus and his fleets reached South America. Among other things, he brought corn seeds back to Europe. Corn became the main food in Spain, Italy, Egypt, and many other Southern European countries in subsequent centuries. Corn contains niacin, but it is tightly bound to its fibers. Cooking corn in boiled water does not release niacin from the fibers. For thousands of years, American Indians living in South America had developed ways to prepare corn by soaking and cooking it in alkaline lime water. At that time, they had no way of knowing that cooking corn in alkaline lime water released niacin from the corn fibers. Because Columbus brought back corn but not the native Indians' recipes, the consumption of niacin-poor corn caused vitamin B3 deficiency and thus a pellagra epidemic in southern Europe. Up until the 19th century, many Southern Europeans suffered from pellagra. In 1937, scientists discovered that niacin was effective in treating pellagra and called it "vitamin B3."

Niacin is involved in the synthesis of NAD and NADP coenzymes. These two coenzymes are essential for enzymatic reactions that convert proteins, lipids, and carbohydrates to energy in the cell. Without NAD and NADP, the body will not be able to produce the energy needed for maintaining the brain, heart, and muscles, as well as other bodily functions.

What Are the Symptoms of Vitamin B3 Deficiency?
- *Pellagra.* The major symptoms of pellagra are dermatitis, dementia, and diarrhea. Severe diarrhea exacerbates deficiencies in niacin and other nutrients. Pellagra patients with dermatitis generally avoid sun exposure and thus are inclined to stay indoors. Niacin deficiency–induced dementia was often misdiagnosed as psychosis. During the 17th–19th centuries, many pellagra patients in Europe were confined to madhouses. There, these patients continued consuming niacin-poor corn, further aggravating pellagra.
- *Tryptophan.* Tryptophan can be converted into vitamin B3 in the body. Tryptophan is a common amino acid found in all protein-rich foods. Many animal-based foods and plant-based foods not only are rich in vitamin B3 but also contain tryptophan. Nowadays, instances of vitamin B3 deficiency are rare.

Prevention and Treatment of Diseases
- *Prevention.* Vitamin B3 may alleviate osteoarthritis.
- *Treatment.* Vitamin B3 may decrease LDL and triglycerides and increase HDL.

Which Food Items Are Vitamin B3 Rich?
A variety of foods contain vitamin B3, including nuts, brown rice, whole wheat, oats, and legumes. Meat, milk, and fish are also excellent

sources of tryptophan. Vitamin B3–fortified foods may include breakfast cereals, bread, rice, and baked goods.

This list of vitamin B3–rich food items is adapted from information provided by the USDA.

FOOD	PORTION	VITAMIN B3 CONTENT, MG	% DAILY REFERENCE VALUE
Tuna	3 ounces	10.0	50.0
Turkey	3 ounces	10.0	50.0
Chicken	3 ounces	9.5	48.0
Salmon	3 ounces	8.5	43.0
Beef	3 ounces	7.3	37.0
Peanuts	1 ounces	3.8	19.0
Spaghetti	1 cup	3.1	16.0
Hyacinth beans	1 cup	2.1	11.0
Bread	1 slice	1.3	6.5
Coffee	1 cup	0.5	2.5

Daily reference value of vitamin B3 is 20 mg according to the 2013 FDA food-labeling guidelines.

What Are the Recommended Dietary Allowances for Vitamin B3?

1–3 years	6 mg
4–8 years	8 mg
9–13 years	12 mg
14–18 years	16 mg (boys); 14 mg (girls)
19 years and older	16 mg (men); 14 mg (women)

The upper daily intake limit of vitamin B3 is 41 mg for men and 35 mg for women.

Vitamin B3 Supplements

- *Dosage.* The most common dosages of vitamin B3 supplements are 100–500 mg, which well exceeds the daily upper limit of 35–41 mg. Common side effects of vitamin B3 include flushing, fever, and itching.
- *Types.* Vitamin B3 supplements contain niacin, nicotinic acid, inositol hexanicotinate, niacinamide, and nicotinamide riboside. Inositol hexanicotinate may lower LDL levels. Niacinamide can mitigate the symptoms of Alzheimer's disease, and nicotinamide riboside lowers LDL and blood glucose levels. These niacin-derived products are less likely to cause flushing or other side effects compared to niacin supplements.
- *Hypercholesterolemia.* Vitamin B3 can mitigate symptoms of hypercholesterolemia and osteoarthritis. The suggested daily dose is 1,000 mg.
- *Melanoma.* High-dose vitamin B3 can prevent melanoma. Australian studies have shown that people who took vitamin B3 supplements reduced their risk of melanoma by 23%. The suggested daily dose of vitamin B3 is 1,000 mg.

Safety Issues

- *Side effects.* High doses of vitamin B3 can cause flushing, itching, nausea, and vomiting, as well as high blood glucose and high blood levels of uric acid.
- *Diseases.* High doses of vitamin B3 increase the risk of type 2 diabetes and hepatitis. People with liver disease, ulcers, gout, or alcoholism should avoid taking high-dose vitamin B3 supplements. The sustained-release dosage form of niacin is also associated with potentially harmful side effects.

What Types of Drugs May Interact with Vitamin B3?

- *Statins.* Statins are the most commonly prescribed drugs to lower blood cholesterol levels. Muscle ache is a common side effect of statin drugs. Vitamin B3 supplementation exacerbates the muscle ache caused by statins.

- *Sulfinpyrazone.* Sulfinpyrazone is used as an antigout medication. Vitamin B3 can interfere with the drug's action.
- *Chemotherapy.* Chemotherapy can reduce blood levels of vitamin B3. Cancer patients who receive chemotherapy should consider taking vitamin B3 supplements.

5

VITAMIN B5 (PANTOTHENIC ACID)

Vitamin B5 is pantothenic acid. In 1933, Roger J. Williams discovered that an acidic water-soluble substance was essential for the growth and proliferation of yeasts. In 1939, scientists confirmed that the chemical structure of this acidic water-soluble substance was pantothenic acid and named it vitamin B5. *Panto* means "everywhere" in Greek, and pantothenic acid is a widely distributed nutrient in animal- and plant-based foods. In 1954, M. B. Hoagland and G. David Novelli found that vitamin B5 was the key precursor for the biosynthesis of coenzyme A, a cofactor that is essential for energy production in the cell and is one of the most important molecules for the survival of all living beings on the planet. Its prominent role in the life process equates to that of DNA. Coenzyme A allows the body to convert proteins, lipids, and carbohydrates from foods into energy. Energy sustains life. Without coenzyme A, no organism can survive on Earth.

What Are the Symptoms of Vitamin B5 Deficiency?
- The major symptoms of vitamin B5 deficiency are adrenal mal-function, dermatitis, enteritis, hair loss, and hepatic encepha-lopathy (liver disease causing a decline in brain functions). Various foods are rich in vitamin B5, so vitamin B5 deficiency is rare. Malnutrition and malabsorption are the main causes of vitamin B5 insufficiency.

Prevention and Treatment of Diseases
- *Treatment.* Vitamin B5 may decrease blood levels of LDL and triglycerides and increase blood levels of HDL. It may also mitigate the morning stiffness and pain associated with rheumatoid arthritis (102).

Which Food Items Are Vitamin B5 Rich?
Vitamin B5 is widely present in a variety of animal- and plant-based foods. Almost all kinds of foods contain vitamin B5. Animal-based foods like fish, eggs, milk, and other dairy products, as well as plant-based foods—such as vegetables, legumes, and whole wheat—are all excellent sources of vitamin B5.

This list of vitamin B5–rich food items is adapted from information provided by the USDA.

FOOD	PORTION	VITAMIN B5 CONTENT, MG	% DAILY REFERENCE VALUE
Beef liver (cooked)	3 ounces	5.60	56.0
Sunflower seeds	1 ounce	2.00	20.0
Trout (cooked)	3 ounces	1.90	19.0
Yogurt	8 ounces	1.60	16.0
Lobster (cooked)	3 ounces	1.40	14.0

FOOD	PORTION	VITAMIN B5 CONTENT, MG	% DAILY REFERENCE VALUE
Avocado	½	1.00	10.0
Sweet potato (cooked)	½ cup	1.00	10.0
Milk	8 ounces	0.87	8.7
Pork (cooked)	3 ounces	0.86	8.6
Chicken (cooked)	3 ounces	0.83	8.3

Daily reference value of vitamin B5 is 10 mg according to the 2013 FDA food-labeling guidelines.

What Are the Recommended Dietary Allowances for Vitamin B5?

1–3 years	2 mg
4–8 years	3 mg
9–13 years	4 mg
14–18 years	5 mg
19 years and older	6 mg (men); 5 mg (women)

There is currently no known toxicity of vitamin B5 and no upper intake limit for vitamin B5.

Vitamin B5 Supplements
- *Dosage.* The most common dosages of vitamin B5 supplements are 300–500 mg.
- *Cholesterol.* Vitamin B5 may lower cholesterol levels in the blood. The suggested daily dose is 1 g.
- *Rheumatoid arthritis.* Vitamin B5 may ameliorate the symptoms of rheumatoid arthritis. The suggested daily dose is 1 g.

Safety Issues

- *Side effects.* High doses of vitamin B5 might interfere with the absorption of vitamin B7 by the intestines.

What Types of Drugs May Interact with Vitamin B5?

- *Oral contraceptives.* Oral contraceptives can lower the blood level of vitamin B5.

6

VITAMIN B6 (PYRIDOXINE)

Vitamin B6 is also known as pyridoxine. In the 1930s, rats were commonly used as laboratory animals to study the nature of human diseases. Scientists noticed that rats developed a skin disease called "rat acrodynia" if fed with semisynthetic feeds containing thiamine and riboflavin but none of the other water-soluble nutrients. In 1934, Paul Gyorgy discovered that the skin disease disappeared if a water-soluble nutrient was added to the semisynthetic feeds. He called this new water-soluble nutrient "vitamin B6." In 1939, scientists confirmed that the chemical structure of vitamin B6 was pyridoxine. In subsequent years, pyridoxine was shown to be involved in the synthesis of PLP and PMP coenzymes.

PLP and PMP coenzymes participate in more than 100 different enzymatic reactions involved in various metabolic conditions, one of which is one-carbon metabolism. One-carbon metabolism has multiple functions in the body, the two most important of which are the methylation of DNA and synthesis of methionine. Vitamin B6, vitamin B9, and vitamin B12 are all involved in one-carbon metabolism. Vitamin B6 deficiency leads to insufficient methylation of DNA, which is a hallmark of cancer cells. In addition, vitamin B6 deficiency can hinder the synthesis of methionine, an essential amino acid. Methionine deficiency induces a high blood level of homocysteine, increasing the risk of cardiovascular diseases such as stroke and heart disease.

What Are the Symptoms of Vitamin B6 Deficiency?
- The major symptoms of vitamin B6 deficiency are peripheral neuropathy (causing damage to peripheral nerves), depression, epilepsy, anemia, and allergies. Many foods contain vitamin B6, so vitamin B6 deficiency is rare. Patients with kidney disease or kidney malfunction are at risk of vitamin B6 deficiency. According to the data from the Centers for Disease Control and Prevention, 10% of the US population is vitamin B6 insufficient.

Prevention and Treatment of Diseases
- *Prevention.* Meta-analysis confirms that vitamin B6 can prevent breast cancer (47), colorectal cancer (56), Parkinson's disease (96), renal cell cancer (100), and venous thrombosis (110). In addition, vitamin B6 may prevent coronary artery disease (57), stroke (108), heart disease (73), and depression (58).
- *Treatment.* Meta-analysis confirms that vitamin B6 can help prevent the recurrence of stroke (108). Vitamin B6 may also reduce vomiting during pregnancy and mitigate symptoms of depression (58).

Which Food Items Are Vitamin B6 Rich?
Vitamin B6 is a nutrient essential to maintaining the normal metabolism of red blood cells and the regulation of immune and neuronal functions. The body cannot produce vitamin B6; therefore, it has to be obtained from foods. Meats—such as chicken, beef, and pork—are

excellent sources of vitamin B6. Fish like cod, salmon, and trout are good sources as well. Many vegetables are also rich in vitamin B6, including bell peppers, spinach, potatoes, and broccoli.

This list of vitamin B6–rich food items is adapted from information provided by the NIH Office of Dietary Supplements.

FOOD	PORTION	VITAMIN B6 CONTENT, MG	% DAILY REFERENCE VALUE
Chickpeas	1 cup	1.1	55
Beef liver	3 ounces	0.9	45
Tuna	3 ounces	0.9	45
Salmon	3 ounces	0.6	30
Chicken breast	3 ounces	0.5	25
Potatoes (cooked)	1 cup	0.4	20
Turkey	3 ounces	0.4	20
Banana	1	0.4	20
Nuts	1 ounces	0.1	5
Spinach	½ cup	0.1	5

Daily reference value of vitamin B6 is 2 mg according to the 2013 FDA food-labeling guidelines.

What Are the Recommended Dietary Allowances for Vitamin B6?

1–3 years	0.5 mg
4–8 years	0.6 mg
9–13 years	1.0 mg
14–18 years	1.3 mg (boys); 1.2 mg (girls)
19 years and older	1.7 mg (men); 1.5 mg (women)

The upper daily intake limit of vitamin B6 is 100 mg.

Vitamin B6 Supplements
- *Dosage.* The most common dosages of vitamin B6 supplements are 50–100 mg.
- *Pregnancy.* Vitamin B6 may alleviate vomiting during pregnancy. The suggested daily dose is 30 mg.
- *Tardive dyskinesia.* Vitamin B6 is effective in treating tardive dyskinesia. Tardive dyskinesias are involuntary movements of the face, tongue, lips, trunk, and extremities caused by long-term medication with an antipsychotic drug, such as aripiprazole. The suggested daily dose of vitamin B6, in this case, is 250 mg.
- *Congenital homocystinuria.* Vitamin B6 may improve the symptoms of congenital homocystinuria patients who have an excess of homocysteine in the urine. The suggested daily dose is 250 mg.

Safety Issues
- *Side effects.* Taking doses of vitamin B6 higher than 2 g daily may be harmful to the nervous system. Symptoms include numbness of extremities, stabbing pain, and, in severe cases, difficulty walking.
- *Diseases.* High doses of vitamin B6 exacerbate the risk of heart disease, stroke, and death in patients with diabetes with kidney disease.

What Types of Drugs May Interact with Vitamin B6?
- *Oral contraceptives.* These can reduce the blood level of vitamin B6. Women who use oral contraceptives should consider taking vitamin B6 supplements.
- *Antihypertensive drugs.* Vitamin B6 enhances the effect of some antihypertensive drugs, such as diltiazem and amlodipine, and interferes with medications for treating Parkinson's disease.
- *Other medications.* Drugs like hydralazine to treat high blood pressure and heart failure, penicillamine to treat rheumatoid arthritis, and theophylline to treat respiratory diseases can cause vitamin B6 deficiency.

7

VITAMIN B7 (BIOTIN)

Vitamin B7 is biotin. The story of biotin is associated with raw egg whites. In 1927, Margarete Boas fed rats only raw egg whites and found that rats suffered from severe dermatitis, hair loss, and neuromuscular malfunctions. She called the disease "egg-white injury." In subsequent years, a water-soluble nutrient was isolated from beef liver. Rats fed this water-soluble nutrient recovered from the disease. In 1942, Vincent du Vigneaud confirmed that the chemical structure of the water-soluble nutrient was biotin, called "vitamin B7." Later, they discovered that raw egg whites contained avidin, a protein that binds tightly to biotin. Almost all biotin in raw egg whites is bound to avidin. Rats cannot absorb biotin that binds to avidin in raw egg whites, so when fed only raw egg whites, they suffered from biotin deficiency. Boiled egg whites would not present such a problem because once boiled, biotin in egg whites is released from avidin.

From an evolutionary point of view, avidin in eggs protects them against bacterial infections. Bacteria need biotin for growth and proliferation. However, biotin bound to avidin makes biotin unavailable to bacteria, guarding eggs against bacterial infections. Avidin in egg whites may allow oviparous animals to survive on Earth.

Vitamin B7 is an essential cofactor for five different carboxylases—enzymes that participate in the fixation of carbon dioxide from the air, activation of histone proteins, and gene expression. Carboxylase enzymes play an important role in transporting glucose into the cell and lowering blood glucose levels to avoid diabetes. Additionally, carboxylase is involved in fat deposition in the dermal layer of the skin, maintaining skin's moisture, elasticity, and smoothness.

What Are the Symptoms of Vitamin B7 Deficiency?
- Vitamin B7 deficiency can lead to a wide range of physiological abnormalities, including growth retardation, nervous system malfunction, skin disorders, depression, fatigue, delusions, numbness, and/or stabbing pain in the hands and feet. Other symptoms related to vitamin B7 deficiency include hair loss and a scaly rash in the eyes, nose, and mouth.

What Are the Causes of Vitamin B7 Deficiency?
- Various foods are rich in vitamin B7; thus, vitamin B7 deficiency is rare. Bacteria living in the human colon also make vitamin B7. Raw eggs contain avidin, which can hinder the absorption of vitamin B7. People who like to eat raw beaten eggs are at risk of vitamin B7 deficiency. Boiled eggs are safe. Vitamin B7 deficiency is common in patients who require long-term parenteral nutrition or who are on anticonvulsant medications.

Prevention and Treatment of Diseases
- *Treatment.* Vitamin B7 supplements may mitigate the symptoms of multiple sclerosis (89) and type 2 diabetes (60) and help avoid brittle nails and hair loss.

Which Food Items Are Vitamin B7 Rich?
Many animal- and plant-based foods contain vitamin B7. Animal-based foods rich in vitamin B7 include internal organs, such as liver

and kidneys. Egg yolks, oats, bananas, soybeans, nuts, milk, and wheat are excellent sources of vitamin B7.

This list of vitamin B7–rich food items is adapted from information provided by the USDA.

FOOD	PORTION	VITAMIN B7 CONTENT, MCG	% DAILY REFERENCE VALUE
Beef liver (cooked)	3 ounces	31.0	10.0
Eggs	1	25.0	8.3
Tomato	1 cup	7.2	2.4
Salmon (cooked)	3 ounces	4.5	1.5
Avocado	1	4.0	1.3
Pork (cooked)	3 ounces	3.0	1.0
Bread	1 slice	3.0	1.0
Cabbage	1 cup	2.0	0.7
Cheese	1 ounce	1.2	0.4
Raspberry	1 cup	1.1	0.3

Daily reference value of vitamin B7 is 300 mcg according to the 2013 FDA food-labeling guidelines.

What Are the Recommended Dietary Allowances for Vitamin B7?

Although vitamin B7 is considered an essential nutrient, bacteria living in the human colon make vitamin B7, which partially meets the body's needs.

1–3 years	8 mcg
4–8 years	12 mcg
9–13 years	20 mcg
14–18 years	25 mcg
19 years and older	30 mcg

There is currently no upper intake limit for vitamin B7.

Vitamin B7 Supplements
- *Dosage.* The most common dosages of vitamin B7 supplements are 2,500–5,000 mcg.
- *Diabetes.* Vitamin B7 can mitigate the symptoms of type 2 diabetes. The suggested daily dose is 7,000–15,000 mcg.
- *Nails and hair.* Many shampoos and nail polishes contain vitamin B7, claiming that it can repair brittle nails and prevent hair loss. Vitamin B7 is a water-soluble vitamin, which cannot penetrate the skin. Salon products containing vitamin B7 are ineffective in repairing brittle nails or preventing hair loss. However, Vitamin B7 taken orally may treat brittle nails and hair loss. The suggested daily dose is 2,500 mcg for six months.

Safety Issues
- *Side effects.* So far, there is no known side effect associated with vitamin B7.
- *Vitamin B5.* High doses of vitamin B5 may interfere with the absorption of vitamin B7 by the intestines.

What Types of Drugs May Interact with Vitamin B7?
- *Anticonvulsant drugs.* Anticonvulsant drugs can lower the blood level of vitamin B7. Patients who take such drugs should consider supplementation with vitamin B7.

8

VITAMIN B9 (FOLIC ACID)

Vitamin B9 is also known as folic acid. In 1941, Henry Mitchell isolated a water-soluble nutrient from spinach leaves. This nutrient was essential for the growth of *Streptococcus* bacteria. He called it folic acid from the Latin word *folium*, meaning "leaves," and found that it could cure megaloblastic anemia, a condition in which abnormally large red blood cells appear in the bloodstream. In the 1950s, scientists discovered that folic acid is involved in many enzymatic reactions. Recognizing its role as an essential nutrient, they named it vitamin B9.

Vitamin B9 participates in one-carbon metabolism involving the methylation of DNA and synthesis of methionine. A sufficient amount of vitamin B9 is needed to avoid incorrect synthesis of new DNA, which is of particular importance during the fetal and infant stages. Incorrect synthesis of DNA could lead to birth defects and growth retardation. The infants of pregnant women who are vitamin B9 deficient have a high risk of birth defects.

What Are the Symptoms of Vitamin B9 Deficiency?
- *Major symptoms.* The major symptoms of vitamin B9 deficiency are lack of appetite, weight loss, weakness, headache, irritability, and anemia. Vitamin B9 deficiency could retard growth in infants and children. Vitamin B9 deficiency during pregnancy can lead to premature births and new babies with neural tube defects.
- *Megaloblastic anemia.* Vitamin B9 deficiency can cause megaloblastic anemia, in which large, irregularly shaped red blood cells called megaloblastic cells circulate in the bloodstream.

What Are the Causes of Vitamin B9 Deficiency?
Insufficient dietary intake is the most common cause of vitamin B9 deficiency. Drinking alcohol and smoking could also lower the absorption of vitamin B9 in the intestines. Cancer and inflammation can deplete the stores of vitamin B9 in the body, resulting in vitamin B9 deficiency. Vitamin B9 is needed for the synthesis of DNA and production of new red blood cells in bone marrow. Vitamin B9 deficiency reduces the production of new red blood cells, leading to anemia.

Prevention and Treatment of Diseases
- *Prevention.* Meta-analysis confirms that vitamin B9 can help prevent breast cancer (47), lung cancer (82), colorectal cancer (56), renal cell cancer (100), bladder cancer (44), and pancreatic cancer (95). In addition, meta-analysis shows that vitamin B9 is effective in preventing hypertension (78), depression (58), chronic kidney disease (52), stroke (108), coronary artery disease (57), venous thrombosis (110), atherosclerosis (39), glaucoma (69), oral cleft (92), neural tube defects (90), recurrent stroke (108), and age-related macular degeneration (84).

- *Treatment.* Meta-analysis confirms that vitamin B9 can treat hypertension (78), depression (58), chronic pancreatitis (54), and atherosclerosis (39).

Which Food Items Are Vitamin B9 Rich?

Vitamin B9 is an essential nutrient for growth and regeneration in the body. Dark-green leafy vegetables like spinach, broccoli, kale, and asparagus and fruits—such as watermelons, oranges, and strawberries—are excellent sources of vitamin B9. Vitamin B9 supplementation curtails the risk of neural tube defects in infants. Therefore, since 1998, many governments have mandated domestic food manufacturing companies to fortify vitamin B9 in breakfast cereals, bread, spaghetti, rice, and the like.

This list of vitamin B9–rich food items is adapted from information provided by the NIH Office of Dietary Supplements.

FOOD	PORTION	VITAMIN B9 CONTENT, MCG	% DAILY REFERENCE VALUE
Beef liver	3 ounces	215	54
Hyacinth beans	½ cup	179	45
Spinach (cooked)	½ cup	155	29
Asparagus (cooked)	4	89	22
Rice (cooked)	½ bowl	77	19
Avocado	½ cup	59	15
Papaya	1 cup	52	13
Corn	½ cup	52	13
Tomato juice	1 cup	49	12
Orange juice	1 cup	47	11

Daily reference value of vitamin B9 is 400 mcg according to the 2013 FDA food-labeling guidelines.

What Are the Recommended Dietary Allowances for Vitamin B9?

1–3 years	150 mcg
4–8 years	200 mcg
9–13 years	300 mcg
14–18 years	400 mcg
19 years and older	400 mcg

The upper daily intake limit of vitamin B9 is 1,000 mcg.

Vitamin B9 Supplements

- *Dosage and types.* The most common dosages of vitamin B9 supplements are 400–800 mcg. Folic acid and folate are the two major types of vitamin B9 supplements. Folic acid is a synthetic product, while folate is naturally produced. Both types are readily absorbed in the intestines.
- *Fortification.* Worldwide, many countries fortify breakfast cereals, bread, and rice with vitamin B9. In the US, the fortification program has proven effective over the years and has successfully reduced vitamin B9 deficiency to only 1% of the population.
- *Pregnant women.* Pregnant women should take a vitamin B9 supplement at a dose of 400 mcg daily immediately after confirming their pregnancies.
- *Hypertension.* Folic acid could lower blood pressure and curtail the risk of stroke. The suggested dose is 800 mcg daily for four years.
- *Depression.* Antidepressants are less effective in patients whose blood levels of vitamin B9 are too low. Supplementation with vitamin B9 at a daily dose of 500 mcg has been found to improve the efficacy of Prozac in patients with depression.

Safety Issues

- *Side effects.* Long-term use of high-dose vitamin B9 could damage the kidneys and increase the risk of prostate cancer. The daily dose of vitamin B9 should not exceed 1,000 mcg.
- *Vitamin B12.* Both vitamin B9 and vitamin B12 are required for the production of new red blood cells in bone marrow. Deficiency of either vitamin B9 or vitamin B12 can cause anemia. Vitamin B9 taken at a daily dose of 400 mcg alone can alleviate the symptoms of anemia. Thus taking vitamin B9 supplements could potentially conceal the hidden problem of vitamin B12 deficiency, leading to permanent damage to the nervous system.

What Types of Drugs May Interact with Vitamin B9?

- Drugs like antacid medications, gallbladder juice inhibitors, diabetes drugs, anticonvulsant drugs, nonsteroidal anti-inflammatory drugs, and antibiotics may reduce the absorption of vitamin B9 by the intestines.
- Methotrexate is a prescription drug that treats cancers and rheumatoid arthritis. Taking vitamin B9 supplements reduces side effects associated with methotrexate without affecting its efficacy.
- Phenytoin is a medication used to treat epilepsy. Vitamin B9 can inhibit the efficacy of phenytoin. Patients who take phenytoin should consult with their physicians before taking vitamin B9 supplements.

9

VITAMIN B12 (COBALAMIN)

Vitamin B12 is cobalamin. In the mid-19th century, many people suffered from pernicious anemia characterized by the appearance of enlarged and irregularly shaped red blood cells in the bloodstream. This was considered a fatal disease until the 1920s. In 1926, George Minot and William Murphy discovered that beef liver was effective in treating patients with pernicious anemia. Together with George Whipple, they shared the 1934 Nobel Prize in Physiology or Medicine for their contribution. In subsequent years, a water-soluble substance isolated from beef liver was called the "extrinsic factor," and a protein produced in the stomach was called the "intrinsic factor." In 1948, scientists confirmed that the chemical structure of the extrinsic factor was cobalamin and named it vitamin B12. The intrinsic factor was required for the absorption of vitamin B12 in the intestines.

Among all vitamins, vitamin B12 has the largest molecular weight and contains cobalt. Vitamin B12 participates in the metabolism of almost all cells in the body. It is an essential cofactor for the enzymatic conversion of homocysteine to methionine. Vitamin B12 deficiency can lead to high blood levels of homocysteine, increasing the risk of cardiovascular diseases. Vitamin B12 is also a cofactor for the enzymatic conversion of lipids and proteins to cellular energy and in the synthesis of new red blood cells.

What Are the Symptoms of Vitamin B12 Deficiency?

Vitamin B12 deficiency can lead to anemia, damage the nervous system, and, in men, lower sperm count. The major symptoms are fatigue, stabbing pain and numbness of the extremities, gait disturbance, and even the inability to walk. According to data from the Centers for Disease Control and Prevention, 2% of the US population and 4% of elderly people in the US are vitamin B12 deficient.

What Are the Causes of Vitamin B12 Deficiency?

- *Malabsorption.* Malabsorption is the major cause of vitamin B12 deficiency. The absorption of vitamin B12 in the intestines is unique. First, stomach acid is required to dissolve and release vitamin B12 from foods. The "free" vitamin B12 then binds the intrinsic factor in the stomach to form a complex that is absorbed by the intestines. Insufficient stomach acid or intrinsic factor could hinder the absorption of vitamin B12 in the intestines, resulting in vitamin B12 deficiency.
- *Atrophic gastritis.* About 10–30% of people aged 60 and older are afflicted by atrophic gastritis. Atrophic gastritis is caused by autoimmune disorders, resulting in immune cells wrongly attacking stomach cells. Atrophic gastritis lowers vitamin B12 absorption, leading to vitamin B12 deficiency. Furthermore, individuals age 60 and older have less stomach acid. Insufficient stomach acid affects the release of vitamin B12 from

ingested foods, reduces the absorption of vitamin B12 in the intestines, and increases the risk of vitamin B12 deficiency.

Which Diseases Are Associated with Vitamin B12 Deficiency?

- *Pernicious anemia.* Vitamin B12 is an essential nutrient for the synthesis of new red blood cells in bone marrow. Vitamin B12 deficiency can cause pernicious anemia, a condition that cannot be reversed by iron supplementation. Anemia often is the earliest sign of vitamin B12 deficiency. Pernicious anemia may be due to vitamin B12 deficiency or lack of intrinsic factor, which is required for vitamin B12 absorption in the intestines. Deficiency of either vitamin B12 or intrinsic factor can lead to pernicious anemia.

- *Nervous system disorders.* Vitamin B12 deficiency triggers numbness in the extremities, memory loss, unconsciousness, and difficulty walking, and in severe cases, it can permanently damage the nervous system. People who take more than 400 mcg of a vitamin B9 supplement a day should be concerned about the potentially hidden problem of vitamin B12 deficiency. Vitamin B9 may cure anemia, but not the underlining problem of vitamin B12 deficiency. Vitamin B12 deficiency often goes unnoticed until the nervous system is permanently damaged.

- *Digestive system retardation.* Stomach surgery or digestive system disorder can cause vitamin B12 deficiency. Lack of appetite and constipation are early signs of vitamin B12 deficiency.

Prevention and Treatment of Diseases

- *Prevention.* Meta-analysis confirms that vitamin B12 can help prevent colorectal cancer (56), renal cell cancer (100), cervical cancer (50), multiple sclerosis (89), depression (58), and venous thrombosis (110).

- *Treatment.* Meta-analysis reveals that vitamin B12 can help treat and prevent recurrent stroke (108).

Which Food Items Are Vitamin B12 Rich?

The human body cannot produce or store vitamin B12; therefore, it needs to be obtained from foods. Vitamin B12 mainly comes from animal-based foods. Plant-based foods such as mushrooms and miso also contain vitamin B12.

This list of vitamin B12–rich food items is adapted from information provided by the NIH Office of Dietary Supplements.

FOOD	PORTION	VITAMIN B12 CONTENT, MCG	% DAILY REFERENCE VALUE
Oyster	3 ounces	84.0	1,400
Beef liver	3 ounces	71.0	1,178
Trout	3 ounces	5.4	90
Tuna	3 ounces	2.5	42
Cod	3 ounces	1.8	30
Beef	3 ounces	1.4	23
Milk	1 cup	1.2	18
Cheese	1 ounce	0.9	15
Eggs	1	0.6	10
Chicken	3 ounces	0.3	5

Daily reference value of vitamin B12 is 6 mcg according to the 2013 FDA food-labeling guidelines.

What Are the Recommended Dietary Allowances for Vitamin B12?

1–3 years	0.9 mcg
4–8 years	1.2 mcg
9–13 years	1.8 mcg
14–18 years	2.4 mcg
19 years and older	2.4 mcg

There is currently no upper intake limit for vitamin B12.

Vitamin B12 Supplements
- *Dosage.* The most common dosages of vitamin B12 supplements are 500–1,000 mcg.
- *Types.* Two major types of vitamin B12 supplements are cyanocobalamin and methylcobalamin. The former is synthetic and the latter naturally produced. In the intestines, cyanocobalamin is converted to methylcobalamin in a two-step process. First, cyanide is removed from cyanocobalamin to produce cobalamin, and then cobalamin is methylated to produce methylcobalamin. In the process, cyanide is released from cyanocobalamin, and though it's only a small amount, cyanide is a toxin. So methylcobalamin is safer than cyanocobalamin, even though the former is more expensive than the latter.
- *Vegetarians.* Vitamin B12 comes predominantly from animal-based foods, not from plant-based ones. Vegetarians should consider taking vitamin B12 supplementation at a dosage of 100 mcg daily or 700 mcg weekly.
- *Elderly.* Supplementation with vitamin B12 is recommended for individuals aged 60 and older, particularly for those who take antacid medications.
- *Cognitive decline.* Vitamin B12 may prevent age-related cognitive decline. The suggested daily dose is 100 mcg.

What Types of Drugs May Interact with Vitamin B12?
- Drugs like omeprazole, ranitidine, colchicine, and metformin reduce the absorption of vitamin B12 through the intestines.

10

VITAMIN C
(ASCORBIC ACID)

Vitamin C is also known as ascorbic acid. Vitamin C deficiency causes scurvy. As early as 3000 BCE, a scurvy epidemic was recorded in Egypt. In 1753, James Lind demonstrated experimentally that fruit consumption could alleviate scurvy in sailors during a long sea voyage. In 1854, the English court enacted laws stipulating that all sailors during long sea voyages be given a daily portion of fruits. In 1928, Albert Szent-Györgyi isolated a six-member carbon compound from the adrenal gland, oranges, and cabbage. In 1932, his research group demonstrated that this water-soluble substance could cure scurvy, and they named it ascorbic acid. Szent-Györgyi was awarded the 1937 Nobel Prize in Physiology or Medicine for his contributions.

Some mammals—such as monkeys, cows, sheep, and dogs—can produce vitamin C in the body. They do not have to rely on foods for vitamin C. Humans cannot produce vitamin C because we do not have an enzyme in the liver required for the de novo synthesis of vitamin C; thus, we need to acquire it from plant-based foods.

Vitamin C is an electron donor, a chemical entity that donates electrons to another chemical entity. All functions of vitamin C in the body are related to this electron donor property. Vitamin C can donate electrons to at least 12 different enzymes that are responsible for many physiological functions. One of these enzymes is involved in the synthesis of collagen. Collagens are the major proteins in the skin, cartilage, tendons, ligaments, and blood vessels.

Vitamin C can also donate electrons to free radicals. After accepting electrons from vitamin C, free radicals are neutralized and can no longer harm the cell. Vitamin C protects DNA, proteins, and lipids in the cell from free radical–induced oxidative damage. Vitamin C participates in many other physiological functions, including accelerating wound healing, repairing and maintaining healthy bones and teeth, and enhancing iron absorption in the intestines.

What Are the Symptoms of Vitamin C Deficiency?

- *Scurvy.* Severe vitamin C deficiency causes scurvy, characterized by subcutaneous bleeding, hair and tooth loss, swollen joints, impaired wound healing, and even death. Nowadays, scurvy is a rare disease restricted only to a high-risk group that includes cancer patients with cachexia, a wasting syndrome in which patients lose weight and experience a decline in overall health and malnutrition. Alcoholics, drug abusers, and institutionalized elderly people are also especially vulnerable.

- *Vitamin C insufficiency.* Vitamin C insufficiency implies the blood level of vitamin C is insufficient, although it has not reached the deficient state. The symptoms of vitamin C insufficiency include dry and cracked hair, periodontal disease, easy bruising, nosebleed, and bacterial infections.

Prevention and Treatment of Diseases

- *Prevention.* Meta-analysis confirms that vitamin C can prevent breast cancer (47), renal cell cancer (100), bladder cancer (44), stomach cancer (107), cervical cancer (50), esophageal cancer (64), endometrial cancer (63), Alzheimer's disease (37), gout (71), stroke (108), cervical intraepithelial neoplasia (51), cataracts (49), exercise-induced bronchoconstriction (65), atrial fibrillation (40), and sleep apnea (106).
- *Treatment.* Meta-analysis confirms that vitamin C can treat breast cancer (47), hypertension (78), cardiovascular disease (48), asthma (38), hemodialysis (75), sleep apnea (106), and hypercholesterolemia (77).

Can Vitamin C Prevent or Treat the Common Cold?

Can vitamin C prevent you from catching a cold? This is still an unsettled question, taking a vitamin C supplement seems to prevent athletes from catching a cold, but it will not protect nonathletes. However, taking a vitamin C supplement soon after catching a cold may alleviate cold symptoms and accelerate the recovery. The recommended daily dose is 1,000 mg of vitamin C.

Which Food Items Are Vitamin C Rich?

Plant-based foods, such as fruits and vegetables, are excellent sources of vitamin C. Fruits—including oranges, grapefruits, lemons, limes, papayas, strawberries, pineapples, cantaloupes, and raspberries—are rich in vitamin C. Vegetables—such as broccoli, kale, potatoes, sweet potatoes, tomatoes, bell peppers, and cauliflower—contain high amounts of vitamin C.

This list of vitamin C–rich food items is adapted from information provided by the USDA.

FOOD	PORTION	VITAMIN C CONTENT, MG	% DAILY REFERENCE VALUE
Red bell pepper	½ cup	95	158
Kiwi	1	91	152
Strawberry	1 cup	85	142
Orange juice	¾ cup	78	130
Orange	1	70	117
Grapefruit juice	¾ cup	66	110
Broccoli (cooked)	½ cup	51	85
Potato	1	17	28
Tomato	1	16	27
Spinach (raw)	1 cup	8	13

Daily reference value of vitamin C is 60 mg according to the 2013 FDA food-labeling guidelines.

What Are the Recommended Dietary Allowances for Vitamin C?

1–3 years	15 mg
4–8 years	25 mg
9–13 years	45 mg
14–18 years	75 mg (boys); 65 mg (girls)
19 years and older	90 mg (men); 75 mg (women)

The upper daily intake limit of vitamin C is 2,000 mg.

Vitamin C Supplements

- *Dosage.* The most common dosages of vitamin C supplements are 50–1,000 mg. Vitamin C supplementation has beneficial effects on health, but high-dose vitamin C supplements can cause diarrhea and other digestive problems. Avoid taking more than 2,000 mg of vitamin C per day.

- *Types.* Various vitamin C supplements are available in the marketplace. Although there are many different kinds, they are all similar in regard to bioavailability. There is no evidence that one product is better than the other in terms of their absorption or efficacy. Ascorbic acid and sodium ascorbate are the two most common vitamin C supplements. Vitamin C palmitate converts to vitamin C and palmitate in the intestines. Some manufacturers claim that their products contain a 100% "reduced form" of vitamin C. The fact is that all vitamin C supplements contain only the "reduced form" if manufactured properly.

- *Liposomal vitamin C.* Liposomal vitamin C is a lipid formulation in which water-soluble vitamin C is encapsulated in liposomes made of phospholipids. The logic behind the design was that the encapsulation of vitamin C in a liposomal form could enhance its absorption in the intestines, thereby elevating the blood level of vitamin C. However, the clinical data so far do not seem to support such claims. If you need to take a vitamin C supplement, choose ascorbic or sodium ascorbate. You do not need to purchase expensive products like liposomal vitamin C.

- *Cataracts.* Vitamin C may prevent cataracts and mitigate the condition. Studies from England have shown that taking a vitamin C supplement at a dose of 250 mg daily for 10 years curtailed the risk of cataracts.

- *Smoking.* Cigarette smoke can deplete vitamin C in the lungs as well as the rest of the body, causing insufficient vitamin C and free radical–mediated oxidative stress. It is imperative that smokers take vitamin C supplementation to avoid vitamin C insufficiency and its deleterious consequences.

- *Hypertension.* Vitamin C supplementation can lower blood pressure, and this beneficial effect is more robust in hypertensive patients. Vitamin C reduces blood pressure through inhibition of endothelin-1, a vasoactive protein that elevates blood pressure.

- *Gout.* Vitamin C supplements may alleviate gout symptoms. The suggested daily dose is 500 mg of vitamin C.
- *Premature mortality.* Vitamin C may decrease the risk of premature death and increase life expectancy. Studies from the US have shown that vitamin C supplementation or sufficient dietary intake of vitamin C could prolong one's life-span. The suggested daily dose is 500 mg of vitamin C.
- *Preeclampsia.* Vitamin C taken together with vitamin E can lower the risk of preeclampsia in pregnant women. Symptoms of preeclampsia include hypertension, edema, and renal problems. The suggested daily doses are 500 mg of vitamin C and 100 IU of vitamin E.
- *Bruises.* Vitamin C supplements can help prevent bruising. The suggested daily dose is 500 mg of vitamin C.
- *Cancers.* High-dose intravenous vitamin C therapy is effective in treating certain types of cancers, particularly in terminally ill cancer patients who have refused any further chemotherapy. (See chapter 47, "Breast Cancer," for details.)

Safety Issues
- *Side effects.* High-dose vitamin C supplementation may increase the risk of cataracts and kidney stones. Vitamin C can be converted to oxalate, which forms oxalate crystals, leading to kidney stones. Studies from Switzerland have shown that taking a vitamin C supplement at a daily dose of 1,000 mg increases one's risk of kidney stones by 66%. Another study from Sweden shows that taking a vitamin C supplement at a dose of 1,000 mg for 10 years increases the risk of cataracts by 25%.
- *Iron.* Vitamin C boosts the absorption of iron by the intestines. People who take iron supplements together with vitamin C supplements need to monitor their blood iron levels to avoid problems associated with iron overload.

What Types of Drugs May Interact with Vitamin C?

- *Oral contraceptives and aspirin.* Both oral contraceptives and aspirin can reduce the blood level of vitamin C.
- *Acetaminophen (Tylenol).* Vitamin C increases the blood level of acetaminophen and exacerbates acetaminophen-induced liver damage. People who take vitamin C supplements together with acetaminophen need to be aware of the potential problems associated with liver damage.
- *Anticoagulants.* Vitamin C decreases the efficacy of anticoagulant drugs such as warfarin and heparin.

11

VITAMIN D (SUNSHINE VITAMIN)

Vitamin D is also known as the sunshine vitamin. The history of vitamin D is associated with rickets. In the late 17th century, Dutch physicians noticed the prevalence of rickets, a condition characterized by bent and deformed bones and enlarged joints in the hands and feet. In severe cases, patients with rickets had difficulty breathing. In the mid-19th century, many countries in Europe were in the midst of the Industrial Revolution, during which factory buildings were widespread and an abundance of coal was burned in public places as well as in houses for cooking and heating. Severe air pollution often blocked ultraviolet light from the sun's rays. In addition, many Europeans worked in sweatshops devoid of sunlight. Rickets became an epidemic.

From the 19th to 20th centuries, there were several major breakthroughs in research on rickets. These included the discovery that city dwellers were more likely to be afflicted by the disease compared to people who lived in the countryside, that the lack of sun exposure caused it, and that fish liver oil could cure it. In 1922, Elmer McCollum confirmed that the lipid-soluble substance in fish liver oil that cured rickets was not vitamin A but an unknown substance he named vitamin D. In 1936, Adolf Windaus confirmed that the chemical structure of vitamin D was calciferol.

Upon sun exposure, human skin produces vitamin D. Strictly speaking, the body produces vitamin D; therefore, vitamin D is not an essential nutrient. Nevertheless, vitamin D produced by the skin is not sufficient for the needs of most people. Intake from foods or supplementation is necessary to ensure optimal health. Vitamin D produced by the skin or from foods is activated in the liver to produce 25-hydroxyvitamin D. Also known as "25(OH)D," 25-hydroxyvitamin D is the major circulating form of vitamin D in the bloodstream, and it is commonly used to assess the blood level of vitamin D. It in turn is further activated in the kidneys to become 1,25-hydroxyvitamin D, the active form of vitamin D, which is involved in hundreds of gene expressions and numerous physiological functions.

What Are the Major Functions of Vitamin D?
- *Calcium homeostasis.* Concentrations of calcium are closely regulated in the body, and calcium homeostasis is related to normal physiological functions in the nervous system, bones, muscles, and many other organs. To maintain good health, it is of foremost importance to carefully control calcium concentration in the body. Vitamin D enhances the deposition of calcium in the bones, while parathyroid hormones release calcium from the bones. The interplay between vitamin D and parathyroid hormones controls calcium concentration in the body.
- *Phosphorus homeostasis.* Similarly, concentrations of phosphorus ions influence many normal physiological functions in muscles, bones, and other organs in the body. When phosphorus levels are low in the blood, vitamin D instructs the intestines to increase absorption of phosphorus ions, and when the phosphorus ion levels are too high, parathyroid hormones

instruct the kidneys to excrete excessive phosphorus ions in the urine.

- *Cell proliferation and differentiation.* Proliferation is a self-replication process by which a cell multiplies and produces more cells, and differentiation is like assigning a given cell specific tasks to perform. When proliferation is dominant, differentiation will be slow, and vice versa. Uncontrollable proliferation can lead to cancer. Vitamin D promotes cell differentiation and prevents cell proliferation to curtail the risk of tumor formation.

- *Immune system.* Many immune cells—including monocytes, macrophages, and T cells—have their own vitamin D activation processes through which the active form of vitamin D influences the gene expression of immune cells. Vitamin D enhances innate immunity (general immune defense) and inhibits autoimmunity (misdirected immune responses). Vitamin D deficiency increases susceptibility to autoimmune disorders.

- *Insulin secretion.* The active form of vitamin D enters pancreatic cells, regulates gene expression in pancreatic cells, and stimulates secretion of insulin from pancreatic cells.

What Are the Symptoms of Vitamin D Deficiency?
Vitamin D deficiency causes rickets in children (103) and osteomalacia in adults.

- *Rickets.* Vitamin D promotes the mineralization of calcium phosphate in the bones, increasing bone density and strength. The bones of children with vitamin D deficiency may grow in length but lack mineralization of calcium phosphate, resulting in soft and porous bones. Such bones cannot support the weight of the body and become bent and deformed. This is known as rickets.

- *Osteomalacia.* Calcium in bones exists in a homeostatic state—an equilibrium of deposition and removal. Vitamin D deficiency causes removal rather than deposition of calcium in the bones, triggering loss of bone density and, in severe cases, resulting in osteomalacia, or soft bone disease, which is characterized by aching pain in the lower back, pelvis, hips, legs, and ribs in adults. Osteomalacia can lead to osteoporosis.

What Are the Risk Factors for Vitamin D Deficiency?

- *Geography.* The closer a place is to the equator, the stronger the intensity of ultraviolet light from the sun. Therefore, people who live closer to the equator have a lower risk of vitamin D deficiency compared to those who live farther away from the equator. Indeed, people who live at the 43rd parallel north and farther are more susceptible to vitamin D deficiency. In those regions, every year from October to April, ultraviolet light from the sun cannot reach the surface of the Earth, so the skin ceases to produce vitamin D, increasing the risk of deficiency.
- *Sun protection.* Except beachgoers and those who love outdoor activities, most people try to avoid sun exposure. Sun umbrellas, hats, long sleeves, long pants, and sunscreen are common remedies to shun sun exposure. Excessive avoidance of the sun can cause vitamin D deficiency.
- *Infants fed with breast milk.* The vitamin D content of breast milk is relatively low. Infants who are born to Asian and African families in the northern hemisphere are at especially high risk of vitamin D deficiency. A daily dose of 400 IU is recommended for infants to avoid vitamin D deficiency.
- *Obesity.* Vitamin D is a lipid-soluble vitamin. Upon absorption in the intestines, vitamin D dissolved in chylomicrons (fat globules) is transported to the liver and other organs in the body. In the bloodstream, vitamin D binds to a vitamin D–binding protein, which is then absorbed by fat tissue. In other words, in obese individuals, vitamin D is mostly stored in fat tissue, while the rest of the body is devoid of vitamin D, causing vitamin D deficiency. Weight loss is the only way to release it from fat tissue and increase vitamin D levels.

- *Chronic kidney disease.* An enzyme in the kidneys is required for final activation of vitamin D in the body, which creates the active form of vitamin D. Chronic kidney disease hinders the activation of vitamin D in the kidneys, resulting in vitamin D deficiency.
- *Enteritis (inflammation of the small intestine).* Inflammatory bowel diseases—such as ulcerative colitis, Crohn's disease, and fat malabsorption—may lower the absorption of vitamin D in the intestines, aggravating the risk of vitamin D deficiency.

Do I Need Sun Exposure?
Vitamin D has a host of health benefits, including maintaining healthy bones and lowering the risk of heart disease, stroke, asthma, inflammation, and autoimmune diseases. Vitamin D also may extend life expectancy.

The amount of sun exposure required to produce an adequate amount of vitamin D depends on the color of your skin and where you live. For example, to produce 1,000 IU of vitamin D in Chicago, Caucasians require 15 minutes, Asians and Hispanics 30 minutes, and Africans 2 hours. The best time for sun exposure is on a sunny day when your shadow is shorter than your height, during which time the skin is most efficiently producing vitamin D. People who live in places at or above the 43rd parallel north can only achieve this from May through September, so in the winter, they may have to rely on intake through vitamin D–rich foods or supplements to obtain adequate amounts of vitamin D.

What Are the Health Reference Values for Vitamin D?
Sufficient blood levels of vitamin D are crucial for maintaining optimal health. If you do not know your vitamin D status, the best way to find out is to measure the 25(OH)D levels in your blood. Health reference values for vitamin D are shown here:

Deficient	< 10 ng/ml
Insufficient	11–19 ng/ml
Normal	> 20 ng/ml
Optimal	25–35 ng/ml
Excess	> 39 ng/ml

If the measurement reveals that your 25(OH)D level is low, how much vitamin D supplement should you take? The rule of thumb is that to increase the blood level of vitamin D by 1 ng/ml, you need to take 100 IU; to increase it by 5 ng/ml, you need to take 500 IU; and so on. The suggested dose is for people of normal weight. Obese people need to take 1.5 times more. Wait at least six weeks to see results.

Prevention and Treatment of Diseases
- *Prevention.* Meta-analysis confirms that vitamin D can help prevent breast cancer (47), lung cancer (82), colorectal cancer (56), blood cancers (45), renal cell cancer (100), bladder cancer (44), melanoma (86), osteoporosis (94), Alzheimer's disease (37), type 1 diabetes (59), type 2 diabetes (60), rickets (103), lupus erythematosus (83), Parkinson's disease (96), autism spectrum disorder (42), cognitive impairment (55), fibromyalgia (67), inflammatory bowel disease (79), multiple sclerosis (89), respiratory infection (101), preeclampsia (97), tuberculosis (109), hypertension (78), rheumatoid arthritis (102), fatty liver disease (66), autoimmune thyroid disease (43), depression (58), gestational diabetes (68), obesity (91), orthostatic hypotension (93), Graves' disease (72), and bone fractures (46).
- *Treatment.* Meta-analysis confirms that vitamin D can help treat chronic obstructive pulmonary disease (53), lupus erythematosus (83), depression (58), asthma (38), hemodialysis (75), and eczema (62).

Which Food Items Are Vitamin D Rich?

Many animal-based foods contain vitamin D, including fish liver oil, fish, beef liver, and eggs. Milk is also an excellent source of vitamin D. Vegans may consider vitamin D–fortified soy milk and fruit juice.

This list of vitamin D–rich food items is adapted from information provided by the NIH Office of Dietary Supplements.

FOOD	PORTION	VITAMIN D CONTENT, IU	% DAILY REFERENCE VALUE
Cod liver oil	1 teaspoon	1,360	340
Swordfish (cooked)	3 ounces	566	142
Salmon (cooked)	3 ounces	447	112
Tuna (cooked)	3 ounces	154	39
Milk	1 cup	120	39
Yogurt	6 ounces	80	30
Sardine (cooked)	3 ounces	46	12
Beef liver	3 ounces	42	11
Eggs	1	41	10
Cheese	1 ounce	6	2

Daily reference value of vitamin D is 400 IU according to the 2013 FDA food-labeling guidelines.

What Are the Recommended Dietary Allowances for Vitamin D?

1–3 years	600 IU
4–8 years	600 IU
9–13 years	600 IU
14–18 years	600 IU
19 years and older	600 IU

The upper daily intake limit of vitamin D is 4,000 IU.

Vitamin D Supplements

- *Dosage.* The most common dosages of vitamin D supplements are 400–5,000 IU, which largely exceed the recommended dietary allowance. Two types of vitamin D supplements are vitamin D2 and vitamin D3. Vitamin D2 comes from plant-based foods and vitamin D3 from animal-based foods. Vitamin D2 and vitamin D3 are similar, although D3 is more potent than D2. Ultraviolet B rays from sunlight trigger the skin to produce vitamin D3, but fish liver oil and deep sea fish are also excellent sources of vitamin D3. Vitamin D supplements in the marketplace predominantly contain vitamin D3.
- *Types.* Vitamin D supplements can be found as tablets, soft gels, and drops. Vitamin D liquid drops are inexpensive and easy to use. One drop usually contains 400 IU of vitamin D3. If a daily dose of 2,000 IU is needed, just use five drops. Vitamin D is tasteless and odorless, so liquid drops can be added directly to meals or beverages.
- *Bone density.* Vitamin D regulates the metabolism of calcium and phosphorus ions in the body. Supplementation with vitamin D can enhance the bone density of teenage girls and help postmenopausal women avoid bone loss. The suggested daily dose is 800 IU of vitamin D3.
- *Bone fractures.* Bone fractures are a major problem for people aged 65 and older. Supplementation with vitamin D can reduce the risk of bone fractures. Studies from Australia have shown that elderly individuals with blood levels of vitamin D in the range of 24–29 ng/ml were the least likely to experience bone fractures, since vitamin D can strengthen bones and muscles. It can also be used by athletes whose blood levels of vitamin D are below 20 ng/ml, which can make them prone to exercise-induced injuries.
- *Insulin resistance.* Obese individuals whose blood levels of vitamin D are below 20 ng/ml have a 12 times higher risk of insulin resistance compared to individuals of normal weight. Insulin resistance is a major risk factor for cardiovascular

diseases, diabetes, and Alzheimer's disease. Vitamin D supplementation can reduce the risk of insulin resistance in obese individuals.

- *Cardiovascular disease.* A high level of C-reactive protein in the blood indicates systemic inflammation in the body, which heightens the risk of cardiovascular diseases. Vitamin D supplementation can lower the levels of C-reactive protein, reducing inflammation and the risk of cardiovascular diseases.

- *Asthma.* Vitamin D supplementation can alleviate pulmonary inflammation, enhance lung function, and control asthma. Supplementation with vitamin D can enhance the efficacy of inhaled corticosteroids in asthmatic patients. The suggested daily dose is 800 IU.

- *Chronic obstructive pulmonary disease.* Supplementation with vitamin D can mitigate symptoms of chronic obstructive pulmonary disease. The suggested daily dose is 2,000 IU.

- *Childhood allergies.* Children and teenagers whose blood levels of vitamin D are below 15 ng/ml have an increased risk of developing childhood allergies. When pregnant women take vitamin D supplements at a daily dose of 800 IU during the last three months of pregnancy, it reduces the risk of childhood allergies in their babies.

- *Fibromyalgia.* Fibromyalgia is a chronic disease characterized by diffuse or sharp pain in joints and muscles. Studies from Austria have shown that supplementation with vitamin D improved symptoms of fibromyalgia in patients. The suggested daily dose is 1,200 IU of vitamin D.

- *Lupus erythematosus.* Vitamin D supplementation can improve symptoms in patients with lupus erythematosus. Adding vitamin D to prescribed medications alleviates the frequency of relapses and enhances immune functions in patients with lupus erythematosus.

- *Depression.* Low blood levels of vitamin D increase the risk of depression in elderly individuals. Supplementation with vitamin D can alleviate depression symptoms in type 2 diabetes patients as well.

- *Dementia.* Elderly individuals whose blood levels of vitamin D are below 10 ng/ml have a greater risk of dementia and Alzheimer's disease. Supplementation with vitamin D at a dose of 500 IU reduces the risk of Alzheimer's disease by 77%. Elderly individuals whose blood levels of vitamin D are higher than 20 ng/ml decrease their risk of Parkinson's disease by 60%.
- *Cancers.* Low blood levels of vitamin D put you at a higher risk of colorectal cancer, breast cancer, melanoma, bladder cancer, and lung cancer. Supplementation with vitamin D improves symptoms of cancer as well as survival rates. The suggested daily dose is 800 IU of vitamin D3.
- *Other diseases.* Low blood levels of vitamin D heighten the risk of rheumatoid arthritis, heart disease, hypertension, and coronary artery disease, shortening life expectancy overall.

Safety Issues
- *Side effects.* Excessive vitamin D can cause hypercalcemia, leading to the formation of kidney stones. Avoid taking more than 10,000 IU of vitamin D per day.
- *Lipids.* Lipids increase the absorption of vitamin D by the intestines. Select a meal with a higher fat content when you are taking vitamin D supplements.

What Types of Drugs May Interact with Vitamin D?
- Anticonvulsant medications, cholesterol-lowering drugs, and chemotherapy can reduce blood levels of vitamin D.

12

VITAMIN E (ALPHA-TOCOPHEROL)

Vitamin E is also known as alpha-tocopherol. In 1922, Herbert Evans studied infertility by feeding rats with his specially formulated feeds. Rats fed with the feeds looked healthy, except pregnant rats. All new broods were dead in the womb. Evans found that by adding vegetables to the feeds, pregnant rats gave birth to healthy broods. He called the lipid-soluble substance isolated from vegetables "factor X." In 1924, Barnett Sure, who also worked on infertility, renamed it vitamin E. In 1936, Evans confirmed that the chemical structure of vitamin E was alpha-tocopherol. *Tocopherol* came from Greek *tokos*, meaning "offspring," and *pherin*, meaning "pregnancy."

Vitamin E from plants consists of eight structurally related chemicals. Among them, alpha-tocopherol is the most important to human health. The lipid-soluble vitamin E is known as a chain-breaking antioxidant. Vitamin E from foods is absorbed in the intestines and distributed through blood circulation to all the cells in the body. In the cellular membrane, vitamin E acts like a guard to get rid of free radicals and prevent free radical–induced chain reactions. Free radicals and other reactive oxygen species can initiate chain reactions that cause oxidative damage to phospholipids and proteins in the cellular membrane, leading to cell death. Vitamin E can terminate this chain reaction.

What Are the Major Functions of Vitamin E?
- *Antioxidant.* Lipid-rich cellular organelles and molecules—such as cell membranes, LDL, and HDL—are susceptible to free radical–induced lipid peroxidation and other related oxidative damage. Lipid-soluble vitamin E can quench free radicals and prevent the lipid peroxidation of cell membranes and molecules in the lipid-rich cellular environment.

What Are the Symptoms of Vitamin E Deficiency?
- Severe vitamin E deficiency is rare. Deficiency symptoms include the inability to stand still, numbness in the extremities, muscle pain and cramps, and retinal malfunction.
- Low blood levels of vitamin E are associated with peripheral neuropathy, ataxia (uncontrollable muscle movement), and retinitis pigmentosa (hereditary retinal degeneration).

Prevention and Treatment of Diseases
- *Prevention.* Meta-analysis confirms that vitamin E can help prevent breast cancer (47), lung cancer (82), renal cell cancer (100), bladder cancer (44), stomach cancer (107), pancreatic cancer (95), prostate cancer (99), cervical cancer (50), endometrial cancer (63), Alzheimer's disease (37), Parkinson's disease (96), fatty liver disease (66), cardiovascular disease (48), heart disease (73), and cataracts (49).
- *Treatment.* Meta-analysis confirms that vitamin E can treat fatty liver disease (66).

Which Food Items Are Vitamin E Rich?
Vitamin E comes from plant-based foods. Vegetable oils—such as wheat germ oil, peanut oil, almond oil, and sunflower oil—are excellent sources of vitamin E. Many vegetables and fruits are also rich in vitamin E, such as asparagus, sweet potatoes, avocados, mangos, and nuts.

This list of vitamin E–rich food items is adapted from information provided by the NIH Office of Dietary Supplements.

FOOD	PORTION	VITAMIN E CONTENT, IU	% DAILY REFERENCE VALUE
Almond	1 ounce	15.0	50
Sunflower oil	1 teaspoon	12.4	41
Safflower oil	1 teaspoon	10.2	34
Hazelnut	1 ounce	9.6	32
Corn oil	1 teaspoon	4.2	14
Peanuts	1 ounce	4.2	14
Olive oil	1 teaspoon	4.2	14
Spinach (cooked)	½ cup	4.2	14
Soybean oil	1 teaspoon	2.4	8
Avocado	1	2.4	8

Daily reference value of vitamin E is 30 IU according to the 2013 FDA food-labeling guidelines.

What Are the Recommended Dietary Allowances for Vitamin E?

1–3 years	9.0 IU
4–8 years	10.5 IU
9–13 years	16.5 IU
14–18 years	22.5 IU
19 years and older	22.5 IU

The upper daily intake limit of vitamin E is 1,000 IU.

Vitamin E Supplements

- *Dosage.* The most common dosages of vitamin E supplements are 20–500 IU. Both International Units (IU) and the weight unit milligram (mg) are often used to quantify vitamin E, with 1 IU being equal to 0.45 mg of natural vitamin E or 0.67 mg of synthetic vitamin E.
- *Types.* The two major vitamin E supplements are natural vitamin E containing d-alpha-tocopherol and synthetic vitamin E containing dl-alpha-tocopherol. Natural vitamin E is better than synthetic vitamin E in terms of bioavailability as well as its retention time in the body.
- *Alzheimer's disease.* Vitamin E can improve the symptoms of Alzheimer's disease. Adding vitamin E to prescribed medications like acetylcholinesterase inhibitors significantly improves daily activities, such as dressing and bathing oneself, in patients with Alzheimer's disease. Vitamin E supplementation can also improve cognitive impairment and prevent its progression to Alzheimer's disease.

Vitamin E Supplements

- Vitamin E can help combat disease in those who are carriers of alpha-tocopherol transfer protein mutant genes, fat malabsorption syndrome, chronic cholestasis, cystic fibrosis, and Crohn's disease.
- Vitamin E can also delay the onset of chronic steatorrhea, such as celiac disease and chronic pancreatitis.

Safety Issues

- *Blood-thinning effect.* High-dose vitamin E can induce a blood-thinning effect and add to the risk of stroke. Patients who take blood-thinning drugs are particularly vulnerable to this effect of vitamin E.
- *Diabetes.* Supplementation with high-dose vitamin E may lead to uncontrollable blood glucose levels in patients with diabetes.

- *Chemotherapy.* Cancer patients who receive chemotherapy should not take vitamin E supplements until they complete their treatment.
- *Shortened life.* Supplementation with high-dose vitamin E could shorten the life-span of elderly people who are in poor health.
- *Blood clotting.* Supplementation with high-dose vitamin E may interfere with the blood-clotting activity of vitamin K.

What Types of Drugs May Interact with Vitamin E?
- Cholesterol-lowering medications that reduce fat absorption can lower vitamin E absorption by the intestines.
- Anticonvulsant drugs may reduce blood levels of vitamin E.

13

VITAMIN K (PHYLLOQUINONE)

Vitamin K is the anticoagulation vitamin. In 1929, Henrik Dam used oil to extract and remove all lipid-soluble substances from animal feed so that it contained only water-soluble substances and then fed that to chickens. He found that the chickens suffered muscle bleeding and slow blood coagulation. Apparently, some molecule in the lipid-soluble substances was important for blood clotting. In 1935, Dam isolated a lipid-soluble substance from the animal feed and called it vitamin K. *K* came from the first letter of the German word *Koagulation*, meaning "blood clotting." In subsequent years, scientists confirmed that the chemical structure of vitamin K was phylloquinone.

Lipid-soluble vitamin K is an essential nutrient for blood coagulation in the body. Vitamin K consists of a group of structurally related naphthoquinones. Among them, vitamins K1 and K2 are most important to human health. Vitamin K1, also known as "phylloquinone," comes from plant-based foods, particularly dark-green leafy vegetables. Vitamin K2, also known as "menadione," is produced mainly by bacteria living in the human colon.

What Are the Major Functions of Vitamin K?

- *Blood coagulation.* Blood coagulation is required to stop bleeding after injury. Vitamin K is an essential cofactor for enzymes participating in the blood coagulation process. Vitamin K deficiency can adversely affect blood coagulation and bring about uncontrollable bleeding.
- *Bone density.* Vitamin K helps maintain bone health. Supplementation with vitamin K augments bone density and curtails the risk of bone fractures in patients with osteoporosis.
- *Calcification of blood vessels.* Vitamin K enhances the activity of matrix Gla proteins, which inhibit calcification of blood vessels and prevent the formation of atherosclerosis.

What Are the Symptoms of Vitamin K Deficiency?

- Symptoms of vitamin K deficiency include nosebleeds, bleeding gums, and/or blood in the urine and stool. Fortunately, deficiency is rare because vitamin K is widely distributed in plant-based foods, and the body is able to recycle oxidized vitamin K through a regenerative oxidation-reduction mechanism. In addition, bacteria living in the colon can produce vitamin K2, at least part of which is available for human use.

What Are the Risk Factors for Vitamin K Deficiency?

- *Anticoagulants.* Oral anticoagulant drugs are the major cause of vitamin K deficiency. Warfarin, a commonly prescribed anticoagulant drug, is an inhibitor of vitamin K epoxide reductase, an enzyme that allows the body to recycle and recover vitamin K. Long-term warfarin users are at a high risk of vitamin K deficiency.
- *Vitamin K–deficient bleeding in newborns.* Bleeding caused by vitamin K deficiency in new babies is a classic example of

vitamin K deficiency–related disease in humans. A number of factors—including low vitamin K in the placenta, defective coagulation factors and germ-free digestive tracts in infants, and low vitamin K in breast milk—can cause vitamin K–deficient bleeding in newborns. Vitamin K–deficient bleeding often occurs during the first week of birth. The American Pediatrics Association recommends that newborns be given an injection of 0.5–1 mg of vitamin K to avoid vitamin K–deficient bleeding.

- *Diseases.* A number of conditions—including liver disease and inflammatory bowel diseases (such as Crohn's disease and ulcerative colitis), as well as the long-term use of antibiotics—can trigger vitamin K deficiency. All these conditions could kill bacteria living in the colon.

Prevention and Treatment of Diseases

- *Prevention.* Vitamin K helps prevent osteoporosis (94), cardiovascular disease (48), and calcification of blood vessels.
- *Treatment.* Vitamin K may treat osteoporosis.

Which Food Items Are Vitamin K Rich?
Dark-green leafy vegetables are excellent sources of vitamin K1. Spinach, broccoli, kale, green beans, oats, and wheat contain vitamin K. Animal-based foods—such as meat, milk, and eggs—also contain vitamin K2. The Japanese food *natto* is rich in vitamin K2 as well.

This list of vitamin K–rich food items is adapted from information provided by the USDA.

FOOD	PORTION	VITAMIN K CONTENT, MCG	% DAILY REFERENCE VALUE
Kale	1 cup	472	590
Swiss chard	1 cup	299	374
Parsley	¼ cup	246	308
Broccoli	1 cup	220	275

continued

FOOD	PORTION	VITAMIN K CONTENT, MCG	% DAILY REFERENCE VALUE
Spinach	1 cup	145	181
Watercress	1 cup	85	106
Lettuce	1 cup	46	58
Peanut oil	1 teaspoon	25	31
Rapeseed oil	1 teaspoon	10	13
Olive oil	1 teaspoon	8	10

Daily reference value of vitamin K is 80 mcg according to the 2013 FDA food-labeling guidelines.

What Are the Recommended Dietary Allowances for Vitamin K?

1–3 years	30 mcg
4–8 years	55 mcg
9–13 years	60 mcg
14–18 years	75 mcg
19 years and older	120 mcg

There is currently no upper intake limit for vitamin K.

Vitamin K Supplements
- *Dosage and types.* The three major types of vitamin K supplements are vitamin K, vitamin K2, and vitamin K7. Unless stated otherwise, vitamin K refers to vitamin K1 (phylloquinone). The most common dosages of vitamin K supplements are 30–1,000 mcg. Vitamin K2 (menaquinone) supplements are more expensive compared to vitamin K1 supplements. Vitamin K7 comes from Japanese *natto*, a food made from fermented soybeans, and supplements of it are the most expensive. The advantage of vitamin K7 is that its half-life in the body is seven to eight times longer than that of vitamin K1. MK-7 (menaquinone-7)

is a form of vitamin K2. The common dosage for MK-7 is in the range of 30–200 mcg.

- *Osteoporosis.* Vitamin K may mitigate age-related bone loss. Studies from the Netherlands have shown that taking 180 mcg of MK-7 daily reduced the risk of bone loss in postmenopausal women. Vitamin K1 at a daily dose of 500 mcg curtailed the risk of osteoporosis.
- *Other diseases.* Sufficient dietary intake of vitamin K may further reduce the risk of coronary artery disease, prostate cancer, and lung cancer.

Safety Issues

- *Side effects.* There is no known side effect associated with vitamin K intake from foods or supplements.
- *Vitamin A and vitamin E.* Taking high doses of vitamin A together with high-dose vitamin E reduces the blood level of vitamin K. High-dose vitamin A decreases the absorption of vitamin K by the intestines, while high-dose vitamin E interferes with the coagulation activity of vitamin K in the bloodstream.

What Types of Drugs May Interact with Vitamin K?

- *Anticoagulants.* Vitamin K may decrease the efficacy of anticoagulant drugs. Patients who take such drugs should not use vitamin K supplements.
- *Other drugs.* Antibiotics and anticonvulsant drugs may reduce blood levels of vitamin K.

PART TWO

Essential Elements

Carbon, hydrogen, oxygen, and nitrogen are the four big elements that make up about 96% of our bodies. Calcium, potassium, sodium, magnesium, and phosphorus are the five essential elements, while iron, zinc, manganese, copper, molybdenum, iodine, chromium, and selenium are eight essential trace elements in the human body. The body cannot produce essential elements; thus it needs to acquire them from food sources to maintain good health and well-being.

Essential elements are called "minerals" or "dietary minerals." Minerals exist in rocks and the soil of the Earth's crust. So far, there are 5,300 known minerals. Nevertheless, it is the pure chemical elements, such as calcium or phosphorus, rather than minerals like limestone or apatite that are needed to maintain optimal health. This book presents a new concept, using the term *essential elements* to replace *minerals*.

14

CALCIUM

Calcium is an essential element. The body contains about one kilogram of calcium, of which 99% is stored in the bones and teeth. The remainder is distributed in various organs and tissues. Calcium is involved in a multitude of important functions, such as the release of neural transmitters and muscle contraction. There is a homeostasis between calcium ions in the bones and calcium ions in the bloodstream. Excessive calcium in blood is actively deposited into the bones, and calcium is readily released from the bones when the blood level of calcium becomes too low. Prolonged calcium insufficiency can bring about osteoporosis.

What Are the Major Functions of Calcium?
- *Bones and teeth.* Bones are in a dynamic state and are constantly being repaired or rebuilt. All the calcium in your bones will be replaced within 8–12 years, but calcium in your teeth will never be replaced once deposited. The interplay

between osteoblasts (bone-forming cells) and osteoclasts (bone-removing cells) in the bones is essential for maintaining bone health. Osteoblasts deposit calcium in the bones, and osteoclasts release calcium from the bones. During the growth phase in childhood, osteoblasts are actively adding calcium to the bones, while in patients with osteoporosis, osteoclasts are actively removing calcium from the bones.

- *Blood coagulation.* Blood coagulation factors require calcium as a cofactor. Binding to calcium enables these blood coagulation factors to adhere to platelets. Without binding to calcium, these blood coagulation factors cannot form blood clots, causing uncontrollable bleeding.

- *Neurotransmitters.* As the action potential (transporting electrical signals from one cell to the next) arrives, calcium ions stored in the neurons are released, which triggers the release of neurotransmitters, such as dopamine, to the neighboring neurons.

- *Muscle contraction.* Muscle cells form muscle fibers, which are comprised of actin and myosin. Actin and myosin display a mutual attraction to each other. The binding of actin to myosin induces muscle contraction. In a resting state, troponin and tropomyosin sandwich themselves between actin and myosin to prevent actin from binding to myosin. When the brain sends a message for muscle contraction, calcium ions are quickly released and bind to troponin. Calcium binding to troponin causes the movement that removes troponin and tropomyosin from between actin and myosin, hastening the binding of actin to myosin and the subsequent muscle contraction.

What Are the Symptoms of Calcium Deficiency?

- The major symptoms of calcium deficiency include fragile bones, impaired vision, atrial fibrillation, and osteoporosis.

What Are the Causes of Calcium Deficiency?
- *Diet.* An unhealthy diet is the main cause of calcium deficiency. According to data from the USDA, 78% of women and 87% of teenage girls are calcium insufficient. Only 55% of men obtain sufficient calcium from foods. Hence it is not surprising that osteoporosis is now a serious health issue in the US.
- *Parathyroid hormone.* Parathyroid hormones regulate calcium concentrations in the blood. Low blood calcium triggers the secretion of parathyroid hormones from the parathyroid gland. Parathyroid hormones then release calcium from the bones and elevate blood calcium levels. When blood calcium is too high, the body will attenuate the secretion of parathyroid hormones. Parathyroid hormone disorder can contribute to problems related to calcium deficiency.

Prevention and Treatment of Diseases
- *Prevention.* Meta-analysis confirms that calcium can help prevent bone fractures (46), preeclampsia (97), and colorectal cancer (56).
- *Treatment.* Calcium supplements help treat hypertension (78).

Which Food Items Are Calcium Rich?
Milk and other dairy products are excellent sources of calcium. Plant-based foods like broccoli, spinach, tofu, and nuts, as well as animal-based foods like eggs, sardines, and salmon, contain high amounts of calcium.

This list of calcium-rich food items is adapted from information provided by the NIH Office of Dietary Supplements.

FOOD	PORTION	CALCIUM CONTENT, MG	% DAILY REFERENCE VALUE
Yogurt	8 ounces	415	42
Sardine	3 ounces	325	33
Cheese	1½ ounces	307	31
Milk	8 ounces	276	28
Tofu (hard)	½ cup	253	25
Salmon	3 ounces	181	18
Tofu (soft)	½ cup	138	14
Cabbage	½ cup	79	8
Orange	1	60	6
Kale	½ cup	47	5

Daily reference value of calcium is 1,000 mg according to the 2013 FDA food-labeling guidelines.

What Are the Recommended Dietary Allowances for Calcium?

1–3 years	700 mg
4–8 years	1,000 mg
9–13 years	1,300 mg
14–18 years	1,300 mg
19 years and older	1,000 mg; 1,200 mg (51 years and older)

The upper daily intake limit of calcium is 2,500 mg (19–50 years old) or 2,000 mg (51 years and older).

Calcium Supplements

- *Types.* Calcium supplements come in different chemical formulations, including calcium carbonate, calcium citrate, calcium malate, calcium lactate, calcium gluconate, and the like. Among them, calcium carbonate is the least expensive—this is the form found in oyster shells and coral. It is easier for the intestines to absorb calcium citrate and calcium malate compared to calcium carbonate. Owing to high molecule weights, calcium lactate and calcium gluconate supplements are mainly available in large tablet sizes, which may contain less calcium per tablet.

- *Dosage.* Calcium contents in calcium supplements often are not clearly stated on the label. For instance, based on their weights, calcium carbonate, calcium malate, and calcium gluconate contain only 40%, 21%, and 9% calcium, respectively. A 1-gram tablet of a calcium gluconate supplement may have only 90 mg of calcium. Read the label carefully for the calcium content of these products when purchasing.
- *Preteen and teenage girls.* During growth and development, girls aged 9–18 should take 500 mg of calcium and 800 IU of vitamin D daily.
- *Women.* Calcium supplementation can attenuate premenopausal syndromes, including mood swings, headaches, overeating, and bloating. It is recommended that premenopausal women take 1 g of calcium daily for three days before menstruation.
- *Bone fractures.* Calcium plus vitamin D supplements prevent bone fractures. It is recommended that postmenopausal women take 500 mg of calcium and 400 IU of vitamin D daily to curtail the risk of bone fractures.
- *Hypertension.* Calcium deficiency elevates the risk of hypertension. Calcium supplementation lowers systolic and diastolic pressure in hypertensive patients.
- *Life-span.* Taking calcium supplements may extend the life-span. Studies from Canada have shown that postmenopausal women who took calcium supplements at a daily dose of 1 g for 10 years had a reduced rate of death from cardiovascular diseases.
- *Cholesterol.* Taking daily supplements of calcium at a dose of 1 g for one year raises "good" cholesterol (HDL) and lowers "bad" cholesterol (LDL) in postmenopausal women.

Safety Issues

- *Overdose.* Daily supplements of calcium at doses greater than 1,500 mg may increase the risk of prostate cancer and heart disease. On the other hand, calcium insufficiency also adds to the risk of prostate cancer.
- *Vitamin D.* Vitamin D enhances calcium absorption in the intestines. It is beneficial to take calcium and vitamin D supplements together. A dose of 500 mg of calcium is absorbed very efficiently by the intestines. If a daily dose of 1,000 mg of calcium is needed, you may take 500 mg twice a day.
- *Diet.* High-sodium and protein-rich diets may trigger overexcretion of calcium in the urine. People who enjoy salty and meaty meals need to be cautious about potential calcium deficiency.

What Types of Drugs May Interact with Calcium?

- *Diuretics.* Diuretic drugs may enhance renal absorption of calcium, leading to problems associated with high blood calcium levels.
- *Digoxin.* Heart failure patients who take digoxin together with calcium supplements may exacerbate the risk of atrial fibrillation.
- *Antibiotics.* Taking calcium supplements may interfere with the absorption of tetracycline and other antibiotics by the intestines.
- *Other medications and supplements.* Antacid drugs, corticosteroids, heparin, iron, manganese, and chromium all lower the absorption of calcium by the intestines.
- *Diabetes.* Metformin interferes with the absorption of vitamin B12 by the intestines in type 2 diabetes patients. Calcium supplementation improves the absorption of vitamin B12. The suggested daily dose is 1 g of calcium.

15

POTASSIUM

Potassium is an essential element. On average, the human body contains about 120 g of potassium, exclusively in the form of potassium ions. Potassium ions are the most abundant cations (or positively charged ions) in the body, followed by sodium ions. Potassium ions are stored inside the cell, while sodium ions are stored outside the cell. Potassium concentration inside the cell is 30 times higher than potassium concentration outside the cell, and sodium concentration outside the cell is 10 times higher than sodium concentration inside the cell. Owing to these concentration gradients of potassium and sodium, each cell holds a tiny electric field and acts like a small battery, negatively charged inside while positively charged outside. The human body comprises 37.2 trillion cells, so we have 37.2 trillion small batteries in the body. About 40% of our daily food intake is used to recharge all these tiny batteries. A healthy body is sustained only when all of them are fully charged. The importance of potassium to human health is beyond description.

What Are the Major Functions of Potassium Ion?

- *Membrane potential.* All cellular membranes, particularly neurons, hold a membrane potential with negatively charged inside and positively charged outside. Membrane potential is about 70 microvolts, through which the semipermeability of the cellular membrane is established. Potassium is actively pumped into the cell, while sodium is actively pumped out of the cell. Potassium and sodium concentration gradients establish the membrane potential, and it is crucial for the existence of all living beings. If potassium and sodium concentration gradients were abolished, the membrane potential would be lost, leading to instant cell death.

- *Cofactor.* Potassium ions serve as cofactors for many enzymes, among which the most important enzyme is sodium-potassium ATPase. Sodium-potassium ATPase is a membrane protein that can convert ATP to ADP and release its energy for muscle contraction and the like.

- *Other functions.* Other cellular functions of potassium include blood pressure control and regulation, the peristaltic movement of the intestines, acid-alkaline balance, and glucose and insulin metabolism.

What Are the Symptoms of Potassium Deficiency?

- Potassium deficiency precipitates hypokalemia, characterized by weakness, fatigue, numbness in the extremities, bloating, nausea and vomiting, constipation, palpitations, and even mental disorders, such as depression, psychosis, and delusion. All these symptoms may contribute to the problem by making it harder to recharge all those tiny batteries and maintain the normal membrane potential of cells in the body.

What Are the Causes of Potassium Deficiency?

- Potassium deficiency often is caused by long-term use of diuretics, alcoholism, severe vomiting, diarrhea, and anorexia.

- Potassium deficiency is rarely caused by insufficient dietary intake.

Prevention and Treatment of Diseases
- *Prevention.* Meta-analysis confirms that potassium supplements can help prevent hypertension (78) and stroke (108).
- *Treatment.* Meta-analysis confirms that potassium supplements can help treat hypertension (78) and stroke (108).

Which Food Items Are Potassium Rich?
Many foods are rich in potassium, including acorns, pumpkins, potatoes, spinach, bananas, oranges, avocados, lima beans, cantaloupes, tomatoes, salmon, and cod. Sweet potatoes, watermelons, and legumes are also excellent sources of potassium.

This list of potassium-rich food items is adapted information provided by the USDA.

FOOD	PORTION	POTASSIUM CONTENT, MG	% DAILY REFERENCE VALUE
Potato	1	926	26
Plum (dried)	½ cup	637	18
Raisins	½ cup	598	17
Plum juice	6 ounces	528	15
Banana	1	422	12
Spinach (cooked)	½ cup	420	15
Orange juice	6 ounces	372	12
Tomato	1	292	8
Sunflower seeds	1 ounce	241	7
Almonds	1 ounce	200	6

Daily reference value of potassium is 3.5 g according to the 2013 FDA food-labeling guidelines.

What Are the Recommended Dietary Allowances for Potassium?

1–3 years	3.0 g
4–8 years	3.8 g
9–13 years	4.5 g
14–18 years	4.7 g
19 years and older	4.7 g

There is currently no upper intake limit for potassium.

Potassium Supplements

- *Type.* In the marketplace, commonly found potassium supplements include potassium carbonate, potassium citrate, potassium gluconate, potassium acetate, and potassium chloride. At least 90% of potassium ingested from foods or supplements is readily absorbed in the intestines. Potassium gluconate has a less bitter taste.
- *Dosage.* When purchasing potassium, pay attention to product labeling. Potassium gluconate supplements may contain only 20% potassium and 80% gluconate. A 500-mg tablet of potassium gluconate may contain only 100 mg of potassium unless stated otherwise on the labeling.
- *Hypertension.* Potassium supplements lower blood pressure. Randomized controlled clinical studies have shown that potassium supplements taken at a dose of 1 g daily for one month lowered blood pressure from 151/93 to 138/88 in the supplement group compared to no significant change in blood pressure in the placebo group. Potassium supplements can be taken with meals to avoid nausea or vomiting.
- *Hypercalcemia.* Potassium supplements mitigate hypercalcemia, a high blood calcium condition that could trigger the formation of kidney stones. Potassium supplementation at a dose of 2 g daily has been found to reduce hypercalcemia by 30%.

Safety Issues
- *Side effects.* Taking potassium supplements at a dose of 18 g daily can give rise to hyperkalemia, a high blood potassium condition characterized by numbness in the extremities, weakness, and temporary paralysis. Other potential side effects of high-dose potassium supplements are nausea, vomiting, and diarrhea.

What Types of Drugs May Interact with Potassium?
- *Hyperkalemia.* Hyperkalemia can be triggered by heart disease drugs, nonsteroidal anti-inflammatory drugs, anticoagulant drugs, and antihypertensive drugs.
- *Hypokalemia.* Hypokalemia can be precipitated by adrenalin, bronchodilators, diuretics, and antibiotics.

16

SODIUM

Sodium is an essential element. The human body contains about 200 g of sodium—about 0.4% of the body's weight. Sodium exists in an ionic form that is distributed widely in the extracellular fluids of all organs and tissues, such as in the blood and lymphatic fluid. Sodium concentration in the human body is equivalent to that in seawater. The main dietary sources of sodium ion are seasonings used in cooking and table salt.

What Are the Major Functions of Sodium Ion?

- *Membrane potential.* Sodium ions and potassium ions help maintain the proper membrane potential in every cell in the body. The membrane potential of the cellular membrane controls the traffic of substances into or out of a cell as well as the transmission of nerve messages from the brain to various parts of the body, such as the heart and muscles.
- *Blood pressure.* Sodium ions participate in regulating blood volume and blood pressure. A high blood sodium concentration

triggers the outflow of intracellular water into the bloodstream and dilutes the blood sodium concentration. On the other hand, the outflow of intracellular water into the bloodstream results in a shortage of water intracellularly and the feeling of thirst. That is why consumption of salty foods will make you feel thirsty. In addition, the outflow of intracellular water into the bloodstream due to a high blood sodium concentration increases the volume of the bloodstream, which exerts extra pressure against the arterial wall and hastens hypertension. Habitual consumption of salty foods can therefore elevate the risk of hypertension.

What Are the Symptoms of Sodium Deficiency?
- The major symptoms of sodium deficiency include headache, nausea, vomiting, and dizziness, as well as, in severe cases, brain swelling, seizures, unconsciousness, and brain damage.

What Are the Risk Factors for Sodium Deficiency?
- *Diuretics.* Sodium deficiency is frequently caused by long-term use of medications such as diuretics, which can diminish the blood sodium concentration, rather than insufficient dietary intake.
- *Athletics.* Heavy perspiration can precipitate the loss of electrolytes such as sodium ions from the bloodstream. For example, triathlon and marathon runners who lose a lot of sodium ions during vigorous competition and drink large amounts of low-sodium water to quench the thirst are vulnerable to severe sodium deficiency, which can, in severe cases, lead to brain swelling, unconsciousness, and even death.

Which Food Items Are Sodium Rich?
Food items that contain high sodium content include table salt, soy sauce, preserved meats, bacon, fast foods, and canned foods.

This list of sodium-rich food items is adapted from information provided by the USDA.

FOOD	PORTION	SODIUM CONTENT, MG	% DAILY REFERENCE VALUE
Chicken noodle soup (canned)	1 cup	1,400	58
Spaghetti (with cheese)	1 cup	1,300	54
French fries (with salt)	8 ounces	1,200	50
Pretzels	2 ounces	1,000	42
Ham	3 ounces	1,000	42
Fish sandwich (with sauce)	1	940	39
Tomato juice (canned)	8 ounces	650	27
Hot dogs	1	510	21
Bread	2 slices	340	14
Whole wheat bread	2 slices	264	11

Daily reference value of sodium is 2,400 mg according to the 2013 FDA food-labeling guidelines.

What Are the Recommended Dietary Allowances for Sodium?

1–3 years	1.0 g
4–8 years	1.2 g
9–13 years	1.5 g
14–18 years	1.5 g
19 years and older	1.5 g

The upper daily intake limit of sodium is 2.3 g.

Safety Issues

- *Side effects.* Too much sodium in salty foods burdens the body. The body needs an extra amount of water to dilute the high blood sodium concentration. To do that, the kidneys inhibit the excretion of water in the urine and reabsorb excreted water back into the bloodstream, causing expansion of the blood volume, which exerts extra pressure against the arterial wall, particularly in the heart and brain, leading to the risk of hypertension, heart disease, and stroke.
- *Stomach cancer.* High consumption of salty foods can induce chronic inflammation in the stomach, increasing the risk of infection by *Helicobacter pylori* bacteria and stomach cancer.
- *Kidney stones.* High dietary intake of sodium can raise the calcium ion concentration in the kidneys and urinary tract and elevate the risk of kidney stone formation.

What Types of Drugs May Interact with Sodium?

- Medications like diuretics, morphine, and antidepressant drugs can cause sodium deficiency.

17

MAGNESIUM

Magnesium is an essential element that exists in an ionic form in biological systems. The magnesium ion is the fourth most abundant cation in the body and the second most abundant cation inside the cell. The human body contains about 25 g of magnesium, of which 60% is stored in the bones and the rest in various organs and tissues. Genetic DNA material is negatively charged, so the binding of cationic magnesium ions stabilizes the structural stability of the anionic DNA. Magnesium ions are also required to support the involvement of 300 different enzymes in various important physiological functions in the body.

What Are the Major Functions of Magnesium?
- *Cellular energy.* Magnesium ions are required to support enzymatic reactions during the conversion of glucose to high-energy ATP in cells. The ATPase enzymes that catalyze ATP to release energy and thus maintain all normal physiological

functions—such as reading, writing, walking, talking, and thinking—require magnesium ions as contributing constituents. Therefore, magnesium ions are needed for the activation and activities of ATP and ATPase that are related to cellular energy production.

- *Bone health.* Magnesium ions participate in maintaining the strength and hardness of the bones. They are present in a crystalline form inside bones as well as in a cationic form on the surface of bones. Magnesium ions present on the surface of bones are in dynamic equilibrium with magnesium ions in the bloodstream. When more blood magnesium ions are needed, the bones release magnesium ions into the bloodstream. When too many magnesium ions are present in the bloodstream, the bones absorb excessive magnesium ions from the bloodstream. Magnesium ions are required for the functions of both osteoblasts and osteoclasts in bone tissue.

- *Blood glucose.* Magnesium ions can enhance cellular insulin sensitivity and lower blood glucose levels. Insulin helps magnesium ions enter the pancreatic cells and enhance insulin production. The interplay between magnesium and insulin regulates the blood level of glucose. Insulin resistance blocks magnesium ions from entering into the cells and furthermore increases urine excretion, leading to magnesium deficiency.

- *Blood pressure.* Magnesium ions prevent calcium ions from entering into endothelial cells in the blood vessels. They act like natural calcium channel blockers. In addition, magnesium ions induce the dilatation of the blood vessels and decrease intracellular sodium concentrations, hence lowering blood pressure.

What Are the Symptoms of Magnesium Deficiency?

- The major symptoms of magnesium deficiency are muscle spasms, atrial fibrillation, and seizure. Although magnesium deficiency is rare, magnesium insufficiency is rather common.

In the US, 65% of people have an insufficient dietary intake of magnesium, and 81% of people aged 71 years and older are magnesium insufficient.

- Certain acute and chronic diseases can give rise to magnesium deficiency. These diseases include digestive disorders and kidney and endocrine malfunctions. Digestive disorders include malnutrition, severe vomiting, acute and chronic diarrhea, and acute pancreatitis. Antacid medications can also lead to magnesium deficiency. Diuretics, hypercalcemia, acute renal failure, alcoholism, and renal toxins, such as cisplatin and amphotericin B, contribute to renal malfunctions. Endocrine malfunctions include type 2 diabetes, phosphate deficiency, hypoparathyroidism, and hyperparathyroidism.

Prevention and Treatment of Diseases
- *Prevention.* Meta-analysis confirms that magnesium supplements can help prevent cardiovascular disease (48), metabolic syndrome (87), colorectal cancer (56), heart disease (73), stroke (108), type 2 diabetes (60), and migraines (88).
- *Treatment.* Meta-analysis confirms that magnesium supplements can help treat hypertension (78).

Which Food Items Are Magnesium Rich?
Many foods contain magnesium. For example, fish, lobsters, legumes, dark-green leafy vegetables, nuts, oats, and tofu are excellent sources of magnesium. Other foods containing magnesium are avocados, bananas, chocolate, and whole wheat.

This list of magnesium-rich food items is adapted from information provided by the USDA.

FOOD	PORTION	MAGNESIUM CONTENT, MG	% DAILY REFERENCE VALUE
Oatmeal	½ cup	96	24
Brown rice (cooked)	1 cup	86	22
Mackerel (cooked)	3 ounces	82	21
Spinach (cooked)	½ cup	78	20
Almonds	1 ounce	77	19
Beets	½ cup	75	19
Peanuts	1 ounce	48	12
Okra	½ cup	37	9
Milk	8 ounces	34	9
Banana	1	32	8

Daily reference value of magnesium is 400 mg according to the 2013 FDA food-labeling guidelines.

What Are the Recommended Dietary Allowances for Magnesium?

1–3 years	80 mg
4–8 years	130 mg
9–13 years	240 mg
14–18 years	410 mg (boys); 360 mg (girls)
19 years and older	420 mg

The upper daily intake limit of magnesium is 350 mg.

Magnesium Supplements

- *Dosage.* The most common dosages of magnesium supplements in the marketplace are 50–500 mg. Read the product labeling carefully when purchasing magnesium to determine the amount of magnesium in each tablet, not just its total weight.

- *Types.* Popular magnesium supplements are magnesium oxide, magnesium chloride, and magnesium malate. Magnesium oxide is the least expensive, but less of it is absorbed by the intestines, and it may cause diarrhea. Magnesium chloride is a good choice if a high daily dose of magnesium supplement is required. In high doses, all magnesium supplements are laxatives, but among them, magnesium hydroxide in particular is most commonly used as a laxative.

- *Type 2 diabetes.* Supplementation with magnesium may decrease the risk of type 2 diabetes. Magnesium ions increase cellular insulin sensitivity. The suggested daily dose is 350 mg for four months.

- *Stroke.* Sufficient dietary intake of magnesium lowers the risk of stroke. Studies have shown that daily consumption of 300 mg of magnesium from foods reduced the risk of stroke by 8%.

- *Heart failure.* Magnesium supplements improve some of the symptoms associated with heart failure. Heart failure patients who took magnesium supplements at a dose of 300 mg for one year had fewer incidences of atrial fibrillation and better survival rates.

- *Lack of exercise.* Magnesium supplements may augment physical strength and activity. Studies from the US have shown that supplementation with magnesium at a dose of 350 mg daily improved walking and shortened the time required to transition from a seated position to standing in elderly people.

- *Migraine.* Magnesium supplements prevent migraines. A randomized controlled trial has shown that supplementation with magnesium diminished the risk of migraines by 40% in migraine patients who took magnesium supplements at a dose of 600 mg daily for 12 weeks.

- *Hearing loss.* Magnesium supplements prevent hearing loss induced by noise. One randomized controlled trial has shown that magnesium supplementation decreases noise-induced hearing loss in participants who take daily magnesium supplements at a dose of 200 mg.

- *Angina.* Magnesium supplements may mitigate certain symptoms associated with angina. The consumption of magnesium supplements at a daily dose of 350 mg for six months made it easier for angina patients to perform daily tasks.
- *Menstruation.* Magnesium supplements prevent menstrual migraines, premenstrual syndrome, and menstrual pain. The recommended daily dose is 400 mg of magnesium chloride taken every day starting three days before the beginning of menstruation.
- *Antacid activity.* Magnesium can be used as an antacid agent. The recommended daily dose is 100 mg of magnesium chloride for patients with stomach hyperacidity.
- *Other diseases.* Magnesium supplements can help treat hypertension, kidney stones, and throbbing pain in the feet during pregnancy. The recommended daily dose is 200 mg of magnesium chloride.
- *Intravenous injections.* Intravenous injections of magnesium ions under a physician's supervision can be used to treat acute asthma, atrial fibrillation, drug overdose, diabetic ketoacidosis, pancreatitis, hyperthyroidism, and hepatitis.

Safety Issues

- *Side effects.* People who take high doses of magnesium supplements may experience side effects that include stomach discomfort, nausea, vomiting, or diarrhea. Avoid taking magnesium supplements above the daily upper limit of 350 mg.
- *Overdose.* High doses of magnesium supplements may lead to exceedingly high blood levels of magnesium, particularly in patients with kidney disease, causing hypotension, fatigue, and atrial fibrillation.
- *Zinc supplement.* High doses of zinc supplements may interfere with the absorption of magnesium by the intestines.

What Types of Drugs May Interact with Magnesium?

- *Antacid drugs.* Antacid drugs, such as proton pump inhibitors, reduce the blood level of magnesium. Long-term antacid drug users should consider taking magnesium supplements. Studies have shown that in spite of taking magnesium supplements, about 25% of long-term antacid users still had a problem with low blood levels of magnesium and needed to discontinue taking proton pump inhibitors.
- *Other drugs.* Digoxin (a heart disease drug), antibiotic tetracycline, oral anticoagulants, and diuretics interfere with the absorption of magnesium by the intestines.

18

PHOSPHORUS

Phosphorus is an essential element. The human body contains about 0.7 kg of phosphorus, of which 90% is stored in the bones and teeth. Phosphorus exists mostly in the form of phosphate in the body. Phosphorus in the bones and teeth is predominantly calcium phosphate. Phosphates are the building blocks that support the double helix structure of DNA in chromosomes, and they are key ingredients in the synthesis of the phospholipids that form lipid bilayers in all cellular membranes. Phosphates are needed for enzymes that participate in energy production in every living organism on the planet.

What Are the Major Functions of Phosphorus?

- *Structural function.* All cell membranes are made of phospholipids, which consist of phosphates and triglycerides. Calcium phosphates contribute to bone density and structure. Phosphates are required for the synthesis of DNA and for maintaining the double helix structure of DNA.

- *Energy storage.* ATP is the basic energy unit of the body, just as the currency is the basis of trade in the marketplace. The cost for a cellular event, such as muscle contraction, can be estimated based on the number of ATP molecules needed for the job, just as the cost for a pair of shoes can be estimated based on the amount of money needed to purchase it. ATP is the "money" or "currency" in the cell, and phosphorus is the key ingredient in its synthesis.

What Are the Symptoms of Phosphorus Deficiency?
- The major symptoms of phosphorus deficiency include neurological disorders, muscle weakness, and anemia. Generally speaking, phosphorus insufficiency rarely occurs due to insufficient dietary intake. Malnutrition, malabsorption of phosphorus, and metabolic abnormalities resulting in the loss of phosphorus via excessive urine excretion are the most likely causes of phosphorus insufficiency.

What Are the Risk Factors for Phosphorus Deficiency?
- *Hunger and refeeding syndrome.* During prolonged starvation, phosphates stored in muscle tissue are released into the bloodstream to keep the blood phosphate level at a relatively normal state. Rapidly refeeding a starved person can lead to an instant rise in blood glucose, which is utilized quickly as a fuel to produce badly needed energy for the hungry body. However, the energy production process consumes a large amount of phosphates due to the synthesis of ATP and other metabolic needs. Phosphates in the blood enter the cells and tissue, causing a precipitous drop in the blood phosphate level. Severe phosphorus deficiency in the blood can give rise to life-threatening sudden cardiac arrest, a phenomenon known as hunger and refeeding syndrome.
- *Premature infants.* Phosphorus deficiency often occurs in premature babies or underweight newborn babies. Phosphorus deficiency prevents the mineralization of calcium phosphates

and hinders the development and growth of infants. The phosphate content of breast milk is adequate for the needs of a normal baby but does not meet the needs of a premature baby. Supplementation of breast milk with phosphate and calcium is important for the health and growth of premature babies.

Which Food Items Are Phosphorus Rich?
Protein-rich foods have high phosphorus content. Animal-based foods—such as beef, pork, chicken, milk, and dairy products—are excellent sources of phosphorus. Plant-based foods—such as nuts, pumpkin seeds, sunflower seeds, flaxseeds, and legumes—are also good sources. In general, phosphorus from animal-based foods is easier for the intestines to absorb compared to that from plant-based foods.

This list of phosphorus-rich food items is adapted from information provided by the USDA.

FOOD	PORTION	PHOSPHORUS CONTENT, MG	% DAILY REFERENCE VALUE
Salmon	3 ounces	315	32
Yogurt	8 ounces	306	31
Milk	8 ounces	247	25
Flounder	3 ounces	244	24
Turkey	3 ounces	217	22
Beef	3 ounces	179	18
Hyacinth beans	½ cup	178	18
Almonds	1 ounce	136	14
Peanuts	1 ounce	108	11
Eggs	1	86	9

Daily reference value of phosphorus is 1,000 mg according to the 2013 FDA food-labeling guidelines.

What Are the Recommended Dietary Allowances for Phosphorus?

1–3 years	460 mg
4–8 years	500 mg
9–13 years	1,250 mg
14–18 years	1,250 mg
19 years and older	700 mg

The upper daily intake limit of phosphorus is 4,000 mg.

Phosphorus Supplements

- *Types.* Sodium phosphate and potassium phosphate are two major phosphorus supplements. Calcium phosphate is commonly used in calcium supplement products.
- *Exercise endurance.* Supplementation with phosphorus can improve exercise endurance. Sodium phosphate taken at a dose of 1 g daily boosts strength and endurance in sports or exercise.
- *Osteoporosis.* Supplementation with phosphorus, specifically calcium phosphate taken at a dose of 500 mg daily, can mitigate the symptoms experienced by patients with osteoporosis.

Safety Issues

- *Side effects.* Supplementation with high-dose phosphorus increases the risk of cardiovascular disease. Taking more than 2 g of phosphorus supplements per day is not recommended.

What Types of Drugs May Interact with Phosphorus?

- Some antacid medications contain aluminum, which can react chemically with phosphorus supplements and form aluminum phosphate, which cannot be absorbed by the intestines.
- Potassium and phosphorus supplements taken together can lead to hyperkalemia (high blood potassium).

19

IRON

Iron is an essential trace element. On average, the human body contains 3–4 g of iron, of which 70% is stored in hemoglobin and myoglobin. Hemoglobin in red blood cells helps carry oxygen and delivers it to organs and tissues via blood circulation. Myoglobin in muscles helps accept, store, and transport oxygen to produce the energy needed for muscle contraction. About 25% of iron is stored in ferritin, an iron storage protein, which is present in nearly every cell in the body and releases iron into the bloodstream when needed.

What Are the Major Functions of Iron?
- *Oxygen transport.* Each heme group in the red blood cell contains four irons. Each iron atom can carry one oxygen molecule. When all the iron atoms in hemoglobin carry oxygen, the color of the blood is bright red, and when only one of the four iron atoms in hemoglobin carries oxygen, the color of the blood is dark red. The former is oxygenated arterial blood,

while the latter is deoxygenated venous blood. Oxygenated arterial blood flows from the heart to all organs and tissues, and deoxygenated venous blood flows back to the heart.

- *Immune functions.* Iron is an essential nutrient for bacteria and viruses to grow and multiply. When bacteria invade the bloodstream, the liver releases hepcidin, a protein that can block iron absorption in the intestines as well as iron released from immune cells into the bloodstream. These combined effects decrease the availability of iron to bacteria or viruses and hamper their growth and multiplication. The overgrowth of bacteria in the bloodstream can lead to sepsis.

- *Energy production.* Iron is an essential cofactor that supports enzymes involved in converting nutrients to cellular energy in the mitochondria of the cells.

- *Antioxidant functions.* Iron-dependent metalloenzymes are involved in degrading hydrogen peroxide and other free radicals produced in cells. In an inflamed cell, hydrogen peroxide can react with iron to generate hydroxyl radical, the strongest oxidant. Iron-dependent catalase enzymes can degrade hydrogen peroxide into oxygen molecules and water and prevent it from generating hydroxyl radicals and other deleterious free radicals.

What Are the Symptoms of Iron Deficiency?

- The major symptoms of iron deficiency include fatigue, dizziness, paleness, hair loss, irritability, and weakness. Iron deficiency is common in teenage girls, premenopausal women, and pregnant women. According to data from the Centers for Disease Control and Prevention, about 9.5% of all females aged 12–29 in the US are iron deficient.

- Iron is essential for bone marrow to produce hemoglobin to make new red blood cells. More than 250 million hemoglobin molecules carry a total of 1 billion oxygen molecules in each mature red blood cell. The human body contains about 20 trillion red blood cells, which carry tremendous amounts of oxygen in the bloodstream. Iron deficiency can lead to anemia.

What Are the Three Stages of Iron Deficiency?
- *Depletion of stored iron.* The body depletes the stored iron, but the blood level of iron is still sufficient.
- *Iron insufficiency.* The stored iron is depleted and the blood level of iron is below normal. Iron insufficiency adversely affects normal physiological functions but has not yet reached the stage of anemia.
- *Iron deficiency anemia.* Hemoglobin content is low in red blood cells, and the total red blood cell count is low as well; these conditions precipitate an inadequate supply of oxygen to organs and tissues, leading to iron deficiency anemia.

Who Is at Risk of Iron Deficiency Anemia?
- *Vegetarians.* The iron content of plant-based foods is relatively low and not easily absorbed by the intestines, so vegetarians are at risk of iron deficiency anemia. Vitamin C enhances iron absorption by the intestines. Sufficient intake of vitamin C from foods and/or supplements may lower the risk of iron deficiency anemia in vegetarians.
- *Infants and children (aged 6 months to 4 years old).* Iron stored in newborns lasts only about 6 months. Adequate intake of iron is important for development and growth in infants and children.
- *Teenagers.* Growing teenagers, especially menstruating teenage girls, need adequate amounts of iron.
- *Pregnant women.* Sufficient dietary intake of iron is crucial for the health of both the fetus and mother during pregnancy.

Prevention and Treatment of Diseases
- *Prevention.* Meta-analysis confirms that iron may help prevent respiratory infection (101) and osteoporosis (94).
- *Treatment.* Iron supplements can treat iron deficiency anemia.

Which Food Items Are Iron Rich?
Animal-based foods, such as meats and fish, and plant-based foods like dark-green leafy vegetables, wheat, and fruits are excellent sources of

iron. Animal-based foods contain heme iron, while plant-based foods contain nonheme iron. The absorption of heme iron is twice as efficient as that of nonheme iron in the intestines.

This list of iron-rich food items is adapted from information provided by the NIH Office of Dietary Supplements.

FOOD	PORTION	IRON CONTENT, MG	% DAILY REFERENCE VALUE
Oysters	3 ounces	8	44
Chocolate	3 ounces	7	39
Beef liver	3 ounces	5	28
Hyacinth beans	½ cup	3	17
Spinach	½ cup	3	17
Tofu	½ cup	3	17
Tomato	½ cup	2	11
Potato	½ cup	2	11
Cashews	1 ounce	2	11
Chicken	3 ounces	1	6

Daily reference value of iron is 18 mg according to the 2013 FDA food-labeling guidelines.

What Are the Recommended Dietary Allowances for Iron?

1–3 years	7 mg
4–8 years	10 mg
9–13 years	8 mg
14–18 years	11 mg (boys); 15 mg (girls)
19 years and older	8 mg (men); 18 mg (women aged 19–50); 8 mg (women aged 51 and older)

The upper daily intake limit of iron is 45 mg.

Iron Supplements

- *Types.* A variety of iron supplements are available. Iron sulfate and iron gluconate are the most common iron supplements. Iron supplements taken with meals can reduce stomach discomfort and improve iron's absorption in the intestines. Vitamin C enhances the absorption of iron in the intestines as well, and it can be taken together with an iron supplement. Heme iron polypeptide is a new type of iron supplement that is odorless and tasteless, and it is easier to absorb compared to iron sulfate.
- *Iron supplementation for children.* Stomach acid is required to dissolve carbonyl iron prior to absorption in the intestines. This acid dissolution step, which is not required for all other iron supplements, slows down the absorption of carbonyl iron in the intestines. The slower absorption rate makes carbonyl iron a safer iron supplement for children to avoid iron overdose.
- *Anemia.* Iron supplements can be used to treat iron deficiency anemia. The recommended daily dose is 100–200 mg for two months.
- *Blood donation.* Iron supplementation can shorten the time required for blood donors to recover from a low hemoglobin level to a normal level. It often takes about 80–150 days for a healthy individual to recover from donating blood. Iron supplements taken at a daily dose of 35 mg can shorten the recovery time to a mere 30 days.
- *Memory.* Iron supplementation can enhance learning and memory. Studies reveal that iron supplementation improves language learning and memory in teenage girls.
- *Attention-deficit/hyperactivity disorder.* Iron supplementation may augment social skills and learning abilities in children with attention-deficit/hyperactivity disorder.
- *Premenstrual syndrome.* Iron supplementation may alleviate symptoms of premenstrual syndrome in women. The recommended daily dose is 20 mg of an iron supplement before menstruation.

- *Menorrhagia.* Women with menorrhagia are likely to lose a large amount of blood during menstruation. Excessive blood loss can give rise to iron deficiency. Supplementation with iron can ameliorate the symptoms in women with menorrhagia.
- *Exercise endurance.* Iron supplementation boosts exercise endurance, especially in woman athletes. The improvement in exercise endurance was even more obvious in iron-deficient woman athletes.

Safety Issues
- *Side effects.* Long-term supplementation with iron can cause the accumulation of excessive iron in the body. Excessive iron can lead to oxidative damage, exacerbating the symptoms associated with atherosclerosis, heart disease, cancers, diabetes, Alzheimer's disease, and Parkinson's disease. According to data from the Centers for Disease Control and Prevention, 29% of men in the US are in danger of excessive iron in the body. One should avoid taking iron supplements of more than 20 mg daily unless a high dose is required for the treatment of iron deficiency anemia.
- *Other essential elements.* Taking high-dose supplements of other essential elements—such as calcium, zinc, magnesium, manganese, or copper—can negatively affect iron absorption in the intestines. Iron supplements should be taken at least two hours apart from other essential element supplements.

What Types of Drugs May Interact with Iron?
- Antacid drugs can lower the absorption of iron in the intestines.
- Iron supplementation can hinder the absorption and efficacy of antibiotics, such as tetracycline.

20

ZINC

Zinc is an essential trace element. In the ancient past, humans already knew that zinc could accelerate wound healing. The human body contains about 2 g of zinc, which is distributed widely in different organs and tissues, including the brain, muscles, bones, kidneys, and liver. A small amount of zinc exists in an ionic state, while more than 95% of zinc is bound to proteins in the body. Zinc is an essential cofactor that supports the functions of more than 300 different enzymes.

What Are the Major Functions of Zinc?
- *Memory and learning.* Zinc plays an important role in memory and learning. Zinc enhances neuron-to-neuron communication in the hippocampus, where memory is stored in the brain. Zinc improves cognitive functions and prevents age-related cognitive impairment.
- *Antioxidant functions.* Zinc possesses antioxidant properties. The brain constitutes only 2% of the body's weight but

consumes 20% of all oxygen and glucose. Glucose metabolism can generate free radicals in neurons. Free radical oxidative damage contributes to the causes Alzheimer's disease and Parkinson's disease. Zinc-dependent enzymes can scavenge and inactivate free radicals and prevent them from causing damage to the brain.

- *Blood pressure control.* Renin-angiotensin system disorder is at least in part responsible for essential hypertension. Zinc enzymes regulate the activity of the renin-angiotensin system to forestall the onset of essential hypertension. Hence zinc deficiency elevates the risk of hypertension.
- *Blood glucose control.* Zinc is required as an essential element for the synthesis of insulin in the pancreas. Zinc deficiency negatively affects insulin production, raises the blood glucose level, and increases the risk of diabetes.
- *Wound healing.* Cell proliferation and regeneration are required for wound healing. Zinc enzymes promote the proliferation and regeneration of neighboring cells in wounded tissue. Zinc deficiency therefore can delay wound healing. In addition to accelerating wound healing, zinc has antibacterial and anti-inflammatory functions.

What Are the Symptoms of Zinc Deficiency?

Insufficient dietary intake is the main cause of zinc deficiency, a condition that occurs fairly often in women, teenagers, infants, and elderly people. Symptoms of zinc deficiency are as follows:

- *Skin and hair.* Zinc deficiency gives rise to acne, eczema, dry skin, hair loss, and delayed wound healing.
- *Oral cavity.* Zinc deficiency induces oral ulcers, and the tongue may be covered in a white coating.
- *Senses.* Zinc deficiency can give rise to night blindness and the loss of smell and taste.
- *Immune system.* Zinc deficiency makes a person more susceptible to gastrointestinal and respiratory infections.

- *Diarrhea.* Zinc deficiency increases the likelihood of frequent diarrhea.
- *Anorexia.* Zinc deficiency may lead to anorexia.
- *Delayed growth.* Zinc deficiency can adversely affect growth in children.

What Are the Risk Factors for Zinc Deficiency?

- *Digestion and absorption retardation.* Digestive diseases can hinder zinc absorption and lead to zinc deficiency. Digestive diseases—such as inflammatory bowel disease, ulcerative colitis, Crohn's disease, and celiac disease—can destroy the structure and integrity of mucosal cells lining the digestive tract, hampering the absorption of zinc in the intestines.
- *Alcoholism.* A low zinc level in the liver and blood and a high zinc level in the urine are common in patients with alcohol-induced cirrhosis. Excessive alcohol consumption disrupts the binding of zinc to albumin proteins, resulting in the presence of free zinc ions in the blood, which are in turn readily excreted via urine, leading to zinc deficiency.
- *Diabetes.* A high level of zinc in the urine is also commonly found in both type 1 and type 2 diabetes patients. Zinc regulates the production of insulin from the pancreas. Zinc deficiency hinders insulin production and exacerbates the condition in patients with diabetes.
- *Infection.* Zinc enzymes are involved in the synthesis of immunoglobulins and support the immune system. People with zinc deficiency are susceptible to bacterial infections. In the developing world, zinc supplementation reduces the incidence of diarrhea and mortality caused by bacterial infections in children.

Prevention and Treatment of Diseases

- *Prevention.* Meta-analysis confirms that zinc can help prevent bladder cancer (44), colorectal cancer (56), Alzheimer's disease (37), respiratory infection (101), rheumatoid arthritis (102), osteoporosis (94), preeclampsia (97), and vitiligo (111).

- *Treatment.* Meta-analysis confirms that zinc can help treat type 2 diabetes (60), type 1 diabetes (59), and metabolic syndrome (87).

Which Food Items Are Zinc Rich?

Many animal-based foods contain zinc. Oysters, beef, pork, and chicken are excellent sources of zinc. Plant-based foods—such as whole wheat, legumes, nuts, and seeds—are good sources of zinc.

This list of zinc-rich food items is adapted from information provided by the USDA.

FOOD	PORTION	ZINC CONTENT, MG	% DAILY REFERENCE VALUE
Oysters (cooked)	3 ounces	38	253
Beef (cooked)	3 ounces	5.0	33
Crab meat (cooked)	3 ounces	4.7	31
Pork (cooked)	3 ounces	3.1	21
Turkey (cooked)	3 ounces	3.0	20
Chicken (cooked)	3 ounces	2.2	15
Cashews	1 ounce	1.6	11
Milk	8 ounces	1.0	7
Almonds	1 ounce	0.9	6
Peanuts	1 ounce	0.9	6

Daily reference value of zinc is 15 mg according to the 2013 FDA food-labeling guidelines.

What Are the Recommended Dietary Allowances for Zinc?

1–3 years	3 mg
4–8 years	5 mg
9–13 years	8 mg
4–18 years	11 mg (boys); 9 mg (girls)
19 years and older	11 mg (men); 8 mg (women)

The upper daily intake limit of zinc is 40 mg.

Zinc Supplements

- *Dosage.* Common dosages of zinc supplements are in the range of 15–100 mg, and the most popular dosage is 50 mg. Many zinc supplements exceed the daily upper limit of 40 mg. Excessive consumption of zinc can lead to copper insufficiency. People who use zinc supplements should be cautious about the potential problems associated with copper deficiency.
- *Types.* Most zinc supplements include zinc oxide, zinc sulfate, zinc acetate, zinc gluconate, and zinc malate. When purchasing zinc, read the product label for the zinc content, not the zinc salt. Zinc gluconate appears to be more readily absorbed than zinc oxide in the intestines.
- *Zinc and copper.* People who take zinc supplements for more than one month need to supplement with copper at a recommended dose ratio of 10:1; for instance, take 10 mg of zinc with 1 mg of copper.
- *Common cold.* Zinc supplements can treat the common cold. Randomized controlled trials have shown that people who took zinc supplements soon after showing symptoms had a decrease in those symptoms: runny nose by 34%, sneezing by 22%, sore throat by 33%, hoarseness by 43%, and coughing by 46%. The recommended daily dose for treating the common cold is 80 mg.

- *Wilson disease.* Supplementation with zinc can alleviate the symptoms of Wilson disease, a rare hereditary copper-storage disorder characterized by abnormal accumulation of copper in the liver, brain, and other organs, leading to psychotic symptoms and hepatic malfunction.
- *Childhood colds.* Daily supplementation with zinc sulfate syrup at a dose of 15 mg may prevent children from catching the common cold, while a dose of 30 mg may treat the common cold in children.
- *Acne.* Zinc supplements can alleviate acne. The recommended daily dose is 30 mg.
- *Age-related macular degeneration.* Supplementation with zinc together with antioxidant vitamins may relieve macular degeneration. Randomized controlled trials have shown that zinc and antioxidant supplementations alleviated the symptoms of patients with age-related macular degeneration. Supplementation with zinc alone seemed effective, but the effect was more profound when taken together with antioxidants, including carotenes, vitamin C, and vitamin E.
- *Sickle cell disease.* Supplementation with zinc can assuage symptoms of sickle cell disease. Studies from India have shown that zinc supplementation given at a dose of 50 mg daily improved development and growth in children with sickle cell disease. Zinc ions augmented the oxygen-carrying capacity of the sickle red blood cell by stabilizing its cell membrane.
- *Attention-deficit/hyperactivity disorder.* Zinc supplements may treat attention-deficit/hyperactivity disorder in children and adults. Randomized controlled trials have shown that supplementation with zinc at a dose of 40 mg daily improved the symptoms of the disorder.
- *Cold sores.* Topical zinc cream may treat cold sores caused by herpes viral infections. Zinc interferes with the reproduction and proliferation of the herpes virus and accelerates wound healing.

Safety Issues
- *Side effects.* The lone side effect of zinc supplements is rare, but it may bring about stomach discomfort.
- *Copper.* Long-term supplementation with zinc may lead to copper deficiency. Excessive zinc levels, combined with copper deficiency, hamper the immune system and lead to anemia and cardiac malfunction. Taking more than the daily upper limit of 40 mg is not recommended.
- *HDL.* Long-term supplementation with zinc at doses greater than 100 mg daily may decrease "good" cholesterol (HDL) and increase the risk of prostate cancer.

What Types of Drugs May Interact with Zinc?
- Antibiotics, such as tetracycline, may negatively affect the absorption of zinc by the intestines.
- Metal chelation agents that treat copper or iron overload may reduce the absorption of zinc in the intestines.
- Anticonvulsants can lead to zinc deficiency.
- Diuretics can increase the renal excretion of zinc in the urine.

21

MANGANESE

Manganese is an essential trace element. The human body contains about 12 mg of manganese, which is stored mostly in the bones as well as in the liver, kidneys, and other organs and tissues. Only a minute quantity of manganese is needed for health and growth, while too much can bring about neurodegenerative disorders such as Parkinson's disease.

What Are the Major Functions of Manganese?

- *Antioxidant functions.* Mitochondria are the "power plants" of cells that produce high-energy ATP molecules. Power production lines in factories often incidentally discharge harmful byproducts, and mitochondria are similar. Deleterious free radicals, such as superoxide anion radicals, are generated during energy production in mitochondria. Nevertheless, mitochondria are equipped with manganese superoxide dismutase, an enzyme that can neutralize and scavenge superoxide anion radicals, thereby eliminating harmful byproducts during energy production.

- *Magnesium function.* Manganese is an essential cofactor that supports the function of various enzymes involved in carbohydrate metabolism, calcium absorption and blood sugar regulation.

What Are the Symptoms of Manganese Deficiency?

- The major symptoms of manganese deficiency are bone deformation, growth retardation, infertility, seizures, nausea, and vomiting. The typical dietary intake of manganese is sufficient to provide a trace amount of manganese for growth and health. Manganese deficiency is rare.

Which Food Items Are Manganese Rich?

Manganese mainly comes from plant-based foods. Manganese-rich plant-based foods include almonds, peanuts, walnuts, dark-green leafy vegetables, sweet potatoes, and tea. Wheat, legumes, and tofu are also excellent sources of manganese.

This list of manganese-rich food items is adapted from information provided by the USDA.

FOOD	PORTION	MANGANESE CONTENT, MG	% DAILY REFERENCE VALUE
Walnuts	1 ounce	1.28	64
Brown rice (cooked)	½ cup	1.07	54
Tea (green)	1 cup	1.00	50
Spinach (cooked)	½ cup	0.84	42
Pineapple (sliced)	½ cup	0.77	39
Almonds	1 ounce	0.65	33

continued

FOOD	PORTION	MANGANESE CONTENT, MG	% DAILY REFERENCE VALUE
Pineapple juice	½ cup	0.63	32
Peanuts	1 ounce	0.55	28
Tea (black)	1 cup	0.48	24
Sweet potato	½ cup	0.44	22

Daily reference value of manganese is 2 mg according to the 2013 FDA food-labeling guidelines.

What Are the Recommended Dietary Allowances for Manganese?

1–3 years	1.2 mg
4–8 years	1.5 mg
9–13 years	1.9 mg (boys); 1.6 mg (girls)
14–18 years	2.2 mg (boys); 1.6 mg (girls)
19 years and older	2.3 mg (men); 1.8 mg (women)

The upper daily intake limit of manganese is 11 mg.

Manganese Supplements

- *Dosage and types.* Common doses of manganese supplements are in the range of 10 to 50 mg. Major manganese supplements contain manganese gluconate, manganese sulfate, or manganese ascorbate. Taking more than 10 mg of a manganese supplement per day is not recommended.

Safety Issues

- *Side effects.* Manganese taken at high doses for long periods can lead to neurological disorders like trembling, shaking, difficulty walking, and facial muscle spasms—symptoms that resemble those of Parkinson's disease.

- *Other essential elements.* Taking iron, copper, zinc, magnesium, or calcium supplements can reduce the blood level of manganese.

What Types of Drugs May Interact with Manganese?
- Antacid medications, laxatives, and antibiotics may interfere with the absorption of manganese by the intestines.

22

COPPER

Copper is an essential trace element. The human body contains about 100 mg of copper. This minuscule quantity of copper is distributed widely in throughout body. It participates in many important physiological functions, including the normal development and growth of the bones, connective tissues, heart, muscles, brain, and many other organs.

What Are the Major Functions of Copper?
- *Oxidation reduction.* Copper can donate or accept electrons, and it is involved in many oxidation-reduction reactions in the body. Copper-dependent enzymes in mitochondria help convert oxygen to water during energy production.
- *Connective tissue.* Connective tissue is the most widely distributed tissue, and it exists in various forms in the body. Its main function is to connect and support the structure and integrity of organs. The most abundant proteins in connective tissue are

collagens, and copper is an essential element for the synthesis of collagens.

- *Oxidative stress.* Oxygen is crucial for life. When inhaled into the lungs, oxygen is involved in the production of free radicals, leading to oxidative damage. Oxidative damage has been attributed in part to the causes of many chronic diseases, such as cardiovascular disease, Alzheimer's disease, and diabetes, among others. Copper-dependent enzymes that exert potent antioxidant properties are widely distributed throughout different organs and tissues to neutralize free radicals and prevent oxidative damage.
- *Central nervous system.* Copper is involved in many physiological functions in the brain, and it is particularly important for the development and growth of the central nervous system. Copper deficiency in infants either during pregnancy or while breastfeeding can cause irreversible damage to the brain, resulting in developmental disorders of the central nervous system.
- *Cardiovascular system.* Copper contributes to maintaining the normal functions of the cardiovascular system. Copper deficiency can give rise to high "bad" cholesterol (LDL), high triglycerides, and hypertension, elevating the risk of cardiovascular diseases.
- *Immune system.* Copper is an essential element for normal functioning of the immune system. Copper deficiency suppresses cellular and humoral immunity and weakens immune functions. Copper-deficient people are prone to bacterial infections. Clinical studies have shown that immune functions in people who were placed on low-copper diets were weakened, as resulting in the inability of white blood cells to kill invading pathogens.

What Are the Symptoms of Copper Deficiency?
- The major symptoms of copper deficiency are anemia, leucopenia, and neutropenia. Additional symptoms include

arthritis, artery disease, skin discoloration, heart disease, and neuropathy. Malabsorption or excessive copper excretion from bile ducts often causes copper deficiency.

- Early signs of copper deficiency are paleness, edema, growth retardation, hair loss, anorexia, diarrhea, and dermatitis.

What Are the Risk Factors for Copper Deficiency?

- High-risk groups for copper deficiency include people undergoing long-term parenteral nutrition therapy without supplementation with copper, premature infants fed only breast milk, newborns with frequent diarrhea, patients with severe burns, hemodialysis patients, and long-term antacid and high-dose zinc supplement users.
- *Menkes disease.* Menkes disease is a hereditary disorder that affects copper metabolism. Boys are more likely than girls to be afflicted by the disease, which, as of today, has no treatment. Patients rarely live more than three years. The disease is caused by mutations in the gene encoding for copper-transporting proteins. An ATP7A gene variant leads to these disorders.
- *Wilson disease.* Wilson disease is a hereditary disorder affecting copper storage in the body. Patients with Wilson disease store too much copper in the liver, brain, and corneas, causing copper-induced multiorgan damage. Chelation therapy is effective in treating Wilson disease, particularly if the treatment starts in childhood. An ATP7B gene variant causes Wilson disease.

Prevention and Treatment of Diseases

- *Prevention.* Meta-analysis confirms that copper can help prevent respiratory infection (101), osteoporosis (94), and vitiligo (111).
- *Treatment.* Meta-analysis confirms that copper can help treat respiratory infection (101) and osteoporosis (94).

Which Food Items Are Copper Rich?

Many animal- and plant-based foods contain copper, including animals' internal organs, shellfish, nuts, and seeds. Oats and whole wheat are also good sources of copper.

This list of copper-rich food items is adapted from information provided by the USDA.

FOOD	PORTION	COPPER CONTENT, MCG	% DAILY REFERENCE VALUE
Beef liver	1 ounce	4,128	201
Oysters	6	2,397	120
Crab meat	3 ounces	1,005	50
Cashews	1 ounce	622	31
Clams	3 ounces	585	29
Sunflower seeds	1 ounce	519	26
Hyacinth beans	1 cup	797	25
Almonds	1 ounce	292	15
Mushrooms	1 cup (sliced)	223	11
Chocolate	1 ounce	198	10

Daily reference value of copper is 2,000 mcg according to the 2013 FDA food-labeling guidelines.

What Are the Recommended Dietary Allowances for Copper?

1–3 years	340 mcg
4–8 years	440 mcg
9–13 years	700 mcg
14–18 years	890 mcg
19 years and older	900 mcg

The upper daily intake limit of copper is 10,000 mcg.

Copper Supplements

- *Dosage and types.* Major copper supplements are copper gluconate, copper picolinate, and copper sulfate. The most common dosages of copper supplements are 1–3 mg.
- *Zinc and copper.* Supplementation with zinc may trigger the loss of copper in the body. Therefore, supplements containing both zinc and copper are common in the marketplace. Typically, the ratio of zinc to copper is 10 to 1 in these supplements (e.g., 10 mg of zinc with 1 mg of copper).
- *Vitamin C.* People who take iron and vitamin C supplements also need to supplement with copper to avoid copper insufficiency. Take these supplements at least two hours apart.
- *Bone density.* Supplementation with copper can prevent bone loss. Randomized clinical trials have shown that a daily dose of 3 mg thwarted the loss of bone density in postmenopausal women.

Safety Issues

- *Side effects.* High blood levels of copper ions increase the risk of coronary artery disease. High blood levels of copper can also reduce the survival rate of patients with chronic heart failure.

23

MOLYBDENUM

Molybdenum is an essential trace element. The human body contains about 5 mg of molybdenum, which is stored mainly in the liver and kidneys, as well as in the bones and teeth. Nitrogen-fixation bacteria can convert nitrogen gas from the air into nitrogen-containing compounds crucial for the survival of animals and plants on the planet. Human existence on Earth can be in part attributed to nitrogen-fixation bacteria. Molybdenum is an essential cofactor that supports enzymes involved in the metabolism of sulfur-containing amino acids in the body.

What Are the Major Functions of Molybdenum?
- *Metabolism of sulfur-containing amino acids.* Molybdenum-dependent enzymes are responsible for the conversion of sulfite into sulfate. This conversion is critical for the production of sulfur-containing amino acids, such as cysteine and methionine, in the body.

- *Uric acid and antioxidant functions.* Molybdenum-dependent enzymes can convert nucleotides into uric acid. Uric acid has antioxidant functions in the blood. However, an excessive amount of uric acid in the blood is known to lead to gout.

What Are the Symptoms of Molybdenum Deficiency?
- Molybdenum deficiency is rare. It is often noticed when an abnormally low amount of uric acid is found in the blood or when there is a shortage of sulfur-containing amino acids, such as cysteine or methionine.

Prevention and Treatment of Diseases
- So far, there is no scientific evidence that molybdenum can prevent or treat diseases.

Which Food Items Are Molybdenum Rich?
Many plant-based foods contain molybdenum, including dark-green leafy vegetables, nuts, legumes, and whole wheat. Animal-based foods—including beef, chicken, liver, and milk—are good sources of molybdenum.

This list of molybdenum-rich food items is adapted from information provided by the USDA.

FOOD	PORTION	MOLYBDENUM CONTENT, MCG	% DAILY REFERENCE VALUE
Hyacinth beans	8 ounces	148	197
Kidney beans	8 ounces	132	176
Black beans	8 ounces	130	173
Almonds	8 ounces	46	61
Chestnuts	8 ounces	42	56
Peanuts	8 ounces	42	56
Cashews	8 ounces	38	51
Yogurt	8 ounces	11	15

FOOD	PORTION	MOLYBDENUM CONTENT, MCG	% DAILY REFERENCE VALUE
Tomato	8 ounces	9	12
Milk	1 cup	9	12

Daily reference value of molybdenum is 75 mcg according to the 2013 FDA food-labeling guidelines.

What Are the Recommended Dietary Allowances for Molybdenum?

1–3 years	17 mcg
4–8 years	22 mcg
9–13 years	34 mcg
14–18 years	43 mcg
19 years and older	45 mcg

The upper daily intake limit of molybdenum is 2,000 mcg.

Molybdenum Supplements

- *Dosage and types.* Molybdenum supplements typically contain sodium molybdate, and its common dosage is 150–500 mcg.
- *Diet.* Dietary intake of molybdenum should be sufficient, and there seems to be no need for molybdenum supplements.

24

IODINE

Iodine is an essential trace element. The human body contains about 15–20 mg of iodine, of which about 70% is stored in the thyroid gland. The remainder is distributed throughout various organs and tissues. The thyroid gland, located right above the collarbone, requires iodine to produce thyroid hormones. The rate of basal metabolism, defined as the number of calories needed at rest, is determined by thyroid hormones. Marine animals and plants provide the major sources of iodine. Before fortifying iodine in table salt, people who lived in inland regions of the world experienced severe iodine deficiency. Iodine deficiency hinders the production of thyroid hormones, giving rise to enlarged thyroid glands and hypothyroidism. Iodine deficiency contributes to brain development disorders and mental disorders in children.

What Are the Major Functions of Iodine?
- *Production of thyroid hormones.* Iodine participates in the production of thyroid hormones T3 and T4. Thyroid hormone

T3 contains three iodine ions, and thyroid hormone T4 contains four. Thyroid hormones control the basal metabolic rate in the body, which is the number of calories needed at rest, like the amount of fuel needed for a car at cruising speed. A fast metabolism, like a car cruising in the fast lane, requires more fuel, and a slow metabolism, like a car in the slow lane, requires less fuel. Iodine deficiency decreases the basal metabolic rate by one-half, while too much thyroid hormone can double the basal metabolic rate. T3 is the active form of the thyroid hormone, and T4 is a precursor to T3. When needed, T4 is converted to T3.

What Are the Symptoms of Iodine Deficiency?

- Iodine deficiency hampers brain development in infants and children and, in severe cases, causes mental disorders in children. Iodine deficiency gives rise to enlarged thyroid glands in adults. Long-term iodine deficiency could lead to thyroid cancer. In the past, people who lived in mountainous regions, such as in Mexico and the Great Lakes region in the US, had a severe iodine deficiency, which was largely resolved after table salt fortified with iodine became available in those regions. Globally, more than 2 billion people still live in an iodine-deficient environment.

Prevention and Treatment of Diseases

- *Prevention.* Iodine supplements may prevent radiation-induced thyroid cancer.
- *Treatment.* Iodine supplements may treat cyclical mastalgia.

Which Food Items Are Iodine Rich?

Shellfish, fish, shrimp, and milk are excellent sources of iodine. Marine plants, such as kelp, are rich in iodine.

This list of iodine-rich food items is adapted from information provided by the NIH Office of Dietary Supplements.

FOOD	PORTION	IODINE CONTENT, MCG	% DAILY REFERENCE VALUE
Cod (cooked)	3 ounces	99	66
Yogurt	1 cup	75	50
Milk	1 cup	56	37
Bread	2 slices	45	30
Shrimp	3 ounces	35	23
Spaghetti	1 cup	27	18
Eggs	1	24	16
Tuna (cooked)	3 ounces	17	11
Corn	½ cup	14	9
Cheese	1 ounce	12	8

Daily reference value of iodine is 150 mcg according to the 2013 FDA food-labeling guidelines.

What Are the Recommended Dietary Allowances for Iodine?

1–3 years	90 mcg
4–8 years	90 mcg
9–13 years	120 mcg
14–18 years	150 mcg
19 years and older	150 mcg

The upper daily intake limit of iodine is 1,100 mcg.

Iodine Supplements

- *Dosage and types.* Doses of iodine supplements commonly range from 150 to 1,000 mcg. Potassium iodine and sodium iodine are the two main products available in the marketplace. Kelp is an excellent source of iodine. Nearly 100% of potassium iodine is absorbed in the intestines.

- *Cyclical mastalgia.* Supplementation with iodine can improve cyclical mastalgia, a condition characterized by painful and swollen breasts during menstruation. A dose of 200 mcg daily before menstruation ameliorated this condition.

Safety Issues
- *Side effects.* Long-term supplementation with high doses of iodine may cause hypothyroidism because excessive iodine blocks thyroid hormone production and gives rise to an enlarged thyroid gland. Sudden intake of high doses of an iodine supplement may also lead to hyperthyroidism in people with iodine deficiency. It is best to avoid taking more than 500 mcg daily of an iodine supplement.

What Types of Drugs May Interact with Iodine?
- *Antithyroid medications.* Taking high-dose iodine supplements together with an antithyroid drug can cause hypothyroidism.
- *Antihypertensive drugs.* Supplementation with iodine may lead to hyperkalemia in hypertensive patients who take angiotensin-converting enzyme inhibitor medications.
- *Potassium diuretics.* Taking potassium diuretics together with potassium iodine may cause hyperkalemia.

25

CHROMIUM

Chromium is an essential trace element. The human body contains about 14 mg of chromium, which is stored mostly in the liver, kidneys, and bones. Chromium exists in two different ionic forms, trivalent chromium ions and hexavalent chromium ions. Trivalent chromium ions are beneficial to health, while hexavalent chromium ions are harmful and toxic chemicals produced by industrial pollution. In this chapter, we will focus mainly on trivalent chromium ions.

What Are the Major Functions of Chromium?
- *Control blood glucose.* Chromium ions can boost insulin functions. They increase insulin sensitivity, aid in glucose entering the cell, and lower blood glucose concentrations.
- *Regulate body weight.* Chronic inflammation is a common symptom of obesity. Obese bodies can produce a high amount of inflammatory mediators. Chromium ions regulate body weight by reducing the amount of inflammatory mediators in

the body. Chromium ions can also facilitate insulin action in the metabolism of carbohydrates, proteins, and lipids.

What Are the Symptoms of Chromium Deficiency?

- The major symptoms of chromium deficiency include anxiety and exhaustion. Consumption of chromium-poor foods is the main cause of chromium deficiency. In addition, a high-sugar diet can trigger the loss of chromium ions from the urine. Chromium deficiency is also related to infection, pregnancy, and a stressful lifestyle.

Prevention and Treatment of Diseases

- *Prevention.* Meta-analysis confirms that chromium ions can prevent type 2 diabetes (60) and obesity (91).
- *Treatment.* Meta-analysis confirms that chromium ions can treat type 2 diabetes (60) and obesity (91).

Which Food Items Are Chromium Rich?

Beef liver, whole wheat, nuts, mushrooms, coffee, tea, and wines (red or white) are rich in chromium. Onions, broccoli, potatoes, green beans, tomatoes, and black pepper are also good sources of chromium.

This list of chromium-rich foods is adapted from information provided by the NIH Office of Dietary Supplements.

FOOD	PORTION	CHROMIUM CONTENT, MCG	% DAILY REFERENCE VALUE
Broccoli	½ cup	11	9.0
Apple juice	1 cup	8	7.0
Potatoes (mashed)	1 cup	3	3.0
Garlic	1 teaspoon	3	3.0
Orange juice	1 cup	2	2.0
Turkey	3 ounces	2	2.0

continued

FOOD	PORTION	CHROMIUM CONTENT, MCG	% DAILY REFERENCE VALUE
Whole wheat	2 slices	2	2.0
Apple	1	1	0.9
Banana	1	1	0.9
Green beans	½ cup	1	0.9

Daily reference value of chromium is 120 mcg according to the 2013 FDA food-labeling guidelines.

What Are the Recommended Dietary Allowances for Chromium?

1–3 years	11 mcg
4–8 years	15 mcg
9–13 years	25 mcg (boys); 21 mcg (girls)
14–18 years	35 mcg (boys); 24 mcg (girls)
19 years and older	35 mcg (men); 25 mcg (women)

There is currently no upper intake limit for chromium.

Chromium Supplements

- *Dosage and types.* Chromium is a popular dietary supplement. Common dosages range from 50 to 1,000 mcg. The major chromium supplements are chromium chloride, niacin chromium, chromium picolinate, high-chromium yeast, and chromium citrate. The recommended dietary allowance of chromium is 35 mcg for men. Since chromium content in foods is generally low and insufficient (see the tables above), chromium insufficiency is common. Supplementation with chromium is relatively safe, as there is no upper daily intake limit. However, taking more than 100 mcg daily of chromium is not recommended.

- *Absorption.* The efficiency of chromium absorption in the intestines is rather poor; less than 2% of chromium from foods is absorbed, and the remainder is excreted from the stools. Among all chromium supplements, chromium picolinate has the highest absorption efficiency.
- *Diabetes.* Supplementation with chromium may ameliorate symptoms associated with type 2 diabetes. Chromium supplements, taken twice daily at a dose of 50 mcg for four months, have lowered fasting glucose levels and insulin levels, as well as levels of HbA1c, in patients with type 2 diabetes.
- *Cholesterol.* Chromium can elevate "good" cholesterol (HDL) blood levels. Supplementation with chromium at a dose of 100 mcg daily boosts HDL levels in patients with hypercholesterolemia.
- *Blood glucose.* Chromium can regulate blood glucose levels. Chromium supplements taken at a dose of 100 mcg daily have raised blood glucose levels in patients with hypoglycemia.
- *Weight loss.* Chromium controls body weight. Supplementation with chromium at a dose of 100 mcg daily has reduced body weight; however, results may vary.

Safety Issues
- *Hexavalent chromium.* Trivalent chromium is an essential trace element, while hexavalent chromium is a byproduct from the chemical and welding industries. Exposure to excessive amounts of hexavalent chromium can lead to stomach ulcers, damage to the liver and kidneys, and even death. When purchasing chromium, read the product label to ensure that it contains no hexavalent chromium.
- *Side effects.* Chromium taken at doses higher than 600–24,000 mcg may cause anemia, thrombocytopenia, and hepatic and renal malfunctions.

What Types of Drugs May Interact with Chromium?
- Antacid medications can reduce the absorption of chromium in the intestines.
- Insulin and nonsteroidal anti-inflammatory drugs can augment chromium's effects on the body. The dosage of chromium supplements needs to be adjusted when taking these medications.

26

SELENIUM

Selenium is an essential trace element. In 1973, scientists discovered that selenium was an essential cofactor for glutathione peroxidase, an enzyme that plays an important role as an antioxidant defense mechanism in the body, and established the significance of selenium in human health. Working together with vitamin E, glutathione peroxidase neutralizes free radicals in the cellular membrane and prevents oxidative damage to the integrity of the cellular structure. The human body contains about 13–20 mg of selenium, of which 30% is stored in the bones and muscles, while the rest is stored in the liver, kidneys, and other organs. About 25 proteins contain a selenium ion as a cofactor. These proteins are called selenoproteins, and they are involved in many important physiological functions, including reproduction, thyroid metabolism, DNA synthesis, and prevention of oxidative stress–induced damage.

What Are the Major Functions of Selenium?

- *Defense against oxidative damage.* Selenoproteins, such as glutathione peroxidase, play an important role in cellular defense against oxidative damage. Glutathione peroxidase can scavenge and inactivate hydrogen peroxide and lipid peroxides produced by pathogens and injured tissues, preventing them from causing oxidative damage to the cells.
- *Immune system.* Selenium can enhance immune functions by activating natural killer cells, enhancing the proliferation of lymphocytes, and increasing the production of interferon-gamma and antibody-producing B cells.
- *Thyroid metabolism.* Selenoproteins participate in the synthesis and metabolism of thyroid hormones T3 and T4. Through their antioxidant properties, selenoproteins attenuate the production of autoimmune antibodies and mitigate the symptoms of hypothyroidism in patients with autoimmune thyroid disease. During the course of normal metabolism, the thyroid gland can produce free radicals and hydrogen peroxide. Selenoproteins, such as glutathione peroxidase, can quench free radicals and degrade hydrogen peroxide, preventing oxidative damage to the thyroid gland.
- *Selenoprotein P.* Selenoprotein P is involved in transporting selenium ions from the liver to other organs and tissues in the body. Each selenoprotein P carries nine selenium ions.
- *Selenoprotein W.* Like glutathione, selenoprotein W has antioxidant properties. It is distributed widely in various organs, including the brain, heart, breasts, and prostate gland.

What Are the Symptoms of Selenium Deficiency?

- Symptoms of selenium deficiency include muscle weakness, muscular dystrophy, and cardiomyopathy. Both animal- and plant-based foods contain selenium, so selenium deficiency is rare.
- *Keshan disease.* Keshan disease precipitates selenium deficiency. Owing to the lack of selenium in the soil, people who lived in

a vast area of China, from the northeast to southwest regions, were afflicted with Keshan disease. Selenium deficiency induces cardiomyopathy. Its symptoms include an enlarged heart, heart failure, and fibrosis, and children and women are most vulnerable to Keshan disease. The Chinese government provided millions of people who lived in the afflicted regions with selenium supplements. Keshan disease has been largely eradicated since 1990.

- *Kashin-Beck disease.* Selenium deficiency in soil also contributes to Kashin-Beck disease. This disease is also most prevalent in China. Kashin-Beck disease affects mostly young people, and symptoms include osteoarthritis and abnormal cartilage growth, causing deformations in the joints and dwarfism. Supplementation with selenium seems to alleviate these symptoms.

Prevention and Treatment of Diseases
- *Prevention.* Meta-analysis confirms that selenium can help prevent bladder cancer (44), Kashin-Beck disease (80), colorectal cancer (56), gestational diabetes (68), rheumatoid arthritis (102), prostate cancer (99), stomach cancer (107), breast cancer (47), preeclampsia (97), and chronic pancreatitis (54).
- *Treatment.* Meta-analysis confirms that selenium can help treat sepsis (105) and autoimmune thyroid disease (43).

Which Food Items Are Selenium Rich?
Foods rich in selenium include plant-based foods—such as Brazil nuts, oats, and whole wheat bread—and animal-based foods like meats, seafood, and milk. The selenium content in soil dictates the amount of selenium present in both plant- and animal-based foods produced in a region. For example, the selenium content in the soil of certain regions in Brazil is very high; therefore, Brazil nuts in general contain high amounts of selenium. Conversely, the soil of certain regions in China, New Zealand, Belgium, and some Northern European countries is relatively low in selenium content. People who live in these selenium-poor

regions of the world should be cautious about their insufficient dietary intake of selenium and potential for selenium deficiency.

This list of selenium-rich food items is adapted from information provided by the NIH Office of Dietary Supplements.

FOOD	PORTION	SELENIUM CONTENT, MCG	% DAILY REFERENCE VALUE
Brazil nuts	1 ounce	544	777
Tuna (cooked)	3 ounces	68	97
Cod (cooked)	3 ounces	32	46
Turkey (cooked)	3 ounces	27	39
Chicken breast (cooked)	3 ounces	24	34
Beef (cooked)	3 ounces	23	33
Sunflower seeds	1 ounce	23	33
Eggs	1	15	21
Bread	1 slice	6	9
Walnuts	1 ounce	5	7

Daily reference value of selenium is 70 mcg according to the 2013 FDA food-labeling guidelines.

What Are the Recommended Dietary Allowances for Selenium?

1–3 years	20 mcg
4–8 years	30 mcg
9–13 years	40 mcg
14–18 years	55 mcg
19 years and older	55 mcg

The upper daily intake limit of selenium is 400 mcg.

Selenium Supplements

- *Dosage and types.* Common dosages of selenium supplements range from 100 to 200 mcg. The major types of selenium supplements include selenite, methylselenocysteine, and selenium extracted from yeasts (containing methylselenocysteine), all of which are readily absorbed in the intestines. The body is quite efficient in absorbing selenium present in foods or supplements.

- *Brazil nuts.* Each Brazil nut contains about 68–91 mcg of selenium. The recommended dietary allowance of selenium is only 55 mcg for adults. Consuming more than two Brazil nuts a day is not recommended in order to avoid an overdose of selenium.

- *Immune system.* Selenium enhances immune functions. Studies from England have shown that supplementation with selenium could boost immune functions in healthy people. In addition, selenium supplements at a dose of 200 mcg daily appear to lower the viral load of AIDS patients.

- *Male infertility.* Selenium supplements may mitigate male infertility. The blood levels of selenium have been found to be low in infertile males. A daily intake of 100 mcg of selenium by men improved the chances of pregnancy for their female partners.

- *Depression.* Selenium may improve symptoms in patients with major depression. Blood selenium content was low in patients with depression. Studies have shown that 100 mcg of selenium taken daily for eight weeks improved the mood and quality of life of patients with depression.

- *Thyroid gland.* Selenium supplementation may alleviate the symptoms of hypothyroidism. Randomized controlled trials have shown that supplementation with selenium at a dose of 200 mcg daily ameliorated the mood and symptoms of patients with Hashimoto's hypothyroidism.

- *Cancer.* Selenium supplementation may prevent cancer. Randomized controlled trials have shown that supplementation with selenium at a daily dose of 200 mcg reduced the risk of prostate cancer by 66%, colorectal cancer by 50%, and lung cancer by 40%, as well as all-cause mortality by 17%.

Safety Issues
- *Side effects.* Daily supplementation with selenium at a dose of more than 900 mcg can cause depression, anxiety, mood swings, nausea, and vomiting. High blood levels of selenium increase the risk of stomach cancer and type 2 diabetes.
- *Inflammatory bowel disease.* Selenium absorption was inadequate in the intestines of patients with Crohn's disease and ulcerative colitis. Such diseases could lead to selenium insufficiency.
- *Prostate cancer.* Prostate cancer patients should not take more than a daily dose of 140 mcg of selenium to avoid exacerbating the symptoms associated with the disease.

What Types of Drugs May Interact with Selenium?
- Antacid drugs, such as proton pump inhibitors, may reduce the absorption of selenium in the intestines.

27

OMEGA-3 FATTY ACIDS

Omega-3 fatty acids are essential nutrients. Dietary intake of omega-3 fatty acids is necessary, since the body cannot produce them. The three major types of omega-3 fatty acids are EPA and DHA (from marine animals and marine plants) as well as ALA (from plants grown in soil). Omega-3 fatty acids are polyunsaturated fatty acids. Omega-6 fatty acids are another type of polyunsaturated fatty acids that exist in plants grown in soil. Omega-3 fatty acids have anti-inflammatory functions, while omega-6 fatty acids possess proinflammatory functions; both functions are important for health and growth. The typical American diet contains 14–25 times more omega-6 fatty acids than omega-3 fatty acids. Hence American diets in general are proinflammatory. The optimal dietary ratio of omega-6 fatty acids to omega-3 fatty acids is 2–3:1. Omega-3 fatty acids play an important role in health, as they have anti-inflammatory properties and the ability to improve cognition and learning, and they can prevent cancers.

What Are the Major Functions of Omega-3 Fatty Acids?

- *Structure and function of the cellular membrane.* If the shape of a cell is like a tiny ball, its surface is covered by a bilayer lipid membrane. Omega-3 fatty acids are important components of the lipids in the cellular membrane, which are involved in regulating membrane fluidity and semipermeability, controlling messages and molecules transported into or out of the cell, and maintaining the normal physiological functions of the cell.
- *Vision functions.* A high amount of omega-3 fatty acids is present in the retina of the eye. Omega-3 fatty acids participate in the conversion of visual images to nerve impulses in the retina before transmitting these impulses to the brain.
- *Immune functions.* Omega-3 fatty acids regulate the immune system in its defense against inflammation caused by bacterial infections. Through modifications of lipid composition in the cellular membrane, omega-3 fatty acids can alleviate inflammatory reactions in the body.

What Are the Symptoms of Omega-3 Fatty Acid Deficiency?

- The major symptoms of omega-3 fatty acid deficiency are rough skin, dry and brittle hair, soft and cracked nails, thirst, frequent urination, insomnia, attention deficit, and depression.

Prevention and Treatment of Diseases

- *Prevention.* Meta-analysis confirms that omega-3 fatty acids can prevent heart failure (74); type 2 diabetes (60); stroke, particularly in women (108); atrial fibrillation (40); cardiovascular disease (48); hypertension (78); breast cancer (47); coronary artery disease (57); cognition impairment in the elderly (55); dry eyes (61); liver cancer (81); and depression (58).

- *Treatment.* Meta-analysis confirms that omega-3 fatty acids can treat type 2 diabetes (60), rheumatoid arthritis (102), cardiovascular disease (48), hemodialysis via lipids (75), attention-deficit/hyperactivity disorder (41), hypertension (78), fatty liver disease (66), coronary artery disease (57), dry eyes (61), schizophrenia in its early stages (104), depression (58), and cognitive impairment of the memory (55).

Which Food Items from Marine Animals Are Rich in Omega-3 Fatty Acid (DHA and EPA)?

Mackerel, lake trout, sardines, herring, and swordfish are excellent sources of omega-3 fatty acids from marine animals (DHA and EPA).

This list of omega-3 fatty acid–rich marine animals is adapted from information provided by the American Heart Association.

FOOD	PORTION	OMEGA-3 FATTY ACID CONTENT, G
Herring	3 ounces	1.81
Salmon	3 ounces	1.48
Sardines	3 ounces	1.19
Oysters	3 ounces	1.18
Swordfish	3 ounces	0.97
Trout	3 ounces	0.84
Flounder	3 ounces	0.48
Crab	3 ounces	0.34
Catfish	3 ounces	0.25
Cod	3 ounces	0.20

Which Food Items from Plants Grown in the Soil Are Rich in Omega-3 Fatty Acid (ALA)?

The best vegetarian sources of omega-3 fatty acids from plants grown in the soil (ALA) are flaxseeds, flaxseed oil, hempseed oil, and linseed oil.

This list of omega-3 fatty acid–rich plant-based foods is adapted from information provided by the USDA.

FOOD	PORTION	OMEGA-3 FATTY ACID CONTENT, G
Linseed oil	1 teaspoon	7.3
Hempseed oil	1 ounce	3.7
Walnuts	1 ounce	2.6
Walnut oil	1 teaspoon	1.4
Rapeseed oil	1 teaspoon	1.3
Peanut oil	1 teaspoon	0.9
Tofu	½ cup	0.2
Strawberries	3 ounces	0.1
Broccoli	3 ounces	0.1
Kiwi	3 ounces	0.1

Is There Any Difference between Omega-3 Fatty Acids from Marine Plants and Animals (DHA and EPA) and Omega-3 Fatty Acid from Plants Grown in Soil (ALA)?

- Omega-3 fatty acids (DHA and EPA) in fish or fish oil or in marine plants such as kelp and algae are essential nutrients that support cognition, vision, and prevention of cardiovascular diseases. Only a small amount of ALA is converted to DHA in the body. Generally speaking, ALA is not as beneficial to health as DHA and EPA. When purchasing omega-3 fatty acids, it is best to select products containing DHA and EPA, not ALA.

Which Food Items Are Rich in Omega-6 Fatty Acids (LA)?

The best vegetarian sources of omega-6 fatty acids (LA) are grape-seed oil, sunflower oil, corn oil, wheat germ oil, and soybean oil.

This list of omega-6 fatty acid–rich foods is adapted from information provided by the USDA.

FOOD	PORTION	OMEGA-6 FATTY ACID CONTENT, G
Safflower oil	1 teaspoon	10.1
Sunflower seed	1 ounce	9.7
Pine nuts	1 ounce	9.4
Sunflower oil	1 teaspoon	8.9
Corn oil	1 teaspoon	7.3
Soybean oil	1 teaspoon	6.9
Walnuts	1 ounce	6.4
Brazil nuts	1 ounce	5.8
Sesame oil	1 teaspoon	5.6
Rapeseed oil	1 teaspoon	5.5

What Are the Recommended Dietary Allowances for Omega-3 Fatty Acids?

1–3 years	0.7 g
4–8 years	0.9 g
9–13 years	1.2 g (boys); 1.0 g (girls)
14–18 years	1.6 g (boys); 1.1 g (girls)
19 years and older	1.6 g (men); 1.1 g (women)

There is currently no upper intake limit for omega-3 fatty acids. However, the FDA recommends that daily intake of omega-3 fatty acids from foods and supplements not exceed 3 g and that daily intake of omega-3 fatty acids from supplements alone not exceed 2 g. WHO suggests that daily dietary intake of omega-3 fatty acids be equal to 1–2% of one's daily calorie requirement, or about 3–6 g.

What Are the Recommended Dietary Allowances for Omega-6 Fatty Acids?

1–3 years	7 g
4–8 years	10 g
9–13 years	12 g (boys); 10 g (girls)
14–18 years	16 g (boys); 11 g (girls)
19 years and older	17 g (men); 12 g (women)

WHO suggests that daily dietary intake of omega-6 fatty acids be equal to 5–8% of one's daily calorie requirement, or 16–25 g.

Omega-3 Fatty Acid Supplements

- *Fish oil versus fish liver oil.* Fish oil is extracted from the meat of marine fishes, which contain omega-3 fatty acids (EPA and DHA) but no vitamin A or vitamin D. Fish liver oil is extracted from the livers of marine fishes, which contain omega-3 fatty acids (EPA and DHA) as well as vitamin A and vitamin D. Compositions of the omega-3 fatty acids in fish oil and fish liver oil are different, as fish oil has a higher content of omega-3 fatty acids compared to fish liver oil. In the winter months, Northern Europeans consume fish liver oil to obtain vitamin D due to lack of sun exposure, while in the summer months, they enjoy sun exposure and consume only fish oil to avoid getting too much vitamin D from fish liver oil.
- *Dosage.* Omega-3 fatty acid supplements have several different formulations, of which the most popular is a soft gel cap containing 200 mg to 1,000 mg. When purchasing omega-3 fatty acid supplements, it is imperative to read the label for the relative amounts of EPA and DHA in each soft gel rather than the total amount of oil in each soft gel. A daily dose of 1 g of omega-3 fatty acids with a meal is sufficient to maintain good health. If a dose of 2 g of omega-3 fatty acids is needed,

you can take 1 g twice a day. Taking more than 2 g of omega-3 fatty acids daily is not recommended.

- *Types.* Omega-3 fatty acid supplements contain natural triglycerides, an ester form of triglycerides, or synthetic triglycerides. Omega-3 fatty acids in fish oil are natural triglycerides. The ester form of triglycerides and synthetic triglycerides are from synthetic fish oil, and their advantage is that they are free of pollutants. The disadvantage is that they lack all other nutrients present in natural fish oil.

- *Krill oil.* Krill oil, which is extracted from krill, is rich in omega-3 fatty acids (EPA and DHA). Krill oil lowers cholesterol and triglycerides and has anti-inflammatory functions, similar to fish oil.

- *Heart.* Supplementation with omega-3 fatty acids may protect heart function, as it lowers triglycerides and blood pressure, increases "good" cholesterol (HDL), and prevents atrial fibrillation and heart disease. Omega-3 fatty acids can also have anticoagulant effects and prevent venous thrombosis.

- *Inflammatory disease.* Omega-3 fatty acids in fish oil have anti-inflammatory functions. As such, they can ameliorate the symptoms observed in the early stages of rheumatoid arthritis, inflammatory bowel disease, and lupus erythematosus.

- *Cancer.* Supplementation with omega-3 fatty acids prevents weight loss in cancer patients undergoing chemotherapy. On average, a cancer patient could lose up to five pounds during a course of chemotherapy. Supplementation with omega-3 fatty acids during chemotherapy not only prevents weight loss; it also increases muscle mass. Long-term supplementation with omega-3 fatty acids was found to lower the risk of breast cancer. Regular consumption of fish may also prevent the recurrence of breast cancer.

- *Depression.* Omega-3 fatty acid supplements can treat depression, particularly supplements in which the EPA content is greater than 60%. Prozac and omega-3 fatty acid supplements

with a high EPA content taken together can effectively mitigate the symptoms of depression.

- *Memory.* Supplementation with omega-3 fatty acids improves
  memory, lowers triglycerides and blood pressure, and raises
  "good" cholesterol (HDL) levels.

- *Life-span.* Studies have shown that people aged 74 and older
  who had higher blood levels of omega-3 fatty acids lived longer and had a lower risk of cardiovascular disease compared to
  those with lower blood levels of omega-3 fatty acids.

- *Venous thrombosis.* Regular consumption of fish and fish oil
  may lower the risk of venous thrombosis. Studies from Nor-
  way have shown that people who consumed fish at least three
  times per week decreased the risk of venous thrombosis by
  22%. People who consumed fish three times per week and also
  took daily omega-3 fatty acid supplements reduced the risk of
  venous thrombosis by 48%.

- *Rheumatoid arthritis.* Supplementation with omega-3 fatty
  acids may prevent rheumatoid arthritis. Studies have shown
  that omega-3 fatty acids taken at a dose of 210 mg daily for
  seven years reduced the risk of rheumatoid arthritis by 52%.

- *Ulcerative colitis.* Supplementation with omega-3 fatty acids
  may lower the risk of ulcerative colitis. Randomized controlled
  trials have shown that omega-3 fatty acid supplements taken
  at doses ranging from 410 to 2,000 mg daily lowered the risk
  of ulcerative colitis by 77%. On the contrary, higher dietary
  intake of omega-6 fatty acids exacerbated the risk of ulcerative
  colitis.

- *Dry eyes.* Supplementation with fish oil may improve dry eye
  syndrome. Studies have shown that a daily dose of 400 mg
  ameliorated dry eyes caused by prolonged computer use.

- *Breast cancer recurrence.* Supplementation with fish oil may
  prevent the recurrence of breast cancer. Women who take fish
  oil supplements have a 32% lower risk of breast cancer. Early-
  stage breast cancer patients who take fish oil supplements have
  a 25% lower risk of breast cancer recurrence.

- *Age-related macular degeneration.* People who consume fish regularly decrease the risk of age-related macular degeneration. Eating fish once a week decreased the risk by 42%.
- *Anxiety.* Supplementation with omega-3 fatty acids may lessen anxiety. Studies have shown that medical students who took 2 g of omega-3 fatty acids daily for 12 weeks curtailed the risk of anxiety by 20%.
- *Suicide.* Low blood levels of omega-3 fatty acids have been linked to a higher risk of suicide. Data obtained from 1,600 US soldiers who had committed suicide revealed that soldiers whose blood levels of omega-3 fatty acids were low had a 62% increased risk of suicide.
- *Psychosis.* Supplementation with omega-3 fatty acids may prevent psychosis. In one study, young people (ages 13–25) with psychotic or schizophrenic tendencies were divided into two cohorts. One cohort received 700 mg of omega-3 fatty acids daily and the other cohort received a daily placebo for a period of one year. The results have shown that while 27.5% of the young people in the placebo cohort developed a psychiatric disorder, only 4.6% of the young people in the omega-3 fatty acid cohort developed one.
- *Muscle strength.* Omega-3 fatty acid supplements may boost muscle strength. Omega-3 fatty acid supplements taken at a daily dose of 3 g for six months have increased muscle mass by 3.5% and muscle strength by 6% in elderly people.
- *Acne.* Supplementation with omega-3 fatty acids may ameliorate acne. A group of acne-afflicted young people (ages 18–33) was divided into two cohorts: one cohort received supplementation with omega-3 fatty acids at a daily dose of 2 g for 10 weeks, and the other received a placebo for 10 weeks. The results revealed that the omega-3 fatty acid cohort's acne outbreaks were reduced by 42% compared to the placebo group.

Safety Issues

- *Side effects.* Fish oil and omega-3 fatty acid supplements are relatively safe. The main complaint is a fishy smell in hiccups.
- *Blood thinning.* Fish oil has a blood-thinning effect. People who take blood-thinning medications, such as warfarin, should be cautious about taking fish oil supplements.
- *Weight gain.* Long-term supplementation with fish oil may cause weight gain.
- *Vitamin A/D.* Avoid taking fish oil together with high doses of vitamin A and vitamin D. Fish oil can increase the absorption of these lipid-soluble vitamins by the intestines and cause high blood levels of vitamin A and vitamin D.

PART THREE

Secrets for Staying Healthy

Recent advances in science provide us with new tips for staying healthy. Through intensive research efforts, we have gained new insights into the molecular and pathological aspects of chronic diseases, such as Alzheimer's disease, heart disease, diabetes, and cancer. However, the root causes of these chronic diseases are still largely unknown. Genetic and environmental factors, as well as their interplay, are known to be associated with chronic diseases. Of environmental attributes, diet and lifestyle are modifiable factors in the prevention of chronic diseases. Diet and lifestyle can even influence the expression of predisposed disease–causing genes. Prevention is the best cure. Most of the drugs developed by pharmaceutical companies to treat chronic diseases are intended to treat only symptoms rather than causes.

Four tips for staying healthy are maintaining an appropriate weight, having a nutrient-balanced diet, learning new things or hobbies, and exercising regularly. All these goals are attainable, as you will see in the following chapters.

28

HOW DOES SUGAR MAKE YOU FAT?

A newborn calf stands wobbly on its own feet and makes a beeline for its mother's udder. Among their innate needs, humans' genes are hard-wired to acquire sugar, salt, and fat. In prehistoric times, humans made long journeys in search of food. Besides filling their empty stomachs, they prided themselves in finding sugar, salt, or fat. People are born with a desire for the sugar in Twinkies and the salt and grease in French fries. But in the 21st century, these have now become a nemesis to our health. Knowledge and willpower are required to conquer these innate needs.

There are at least 61 different names for sugar, among which *sucrose* is the one most widely used in food and beverages. Sucrose, a disaccharide, is made from glucose and fructose. Glucose is needed for energy production in every cell in the body. On the other hand, fructose is metabolized only in the liver. All fructose from food and beverages eventually will end up in the liver, where fructose is converted to fat, some of which is stored in the liver, and the rest of it is shipped to the adipose tissues via blood circulation. Fat stored in the liver can bring about fatty liver disease, and fat in the bloodstream and elsewhere increases triglycerides and causes weight gain. This is why sugar makes you gain weight even if you avoid eating fatty foods.

In 1972, English physiologist and nutritionist John Yudkin published a book titled *Pure White, Deadly: The Problem of Sugar*. In his book, Yudkin explicitly warned readers about the danger of sugar to health and how high consumption of sugar could lead to a host of diseases, including tooth decay, obesity, diabetes, and heart disease. Yudkin's book and his warnings pertaining to sugar intake caused concerns in the US food industry. To neutralize the effects of Yudkin's findings on US consumers, the food industry hired academic nutritionists to discredit him. For example, the food industry hired certain individuals in the audience to challenge and interrupt Yudkin's presentation every time he spoke about his research work on the negative effects of sugar on health. At the time, their strategy proved successful. Despite his great efforts to warn the public about the effects of sugar, the media and consumers largely ignored Yudkin's book and its messages in the 1970s. Annual sugar consumption per capita in the US increased from 80 pounds in 1970 to 150 pounds in 2010.

In 2009, Robert Lustig, professor of pediatric endocrinology at the University of California in San Francisco, observed an alarming number of children from eight to nine years of age in his clinic who were afflicted with obesity and diabetes. He could no longer just continue his clinic work and keep silent on the role of sugar in childhood obesity. Lustig started speaking out about the unhealthy effects of sugar. His recorded speech "Sugar: The Bitter Truth" has been viewed 6 million times on YouTube. The food industry again hired academic nutritionists and mounted vicious attacks against Lustig. However, unlike the situation with Yudkin in the 1970s, consumers did become more aware of the harmful effects of sugar on their bodies. Even the mainstream media joined the bandwagon and increased their coverage of the danger of sugar to health.

Nevertheless, Americans like sweets. About one-half of the US population is overweight, and one-third of the population is obese. A can of coke contains 39 g of sugar, and each American consumes 126 g of sugar a day. The recommended dietary allowance of sugar is only 35 g for men and 24 g for women according to the American Heart Association, so sugar consumption in the US is way over the amount they deem healthy. Sugar is the cause of a host of chronic diseases, including obesity, hypertension, diabetes, heart disease, stroke, and cancer, and it's also a significant cause of weight gain.

29

WHY SHOULD PATIENTS WITH AUTOIMMUNE DISEASES NOT EAT MEAT?

Autoimmune diseases include rheumatoid arthritis, lupus erythema-tosus, ankylosing spondylitis, and the like. Autoimmune disorders are caused by the immune system attacking organs and tissues, mistaking them as foreign. Why does eating meat exacerbate autoimmune disorders? Proteins from animal-based foods are degraded to amino acids and oligopeptides in the digestive tract. Oligopeptides are small pieces of undigested proteins that cannot be absorbed by the intestines. In a healthy individual, these oligopeptides are excreted in the feces. On the other hand, in an individual who has leaky gut syndrome manifested by intestinal tight junction malfunction, these oligopeptides may pass through the gap created by that tight junction malfunction in the intestinal wall and enter the bloodstream. Leaky gut syndrome is common among patients with autoimmune disease. When an oligopeptide from animal protein enters the bloodstream, it can provoke an immune response. Immune cells start producing antibodies against invading oligopeptides, and if the amino acid sequence of the oligopeptide resembles that of a protein in the kidneys, the newly formed antibody may attack the kidneys, mistaking them as foreign, and cause renal damage. Likewise, if the amino acid sequence of the oligopeptide resembles that of a protein in the knee, the newly produced antibody may attack the knee and cause arthritis.

Why does eating vegetables not aggravate autoimmune disorders? Plants, such as vegetables, are genetically distinct from humans. None of the amino acid sequences of proteins from vegetables resemble those in humans. Even though the human body may produce antibodies against oligopeptides from vegetables, these antibodies will not attack the kidneys or knees because no plant-like protein exists in the human body. So patients with autoimmune disorders should eat more vegetables rather than meat. If meat is needed in a diet, fish or shellfish—species that are distant from humans in the evolutionary tree—are recommended.

30

WHO'S COMING TO THE PARTY? FREE RADICAL, A PERSONA NON GRATA

Imagine a ballroom where waltz music is playing and couples are dancing gracefully. A sign posted at the entrance reads, "Singles Not Allowed." Unexpectedly, a single man shows up at the entrance, ignores the objection from the security guard, and forces himself onto the dance floor. Once there, he quickly grabs a female partner from a couple and dances away. The angry male who lost the partner grabs a female partner from another couple, and the vicious cycle repeats itself. What was once a graceful dance party has now become chaotic. This scene resembles a destructive event caused by a free radical. That single man (who also could have been a woman) is like a free radical, the dance floor is the cell, and the couples are proteins in the cell. This example illustrates how a free radical can initiate a destructive chain reaction inside a cell. If this event occurs simultaneously in millions of cells rather than just a single cell within the brain, liver, heart, or kidneys, it is not hard to imagine the deleterious effects of free radicals on our bodies.

31

WHAT ARE FREE RADICALS?

A free radical is a molecule that contains an unpaired electron. Although many types of free radicals exist, all of them are derived from the same free radical, the superoxide anion radical ($\cdot O_2^-$). Mitochondria are cellular organelles that produce superoxide anion radicals as byproducts during energy production, and they are the power plant of the cell. Ingested food is degraded to simple nutrients, such as glucose, amino acids, and fatty acids, in the intestines. Glucose is converted to energy in mitochondria, where electrons are generated. Oxygen serves as an electron acceptor in mitochondria. With the aid of enzymes, each oxygen molecule can accept four electrons and convert to a water molecule. Therefore, oxygen is essential for energy production in mitochondria. This is why we need to breathe—in order to bring oxygen molecules to mitochondria for energy production in every cell in the body.

Incidentally, electrons generated during energy production can stray or become lost in the mitochondria, similar to the power lost when electricity is transported through high-voltage power lines in our communities. The stray or lost electron can react with oxygen molecules to produce superoxide anion radicals, which are the origins of all other free radicals in the cell. All other free radicals, including peroxide and hydroxyl radicals, are derived from superoxide anion radicals. To circumvent this potential free radical problem, mitochondria are equipped with two powerful enzymes, superoxide dismutase and catalase. The former converts superoxide anion radicals to hydrogen peroxide, while the latter converts hydrogen peroxide to water and oxygen.

In small amounts, hydrogen peroxide works as a cellular messenger. Hydrogen peroxide can enter a cell nucleus and promote expression of antioxidant-related genes and boost production of antioxidant enzymes. Here, hydrogen peroxide acts as part of the body's natural defense mechanism against free radical–induced oxidative damage to organs and tissues.

On the other hand, in large amounts, hydrogen peroxide can be harmful to the body. Excessive hydrogen peroxide can react with metal ions, such as ferrous ions, in the cell, which is called a "Fenton reaction."

$$Fe^{+3} + H_2O_2 \rightarrow Fe^{+3} + OH^- + \cdot OH$$

The Fenton reaction generates hydroxyl radicals (OH^-), the most potent and harmful free radicals known to humankind. Hydroxyl radicals are the strongest oxidants and possess an extremely high reactivity toward biomolecules, such as lipids, proteins, or nucleic acids. They work by stealing electrons from these biomolecules. Losing electrons precipitates structural instability in proteins, lipids, and DNA and eventually causes the structural collapse of these biomolecules, which then generates even more free radicals. This is known as the chain reaction of a free radical. The chain reaction initiated by hydroxyl radicals and the like can lead to oxidative damage to organs and tissues. Oxidative damage is the major cause of chronic diseases, including cardiovascular disease, diabetes, Alzheimer's disease, heart disease, chronic inflammation, atherosclerosis, and cancers.

Author's note: Using electron spin resonance spectroscopy, I demonstrated experimentally for the first time the existence of hydroxyl radicals in a biological system when I was a graduate student in Honolulu, Hawai'i. In the next chapter, I will briefly present a personal account of my hunt for the hydroxyl radical.

32

A PERSONAL STORY OF THE HUNT FOR THE HYDROXYL RADICAL

In autumn 1975, I was a second-year graduate student, sitting in a class on ESR (electron spin resonance) spectroscopy taught by the late Professor Lawrence Piette at the University of Hawai'i. ESR is a form of spectroscopy in which a strong magnet and a microwave device are combined to detect and analyze chemical and physical properties of unpaired electrons in either free radicals or transition metals.

After spending time in two different professors' labs during the preceding summer, I still had no idea what I was going to study specifically. A second-year student was supposed to have made up his mind about the topic of his dissertation. But in the class, when Dr. Piette showed how ESR could be used for fingerprinting and identifying the chemical structure and physical properties of free radicals, I was immediately attracted to the beauty and precision of spectroscopy. It could potentially be utilized to discover new species of free radicals, and that was what I wanted to do. That was the epiphany of my life.

I met with Dr. Piette after the class. He showed me his lab, and for the first time, I saw the ESR spectrometer. It was a big lab filled with people from all different corners of the world: French, Italian, Filipino, and Russian, among others. Anatoly, a Russian scientist, was about to finish a two-year fellowship and planned to return to Russia a month later. Dr. Piette asked me to spend time with Anatoly to learn about his work, and if I liked it, I could take over and continue his line of research. Anatoly had spent two years hunting for hydroxyl radicals in biological systems. The hydroxyl radical is the most reactive free radical ever known to humankind. It can be generated by ionized radiation, like an X-ray, or chemical processes, like the Fenton reaction. At that time, no one believed that such a highly reactive free radical could exist in a living system. Anatoly aimed to prove that hydroxyl radicals could indeed exist in living systems, but repeatedly, he was disappointed, as his search showed nothing. However, his research hinted that hydroxyl radicals were lurking somewhere in living systems; he just could not get close to them.

Anatoly shook his head when I told him that I wanted to continue his line of research after he left the country. He told me that I should reconsider my decision because the hunt for the hydroxyl radical was so elusive that I might not be able to complete my PhD dissertation. All my life, I had become particularly excited when people told me that this or that could not be done; thus I decided to take the plunge into the unknown.

After many months of disappointment, I finally realized that some chemicals used in a buffer solution could potentially intercept the production of hydroxyl radicals and form different adducts, thereby eluding detection. Giovanni, our Italian organic chemist in residence, had just synthesized a new spin trap. By changing the buffer system and using the new spin trap, I was able to fingerprint and identify a hydroxyl radical in a biological system using ESR spectroscopy. This was the first time in the history of science that the production of hydroxyl radicals had been proved to exist in a living system. That was an exciting time! Our first paper on hydroxyl radicals was published in 1977. Since then, tens of thousands of papers have been published on hydroxyl radicals, linking them to the cause of oxidative damage and a host of diseases and conditions, such as neurodegenerative diseases, cancer, diabetes, inflammation, cardiovascular diseases, and aging.

33

WHAT ARE ANTIOXIDANTS?

An antioxidant can be an enzyme or a small molecule capable of neutralizing free radicals. It can be divided into two major types, intrinsic or extrinsic.

- Intrinsic antioxidants include antioxidant enzymes such as superoxide dismutase and catalase and antioxidant molecules like glutathione and uric acid.
- Extrinsic antioxidants include antioxidant vitamins from foods, such as vitamin C, vitamin E, and phytochemicals.

When the number of free radicals produced exceeds those of antioxidants in the body, it causes oxidative stress, which can lead to oxidative damage. As we age, the body produces more free radicals but fewer antioxidants. Aging is a result of free radical–induced oxidative damage, causing wrinkled skin and weakened bones. To age gracefully, you need to boost antioxidant capacities in the body. Eating more fruits and vegetables can enhance your antioxidant capacities. However, if higher antioxidant contents are needed to prevent or treat diseases, antioxidant vitamins derived from fruits and vegetables may not be sufficient. For example, one orange contains only about 51 mg of vitamin C. If you need 500 mg of vitamin C twice daily to treat the common cold, you will have to eat 20 oranges, a task that seems almost impossible. Therefore, to boost antioxidant contents to treat the common cold, supplementation with vitamin C is needed. On the other hand, vitamin A, vitamin E, and vitamin D are lipid-soluble vitamins, which can be retained in the body for a long time. Supplementation with these lipid-soluble vitamins at high doses could be harmful to the body. This book intends to show you how to use vitamin supplements correctly to prevent and treat chronic diseases and to maintain optimal health.

Glutathione is known as the mother of antioxidants. Every cell in the body needs glutathione to defend against free radical–induced oxidative damage. Glutathione is lost during reactions with free radicals. Cells that produce more free radicals have lower levels of glutathione and a weakened defense mechanism against free radical attacks. In addition to scavenging free radicals, glutathione has other important functions, including binding and neutralizing toxins—such as mercury, cadmium, lead, arsenic, insecticides, and herbicides—as well as detoxifying drugs in the liver. Toxic chemicals from foods or air pollution will eventually all end up in the liver. The liver is the body's detox center. It is therefore not a coincidence that among all organs, the liver contains the highest amount of glutathione. Glutathione reacts with lipid-soluble toxins and converts them to water-soluble moieties in the liver. Those are then discharged through the bile ducts into the intestines and excreted in feces. Again, glutathione is lost in the process, and its stores in the liver can be depleted if not continually replenished.

The other important function of glutathione is to rejuvenate vitamin C and vitamin E in the cell. In the process of neutralizing free radicals, these antioxidant vitamins are converted from active forms to inactive forms. But glutathione can convert vitamin C or vitamin E from inactive forms back to active forms. In other words, glutathione recycles vitamin C and vitamin E in the cell, and that is why it is called the mother of antioxidants.

Glutathione deficiency is common among all patients afflicted with chronic diseases, including Alzheimer's disease, Parkinson's disease, autism spectrum disorder, heart disease, chronic infections, diabetes, autoimmune disease, kidney disease, arthritis, and chronic pancreatitis. Chronic diseases deplete the glutathione contents of the body. How to replenish glutathione in patients with chronic diseases thus becomes an important health question.

Glutathione is made up of three amino acids: glutamine, cysteine, and glycine. Among these three amino acids, the sulfur-containing cysteine is the most interesting one, as it can adhere to a toxin or a drug, like glue on the surface of a flyswatter. Due to its importance in health and sickness, several glutathione supplements are available in the marketplace claiming to boost the body's glutathione content. However, none of these supplements can really raise the glutathione content of the body. The reason is simple. Glutathione is an oligopeptide, which is degraded readily in the digestive tract to glutamine, cysteine, and glycine, and only a small amount of it may actually be absorbed and enter the bloodstream. Supplementation with glutathione therefore is not the right way to boost glutathione levels. One can only achieve this through proper diet and regular exercise. Proper diet means eating the right kinds of food, containing adequate amounts of the right ingredients needed to produce glutathione. Fortunately, fruits and vegetables, as well as meats, contain plentiful amounts of both glutamine and glycine. Thus you need only search for foods that contain high amounts of sulfur-containing cysteine. Cysteine-rich foods include garlic, onions, ginger, broccoli, spinach, tomatoes, and cabbage. Regular consumption of these cysteine-rich foods can boost glutathione production in the body. In addition to eating the right kinds of foods, exercise enhances the body's ability to generate glutathione. Proper diet provides the ingredients and regular exercise provides the capacity to boost glutathione levels. Adequate glutathione levels are needed to prevent chronic diseases and maintain good health.

34

HOW DOES EXERCISE BENEFIT BRAIN HEALTH?

Everyone knows that exercise benefits health. Exercise burns calories, controls body weight, lowers blood pressure, prevents cardiovascular disease, improves quality of sleep, and boosts sexual desire. However, how does exercise benefit brain health?

Exercise can have beneficial cognitive, psychological, and neurological effects on brain health.

- **COGNITIVE EFFECTS.** In prehistoric times, running was not a hobby but a survival skill. Humans during hunter-gatherer times ran with a specific purpose in mind: to hunt prey or to escape from danger. Clear thinking is required to survive in such a crucial moment. It's what allowed prehistoric humans to catch prey and relieve hunger, and without clear thinking, they could have become pieces of meat to larger predators. So running can improve cognition and critical thinking skills, because knowing how to run meant life or death in hunter-gatherer times.

The brain volume of monkeys living in trees is about 300 cc. The brain volume of humans is about 3,000 cc. Archaeologists claim that running was the main reason that human brain volume increased tenfold, particularly in the forehead region, compared to that of tree-dwelling monkeys. Runners indeed have slightly larger foreheads. Running can have numerous benefits on brain health, as it can improve thinking, memory, attention, problem-solving skills, and IQ.

- **PSYCHOLOGICAL EFFECTS.** Exercise raises one's ability to resist stress and decreases episodes of emotional outbursts due to minor frustrations or setbacks. Exercise can induce the brain to produce GABA cells, the neurons that can inhibit mental pressure from daily activities. Exercise also enhances the brain's ability to release dopamine and serotonin. Both neurotransmitters control the reward/pleasure centers in the brain, evoking a pleasant mood and having a calming effect on one's emotions, thus reducing the risk of anxiety and depression.

- **NEUROLOGICAL EFFECTS.** You might have heard that the total number of neurons in the brain is fixed at birth, and as you age, the number of neurons gradually dwindles, which is why your memory gets worse. The above presumption is outdated and has been proven wrong. Regardless of how old you are, you can still regenerate your neurons and produce new ones in the brain. Regular exercise stimulates the brain to produce brain-derived neurotropic factor, or BDNF, a neuronal nutrient that nourishes the nervous system and enhances neurogenesis to produce new neurons in the brain. BDNF can also promote the growth of new synapses, which in turn increase cognition and memory.

Jogging and speed walking are the two most highly recommended forms of exercise. Simply go out and jog twice weekly for 45 minutes or speed walk twice weekly for one hour, and continue to do so for 6 months. Among other things, you will notice an increase in your stamina and strength, as well as improvements in your memory and cognition.

35

WHY ARE FRUITS AND VEGETABLES GOOD FOR YOUR HEALTH?

In childhood, you were told countless times to "eat your vegetables." Eating fruits and vegetables is good for your health. But why?

Plants contain phytochemicals, or plant-derived chemicals. So far, more than 5,000 phytochemicals have been identified, of which vitamin C and vitamin E are well known. The functions and mechanisms of action of these two phytochemicals have been well researched and documented. Vitamin C and vitamin E are known as essential nutrients. However, we still have limited knowledge of the functions and mechanisms of the actions of thousands of other phytochemicals derived from vegetables and fruits.

Rooted deeply in the soil, plants are immobile and cannot move around. Unlike animals, they cannot just run away when threatened or in danger. To protect themselves against insects and other pathogens, the flowers, leaves, stems, and roots of plants contain insecticides and pesticides, collectively called phytochemicals. These phytochemicals can ward off bacteria and viruses and prevent damage by insects. Phytochemicals allow immobile plants to cope with adverse environmental conditions. From an evolutionary viewpoint, animals—particularly humans—evolved and adopted the natural defense mechanisms of phytochemicals in plants to cope with unfavorable environmental conditions. Phytochemicals became part of the cellular alarm system in the human body. As phytochemicals enter the cells, an alarm bell rings, signaling an immediate danger. Once inside a cell, phytochemicals activate transcription factors, which then move from the cytoplasm into the nucleus, where transcription factors trigger the expression of antioxidant genes in chromosomes and produce a host of antioxidant enzymes. Thus phytochemicals serve as cellular messengers to activate and strengthen antioxidant functions in the cell.

The phenomenon in which a small quantity of phytochemicals can induce profound amplification in cellular antioxidant functions is called "hormesis." Hormesis is a normal biological phenomenon characterized by low-dose stimulatory and high-dose inhibitory effects. For example, a small amount of vitamin A enhances vision, but a high amount can lead to anorexia, headaches, and lethargy. In toxicology, this phenomenon is called a "biphasic" reaction. Many known chemicals exhibit biphasic reactions in the body, including hydrogen peroxide, nitric oxide, and curcumin, and so does exercise. That's right—exercise also exhibits biphasic hormetic effects. Proper exercise improves cognition and strengthens muscle. Nevertheless, extreme exercise can be harmful to the body.

Phytochemicals are not easily absorbed in the intestines, and only a small quantity from food sources enters the bloodstream. The various colors of different parts of plants—red, yellow, green, blue, purple, and the others—are derived mainly from phytochemicals. It is best to include different colors of vegetables and fruits in your diet. Not only will this provide sufficient amounts of vitamin A, vitamin C, and vitamin E, but it will enhance the body's antioxidant capacity and immune functions.

36

WHAT IS AGING?

Aging is an innate biological phenomenon. Birth, aging, sickness, and death are life stages from which no one is spared. Average life expectancy is now 70–80 years. With no major illness before age 60, chances are great that you might live to celebrate your own centenarian birthday. But how do we age? And why do some people age gracefully and others look old at the same age others are in their prime? We all hope that by the time we reach 70, we still look fit, feel healthy, are agile and mentally sharp, and are doing what we like to do.

In the 1950s, Denham Harman hypothesized that free radicals caused human aging. Harman became the guru of the free radical theory of aging. Since then, the free radical theory of aging has been modified and updated; the newest version postulates that a low amount of free radicals is beneficial, whereas an excessive amount of free radicals accelerates aging. The current theory resonates with the concept of hormesis mentioned in the previous chapter.

Although oxygen from inhaled air is required for energy production, it generates free radicals as unwanted byproducts. This is a drawback, the price we pay for utilizing oxygen in energy production in mitochondria. In youth, our bodies produce a sufficient amount of antioxidant enzymes to neutralize and scavenge these unwanted free radicals, preventing oxidative damage. As we age, our bodies produce fewer antioxidant enzymes; therefore, we are unable to get rid of these unwanted free radicals, leading to free radical–induced oxidative damage. If this accumulated damage occurs in the skin, it will wrinkle. If it occurs in the eyes, your vision will diminish, and if in the hair, your hair will turn gray and fall out. This is aging in action! The extent of the accumulated damage is associated with the body's antioxidant capacity. Greater antioxidant capacity in the body decreases the accumulated damage incurred by free radicals. Contrary to that, if the antioxidant capacity in the body is low, you will age faster. Regular consumption of fruits, vegetables, nuts, and fish can boost antioxidant capacity.

Aging is associated with numerous physiological changes in the body. The following discussion focuses on physiological changes attributed to genetics, vitamin insufficiency, and physical activity to try to answer the question of why some people age prematurely and others remain healthy and active late in life.

- **GENETIC FACTORS.** Scientific advances have contributed to extending life expectancy. In 1900, the average life expectancy of an American was only 47 years, while the average life expectancy in 2017 is 78 years. The life expectancy in Japan is now 83 years, and more than 60,000 Japanese are over 100 years old. It is now a distinct possibility that you may live to be 100. However, if you want to live to 110 and beyond, you will need to possess longevity genes from your parents and grandparents. The longest-lived human being was Jeanne Calment, a French woman who lived to be 122 years old. Currently, the longest-living individual is Nabi Tajima, a Japanese woman aged 117. Longevity is associated with genetics. Your chance of living beyond 100 is greatly improved if your parents or grandparents lived more than 100 years.

Every cell in the body contains 23 pairs of chromosomes. The end of each chromosome contains a special segment of DNA called a "telomere." Telomeres protect chromosomes, just like small pieces of plastic protect the ends of shoelaces. Telomeres become shorter each time cell division occurs. A cell dies when telomeres at each end of the chromosome are depleted. People with long telomeres in their chromosomes live longer lives. How to extend the length of telomeres is one of the hottest topics in life-extension research, but a nutrient-balanced diet plus regular exercise can slow down the shortening of telomeres in a chromosome. Although genes play important roles in aging, proper diet, lifestyle, and willpower are also crucial factors in achieving longevity.

- **VITAMIN INSUFFICIENCY.** Facial wrinkles and postural abnormalities are two common signs of aging. Regardless of age, no one wishes to see wrinkles in the face or elsewhere in the body. The appearance of wrinkles is due to a combination of many biochemical changes in the skin, among which is the lack of newly synthesized collagen in the dermis layer of the skin, caused by insufficient vitamin C. Vitamin C is an essential nutrient needed for the synthesis of collagen, a protein that is the main component of the dermis layer. The collagen content is high in the dermis layer in healthy and young skin, which gives rise to the skin's elastic, smooth feeling. To possess younger and healthier-looking skin, you will need to eat adequate amounts of fruits and vegetables—and better yet, some extra vitamin C supplement.

  Postural abnormalities are often caused in part by incorrect posture when standing or sitting, as well as insufficient vitamin D and calcium. Vitamin D and calcium are important for bone strength and bone density. Insufficient dietary intake of vitamin D and calcium can lead to osteoporosis and postural changes—and even to shorter stature. When we age, our skin produces less vitamin D. Dietary intake of vitamin D and supplementation with vitamin D are crucial for preventing bone loss and posture abnormality, particularly in older people. Older people are often unaware of problems related to osteoporosis and vitamin D deficiency until after accidentally falling and fracturing a bone.

Vitamin D deficiency is a global public health issue. Due to the avoidance of sun exposure, even people who live near the equator are in danger of vitamin D deficiency. If you become shorter or hunched, which is a physical sign of aging, you probably are vitamin D deficient. It is imperative that you get tested and start taking vitamin D supplementation if necessary.

- **PHYSICAL STRENGTH.** Aging weakens the muscles and physical strength. In your mind, you may wish to take part in certain sports or activities, but physically, it just may not be possible. Nevertheless, you can regain physical strength through training, exercise, and sheer determination.

The second law of thermodynamics deals with entropy or randomness. Entropy implies that everything in life eventually will approach infinite randomness. At youth, the molecules in the human body are arranged in an orderly manner, with minimal randomness. At an older age, the molecules in the human body are in disarray, with increased randomness. The appearance of wrinkles in the skin or losses in eyesight are signs of the increased randomness of the molecules in the skin or the eyes. Aging and disease accelerate the randomness of the molecules in the body. All things that are living and nonliving in the universe will eventually meet their demise and approach infinite randomness. Aging is a biological example of entropy in action. Human aging, like everything else, obeys the laws of the universe. Keeping the molecules in the body in order is the key to slowing down the aging process.

PART FOUR

Prevention and Treatment of Diseases and Conditions

Researchers worldwide have employed meta-analysis to sort through published clinical data and determine whether vitamins and essential elements are effective in treating or preventing chronic diseases. Searching PubMed's database and other medical databases reveals that in the past decade, hundreds of meta-analysis papers have confirmed the efficacies of vitamins and essential elements in prevention and treatment of more than 75 chronic diseases and conditions. These clinically proven remedies have been tested in hundreds of trials involving millions of participants worldwide. This treasure trove of natural remedies is hidden in the vast scientific literature and is not accessible to the public.

This book is intended to increase the reader's awareness of these clinically proven remedies. The benefits and efficacies of vitamins and essential elements in the prevention and treatment of diseases and conditions described here in part 4 are based solely on the conclusions drawn by meta-analysis of clinical research articles.

These human diseases and conditions—including Alzheimer's disease, autism, breast cancer, diabetes, heart disease, hypertension, Parkinson's disease, and others—are presented alphabetically from chapters 37 to 111.

37

ALZHEIMER'S DISEASE

Alzheimer's disease is a chronic neurodegenerative disease. Memory loss and cognitive decline are noticeable in the early phases of the disease, and as the disease progresses, a patient loses his ability to perform daily activities, such as eating meals or putting on clothes. Dementia is characterized by loss of cognitive functions, including thinking, memory, and problem-solving abilities. Alzheimer's disease is the most severe form of dementia. About 80% of dementia cases are caused by Alzheimer's disease, which is now ranked the third-highest cause of death in elderly people. The first and second are cardiovascular disease and cancer. In the US, 5 million people are afflicted with Alzheimer's disease. Thus far, there is no effective treatment for the disease.

What Are the Symptoms of Alzheimer's Disease?
- *Memory decline.* Alzheimer's patients experience short-term memory decline that worsens progressively. Patients may

repetitively ask the same questions and forget familiar names, places, events, or dates.

- *Cognitive decline.* Cognitive functions include problem-solving skills, judgment, and logical-reasoning abilities. Patients with Alzheimer's disease can easily get lost or misplace things; for example, they may place their reading glasses in the refrigerator.
- *Depression.* Depression is common in Alzheimer's patients. They become irritable, lose empathy, and display unreasonable hostility.
- *Speech impediment.* Alzheimer's patients tend to forget common and frequently used words. To cover up these shortcomings, they often choose an incorrect or unrelated word to substitute for forgotten words in conversation; therefore, it becomes harder to comprehend them and understand their intentions.
- *Bizarre behavior.* Alzheimer's patients' behaviors and daily activities become strange; for example, they may urinate in improper places or steal things from people.

What Are the Risk Factors for Alzheimer's Disease?

- *Age.* Age is a major risk factor for Alzheimer's disease. One in nine people over age 65 and one in every three people over age 85 suffer from Alzheimer's disease. The older a person is, the higher his or her risk of developing Alzheimer's disease.
- *Family and genetics.* Your risk of Alzheimer's disease will be higher if a parent or sibling has the disease. About 70% of Alzheimer's disease cases are linked to genetics. A multitude of genes, including ApoE and BDNF gene polymorphic variants, have been identified to be associated with Alzheimer's disease. ApoE genes regulate cholesterol metabolism in the brain, and BDNF genes encode brain-derived neurotropic factors, proteins that enhance neurogenesis and improve learning and memory. Mutations of these genes heighten the risk of Alzheimer's disease.

- *Head trauma.* People with head trauma earlier in life have an elevated risk of Alzheimer's disease at older ages. Head trauma can cause comas, confusion, and forgetfulness, and it can affect speech, vision, and personality. A person can recover from mild head trauma. However, severe head trauma, particularly at older ages, may lead to Alzheimer's disease.
- *Hypertension.* Hypertension can lead to stroke, atherosclerosis, heart disease, diabetes, obesity, and hypercholesterolemia, all of which are risk factors for Alzheimer's disease. Hypertension can also cause the narrowing of the arterial wall, which diminishes the supply of nutrients and oxygen to the brain and increases the risk of Alzheimer's disease.
- *Heart disease.* Heart disease and other heart-related illnesses can cause insufficient blood perfusion to the brain, exacerbating the risk of Alzheimer's disease.
- *Stroke.* A stroke damages the brain's structure, causing endothelial dysfunction and permeability changes in the blood-brain barrier. Endothelial dysfunction of the arterial vessel in the brain is linked to Alzheimer's disease. The symptoms of endothelial dysfunction often appear before the onset of dementia and neurodegenerative disease. Permeability changes in the blood-brain barrier can lead to insufficient perfusion of the brain tissue, resulting in the accumulation of beta amyloid peptide in the brain. That accumulation further damages the neurons and heightens the risk of Alzheimer's disease. Stroke survivors have an increased risk of Alzheimer's disease.
- *Diabetes.* Patients with diabetes have a greater risk of Alzheimer's disease compared to individuals without diabetes. Insulin resistance and insulin deficiency cause the brain to produce beta amyloid peptides and phosphorylated tau proteins, both of which are markers of Alzheimer's disease. Because the pathology of Alzheimer's disease resembles that of type 2 diabetes, Alzheimer's disease is often called "type 3 diabetes."
- *Obesity.* Obesity increases the accumulation of beta amyloid peptides and tau proteins in the brain, which are toxic

proteins that are harmful to the neurons. If obesity persists over 10–20 years, the accumulation of these toxic proteins in the brain can lead to cognitive impairment, dementia, and Alzheimer's disease.

What Is the Association between Vitamin A and Alzheimer's Disease?

- Vitamin A regulates the development and growth of neurons from infancy to adulthood. Supplementation with vitamin A can enhance cognition, memory, and brain plasticity in children and adults.

- Vitamin A from food intake enters the brain through the blood-brain barrier. However, the permeability of the blood-brain barrier is often compromised in patients with Alzheimer's disease, thus preventing the transport of vitamin A to the neurons and causing vitamin A deficiency in the brain. Vitamin A deficiency diminishes antioxidant capacity and exacerbates oxidative damage to the brain, leading to Alzheimer's disease.

What Is the Association between Vitamin C and Alzheimer's Disease?

- Vitamin C insufficiency heightens the risk of epilepsy in patients with Alzheimer's disease. The brains of Alzheimer's patients are in an oxidized state, which makes patients prone to developing epilepsy. Vitamin C insufficiency can worsen the brain's oxidized state and increase the risk of epilepsy in Alzheimer's patients.

- Vitamin C, an electron donor, maintains brain tissue in a reduced state and boosts the antioxidant capacity in the brain. About 30% of Americans are vitamin C insufficient. The percentage of vitamin C–insufficient elderly individuals who live in nursing homes and assisted-living housing facilities is much higher compared to that of healthy elderly individuals. Vitamin C insufficiency increases the risk of Alzheimer's disease.

What Is the Association between Vitamin D and Alzheimer's Disease?

- Blood levels of vitamin D are lower in Alzheimer's patients compared to that of healthy individuals. Low blood levels of vitamin D are associated with a decline in cognitive functions and memory. Vitamin D protects neurons, mitigates cognitive impairment, and reduces the risk of Alzheimer's disease. Vitamin D deficiency alters the neural circuitry in the prefrontal cortex of the brain.

- Low blood levels of vitamin D during the young adult years increase the risk of Alzheimer's disease in old age. Studies have shown that people whose blood levels of vitamin D were low in young adulthood had a high risk of Alzheimer's disease 30 years later. On the contrary, people whose blood levels of vitamin D were high in young adulthood had a low risk of Alzheimer's disease 30 years later.

- Low blood levels of vitamin D increase the risk of Alzheimer's disease in elderly people. Studies have shown that vitamin D deficiency increased the risk of Alzheimer's disease threefold in elderly people.

- Vitamin D regulates brain functions, including the growth and differentiation of neurons and signal transmission in the brain. Vitamin D deficiency can lead to growth retardation as well as signal transmission disorders, increasing the risk of Alzheimer's disease.

What Is the Association between Vitamin E and Alzheimer's Disease?

- Blood levels of vitamin E are lower in Alzheimer's patients compared to that in healthy individuals. Low blood levels of vitamin E are associated with poor memory and cognitive functions in elderly people. Centenarians who have sufficient blood levels of vitamin E often show excellent memory capacity.

- Vitamin E has antioxidant functions. It quenches free radicals, prevents oxidative damage to cellular membranes in the neurons, and reduces the risk of cognitive impairment and Alzheimer's disease.
- Supplementation with vitamin E alleviates the symptoms of Alzheimer's disease, including improving one's ability to perform daily activities and reducing the need for nursing assistance.
- Studies that used MRI revealed that vitamin E supplementation decreased brain atrophy in Alzheimer's patients.

What Is the Association between Zinc and Alzheimer's Disease?
- Zinc is required for stabilizing the three-dimensional structure of proteins in the brain. Zinc deficiency can cause the destabilization of protein structures due to incorrect protein folding. Incorrect protein folding produces deformed proteins. Not only are these deformed proteins unable to perform their physiological functions, but they also tend to form aggregates in the neurons and cause neuronal death. Zinc deficiency increases the risk of Alzheimer's disease.
- Zinc ions have both antioxidant and anti-inflammatory qualities. Alzheimer's disease is a chronic inflammatory disease caused in part by oxidative damage to the brain, so zinc deficiency aggravates oxidative damage to the brain.

Meta-analysis
- *Antioxidant vitamins.* Seven research papers investigated the association between antioxidant vitamins and Alzheimer's disease. The meta-analysis confirmed that sufficient dietary intake of antioxidants reduced the risk of Alzheimer's disease. Vitamin E, vitamin C, and beta-carotene decreased the risk of Alzheimer's disease by 24%, 17%, and 12%, respectively.
- *Vitamin D.* Ten research publications studied the relationship between vitamin D and Alzheimer's disease. The meta-analysis confirmed that individuals with vitamin D deficiency had a

greater risk of dementia, as well as Alzheimer's disease, compared to those with sufficient amounts of vitamin D.

- *Zinc.* A meta-analysis of 27 research articles that included 1,356 Alzheimer's patients and 2,073 healthy controls investigated the relationship between zinc and Alzheimer's disease. The result confirmed that Alzheimer's patients had significantly lower blood zinc levels compared to healthy controls.

Recommendation

- *Prevention.* For people at risk of dementia and Alzheimer's disease, take daily 2,000 IU vitamin A (1), 200 mg vitamin C (10), 800 IU vitamin D3 (11), 30 IU vitamin E (12), and 10 mg zinc (20).
- *Treatment.* For dementia and Alzheimer's patients, take daily 5,000 IU vitamin A (1), 500 mg vitamin C (10), 2,000 IU vitamin D3 (11), 100 IU vitamin E (12), and 20 mg zinc (20).

38

ASTHMA

Asthma is caused by an oversensitive and reactive immune system. Triggered by sensitive substances in the air, the bronchi and lungs secrete copious mucus, resulting in chest discomfort, coughing, and difficulty breathing. Asthmatic children are often physically weak and susceptible to infections. They are inclined to avoid outdoor activities, which would further worsen asthmatic symptoms. Asthma is the leading cause of emergency care, inpatient care, and skipping or missing classes during childhood. If untreated, childhood asthma may persist over years and even into adulthood. It is estimated that 25 million people suffer from asthma in the US, including 7 million children aged 18 and under.

What Risk Factors Trigger or Exacerbate Asthma?
- Influenza viruses from the common cold
- Particulate matters in air pollution, such as PM2.5, PM10, and cigarette smoke

- Dust mites, pet dander, and pollens
- Exercise and other vigorous physical activities
- Temperatures that are too hot or too cold

What Are the Risk Factors for Asthma?

- *Allergies.* Asthma is not a single disease but a collection of syndromes, including bronchoconstriction, caused in part by allergens. Allergens that are known to trigger bronchoconstriction are milk, eggs, nuts, fish, shrimp, and peanuts. Allergic reactions can lead to asthmatic attacks.
- *Cigarette smoking.* About 25% of asthmatic patients are habitual smokers. Smoking damages lung function and aggravates the symptoms of asthma. Smoking diminishes the efficacy of corticosteroid, a common medication to treat asthma.
- *Air pollution.* Air pollution induces the inflammation of the bronchi and exacerbates asthma. Asthmatic children are particularly susceptible to air pollution. Pollutants weaken immune functions and increase the frequency of asthmatic attacks.
- *Viral infection of the respiratory tract.* Viral infection of the respiratory tract can worsen the symptoms of asthmatic children. Syncytial virus, rhinovirus, metapneumovirus, and coronavirus are known to infect the respiratory tract in children.
- *Obesity.* Obesity causes chronic inflammation in the respiratory tract and reduces pulmonary function, increasing the risk of asthma.
- *Family and genetics.* Genes are linked to asthma. ORMDL3 gene mutations cause the accumulation of eosinophils and induce allergic inflammation in the bronchi. Children with ORMDL3 gene mutations have a higher risk of childhood asthma.

What Is the Association between Antioxidant Vitamins and Asthma?

- Antioxidant vitamins neutralize free radicals in the bronchi and lung tissue and prevent oxidative damage–induced pulmonary inflammation.
- Blood levels of vitamin A and vitamin C are lower in asthma patients compared to healthy controls.
- Vitamin A can quench singlet oxygen, a reactive oxygen species that can induce bronchoconstriction. Supplementation with vitamin A alleviates the symptoms of bronchoconstriction in asthmatic patients.
- Vitamin C reduces exercise-induced bronchoconstriction, a condition that frequently occurs during sports activities. Supplementation with vitamin C at a dose of 500 mg before engaging in sports activities can reduce exercise-induced bronchoconstriction.

What Is the Association between Vitamin D and Asthma?

- The intensity of ultraviolet B from the sun's rays becomes weaker when one is away from the equator. People who live far away from the equator have a greater risk of asthma because of lack of sun exposure. Sun exposure causes the skin to produce vitamin D and decreases the risk of asthma. Lower blood levels of vitamin D are associated with weaker lung function and increased risk of asthma.
- Glucocorticoid drugs are commonly prescribed medications for treating asthma. Low blood levels of vitamin D decrease the efficacy of glucocorticoid drugs.
- Low blood levels of vitamin D during pregnancy increase the rate of respiratory infections in newborn babies. Children with low blood levels of vitamin D have weaker lung function, hoarse voices, and a higher incidence of asthma. Low blood levels of vitamin D also reduce the efficacy of glucocorticoid drugs in asthmatic children. Higher doses are often needed to control asthmatic symptoms.

- Inflammatory cytokines activate B cells to secrete immunoglobulin IgE. High blood levels of immunoglobulin IgE exacerbate the symptoms of asthma. Vitamin D inhibits the production of inflammatory cytokines and reduces asthmatic symptoms.

Meta-analysis

- *Vitamin A and vitamin C.* Forty clinical research papers studied the relationship between antioxidant vitamins and asthma. The meta-analysis confirmed that sufficient dietary intake of vitamin A and vitamin C significantly reduced the number and severity of asthmatic attacks.
- *Vitamin D.* A meta-analysis of eight randomized controlled trials that included 573 children ages 3–18 with asthma explored the association between vitamin D and asthma. Supplementation with vitamin D at a dose of 1,000 IU daily reduced the number of episodes of asthmatic attacks in children.

Recommendation

- *Prevention.* For children at risk of asthma, take daily 1,000 IU vitamin A (1), 80 mg vitamin C (10), and 400 IU vitamin D3 (11).
- *Prevention.* For adults at risk of asthma, take daily 2,000 IU vitamin A (1), 200 mg vitamin C (10), and 800 IU vitamin D3 (11).
- *Treatment.* For children with asthma, take daily 4,000 IU vitamin A (1), 300 mg vitamin C (10), and 1,000 IU vitamin D3 (11).
- *Treatment.* For adults with asthma, take daily 5,000 IU vitamin A (1), 500 mg vitamin C (10), and 2,000 IU vitamin D3 (11).

39

ATHEROSCLEROSIS

Atherosclerosis is a chronic cardiovascular disease characterized by the accumulation of plaques in the wall of the arterial vessel. The main ingredients of plaque are fat, cholesterol, calcium, and other substances, all of which come from the bloodstream. This narrows the arterial wall, diminishing blood flow. Severe atherosclerosis is the major cause of heart attack and stroke. About 4.6 million Americans suffer from atherosclerosis.

What Are the Symptoms of Atherosclerosis?
The thickening of the middle layer in the intima of the carotid artery is a sign of atherosclerosis. The thickness of the middle layer in the intima of the carotid artery can be measured using ultrasound. If the thickness is more than one millimeter, it is indicative of atherosclerosis. Other than that, no symptoms are associated with early stages of atherosclerosis.

What Are the Causes of Atherosclerosis?

Atherosclerosis is a gradual and progressive disease that can start at a young age and worsen in adulthood. Injuries to the arterial wall lead to the accumulation of fat, cholesterol, calcium, and other substances in the wounded region, triggering plaque formation. When the plaque ruptures and causes bleeding, platelets adhere to the surface of the plaque and form a blood clot. Blood clots are the causes of heart attack and stroke. Smoking, hypertension, hypercholesterolemia, high triglycerides, and high blood glucose are the major risk factors for atherosclerosis.

What Are the Risk Factors for Atherosclerosis?

- *Smoking.* Smoking is an avoidable risk factor for atherosclerosis. Cigarette smoke contains thousands of different chemicals, some of which enter the bloodstream, travel to the lungs, and damage the endothelial layer of the arterial wall. The injured endothelial layer is prone to plaque formation and atherosclerosis. Nicotine in the smoke stimulates the vascular system to produce catecholamines, which increase the heartbeat, blood pressure, and the coagulation function of platelets.
- *Hypertension.* Hypertension exerts extra pressure on the arterial wall. This constant extra pressure can damage the endothelial layer and induce thickening in the muscle layer of the arterial wall, resulting in endothelial dysfunction. Endothelial dysfunction increases the risk of plaque formation and atherosclerosis.
- *High triglycerides.* Atherosclerosis is a chronic inflammatory disease. High blood levels of triglycerides can activate mononuclear leukocyte recruitment mechanisms and exacerbate the inflammation of the arterial wall, leading to oxidative damage and the risk of atherosclerosis.
- *Hypercholesterolemia.* High blood LDL, or "bad" cholesterol levels, increase the incidence of atherosclerosis. High LDL levels trigger the immune system to produce inflammatory cytokines and free radicals, leading to the oxidation of LDL.

Macrophages engulf oxidized LDL, forming foam cells in the endothelial layer of the blood vessel. Taking in high amounts of oxidized LDL causes the death of the foam cell, which releases oxidized lipids, cholesterol, and other substances, all of which contribute to the formation of plaques and atherosclerosis.

- *Overweight/obesity.* Being overweight or obese comes with a higher risk of atherosclerosis. Obesity worsens endothelial dysfunction. Consequently, blood vessels produce less nitric oxide, which acts as a strong vasodilator. The lack of nitric oxide reduces the elasticity of the arterial wall and increases one's chances of suffering from atherosclerosis.
- *Sugar consumption.* Fructose from foods enters the blood-stream and travels to the liver, where it is converted to fat. Fat is stored in the liver or transported back to the bloodstream, resulting in high triglyceride levels in the bloodstream. Since high sugar consumption causes high blood triglyceride levels, this is another risk factor for atherosclerosis.
- *Lack of exercise.* Lack of regular exercise and physical activity can lead to overweight, obesity, hypertension, high triglycer-ides, and hypercholesterolemia, all of which are risk factors for atherosclerosis. Regular exercise can boost endothelial func-tions and reduce the risk of atherosclerosis.
- *High-salt diet.* Habitual consumption of salty foods increases the risk of atherosclerosis. High blood sodium contents trig-ger the immune cells to produce free radicals in the bloodstream, leading to oxidative damage and endothelial dysfunction of the blood vessels. A high-salt diet can also lead to hypertension. Endothelial dysfunction and hypertension are risk factors for atherosclerosis.

What Is the Association between Vitamin B9 and Atherosclerosis?

- Vitamin B9 improves the endothelial functions of the blood vessels. Vitamin B9 deficiency leads to endothelial dysfunc-tion and increases the risk of atherosclerosis.

- Vitamin B9 can lower homocysteine levels in the blood, while deficiency raises them. High blood homocysteine levels are a risk factor for atherosclerosis and other cardiovascular diseases.

Meta-analysis

- *Vitamin B9.* Ten randomized controlled trials conducted with 2,052 people studied the relationship between vitamin B9 and atherosclerosis. Ultrasound was used to measure the thickness of the middle layer in the intima of the carotid artery of each participant. Analysis confirmed that vitamin B9 supplements reduced the thickness in the middle layer of the carotid artery compared to a placebo. Overall, vitamin B9 supplementation alleviates the symptoms of atherosclerosis.

Recommendation

- *Prevention.* For people at risk of atherosclerosis, take daily 400 mcg vitamin B9 (8).
- *Treatment.* For atherosclerosis patients, take daily 800 mcg vitamin B9 (8).

40

ATRIAL FIBRILLATION

Atrial fibrillation is characterized by a rapid and irregular heartbeat. The duration of each episode can be transitory or long-lasting. A normal heartbeat ranges from 60 to 100 beats per minute, but the heartbeat of patients with atrial fibrillation ranges from 100 to 175 beats per minute. Atrial fibrillation can lead to blood clots, stroke, heart failure, and other heart diseases. It is estimated that 2.7 million people suffer from atrial fibrillation in the US every year.

What Are the Symptoms of Atrial Fibrillation?
- Trembling hands
- Heart palpitations
- Shortness of breath
- Anxiety
- Fatigue

- Dizziness
- Excessive sweating
- Chest pain

What Are the Risk Factors for Atrial Fibrillation?

- *Strenuous exercise.* Extreme and vigorous exercise can increase the risk of atrial fibrillation. Proper exercise is beneficial to cardiovascular functions. However, extreme types of exercise, such as marathons and triathlons, may damage the heart muscle and induce atrial fibrillation. Long-term extreme exercise can cause irregular heartbeat, heart inflammation, and an enlarged atrium. About 20% of athletes who performed extreme physical activities experienced atrium enlargement and atrial fibrillation.
- *Heart disease.* Heart disease increases the risk of atrial fibrillation. Patients with heart disease often have cardiac muscle fibrosis, which can cause atrial fibrillation.
- *Alcoholism.* A moderate amount of alcohol, particularly red wine, is good for heart health. Heavy consumption of alcohol, on the other hand, can lead to an irregular heartbeat. Although the effects of alcohol on health vary individually, long-term heavy alcohol consumption has deleterious effects on the heart, and it can lead to atrial fibrillation.
- *Hypertension.* Hypertension is a major risk factor for atrial fibrillation. Hypertensive patients with atrial fibrillation have an elevated risk of other cardiovascular diseases. High blood pressure exerts extra pressure on the atrium and causes atrium enlargement. Hypertension can also activate the renin-angiotensin-aldosterone system, induce atrial fibrosis, damage the electrical system of the heart, and increase the risk of atrial fibrillation.
- *Sleep apnea.* Irregular heartbeat is common in people with sleep apnea. Sleep apnea is characterized by repetitive hypoxia that damages the cardiovascular system and induces the production of inflammatory cytokines, both of which are risk factors for atrial fibrillation.

- *Obesity.* Obesity is associated with hypertension, sleep apnea, and cardiovascular disease, as well as pericardial fat, all of which can damage the electrical system of the heart, cause structural changes in the atrium, and increase the incidence of atrial fibrillation.
- *Smoking.* Cigarette smoke contains nicotine, carbon monoxide, and polycyclic aromatic hydrocarbons, all of which can induce endothelial dysfunction, cause atherosclerosis and irregular heartbeat, and increase the incidence of atrial fibrillation.

What Is the Association between Vitamin C and Atrial Fibrillation?

- Atrial fibrillation triggers cardiac cells to produce free radicals and induces oxidative damage to the heart tissue, which further exacerbates atrial fibrillation. Vitamin C can neutralize free radicals, break this vicious cycle, and mitigate the symptoms of atrial fibrillation.
- Supplementation with vitamin C at a dose of 500 mg daily can alleviate the symptoms of atrial fibrillation.

What Is the Association between Omega-3 Fatty Acids and Atrial Fibrillation?

- Omega-3 fatty acids have anti-inflammatory functions because they inhibit atrium fibrosis, which is an early sign of atrial fibrillation.
- Atrial fibrillation is a common outcome of heart surgery. Blood levels of omega-3 fatty acids are low in patients with heart disease, and supplementation after heart surgery reduces the risk of arterial fibrillation.

Meta-analysis

- *Vitamin C.* Fifteen research papers investigated vitamin C and atrial fibrillation in 1,738 post–heart surgery atrial fibrillation patients. The result confirmed that supplementation with vitamin C after heart surgery significantly curtailed the risk of the recurrence of atrial fibrillation.

- *Omega-3 fatty acids.* Six research papers studied the relationship between omega-3 fatty acids and atrial fibrillation in 928 heart surgery patients. Supplementation with omega-3 fatty acids after heart surgery was found to significantly reduce the risk of atrial fibrillation.

Recommendation

- *Prevention.* For people at risk of atrial fibrillation, take daily 200 mg vitamin C (10) and 1 g omega-3 fatty acids (27).
- *Treatment.* For atrial fibrillation patients, take daily 500 mg vitamin C (10) and 2 g omega-3 fatty acids (27).

41

ATTENTION-DEFICIT/ HYPERACTIVITY DISORDER

Attention-deficit/hyperactivity disorder (ADHD), characterized by attention deficit and hyperactive behavior, is a developmental disorder of the central nervous system resulting in a mental disorder. ADHD often starts in children aged 3–6, and it can persist throughout the teenage years and even into adulthood. It is estimated that 6.4 million children are afflicted with ADHD in the US. According to the World Health Organization, ADHD affects 7% of children and 2–5% of all adults worldwide.

What Are the Symptoms of ADHD?
- *Talking incessantly.* Individuals with ADHD talk in a continuous manner and frequently interrupt others during

conversations. They lack interest in listening, or they have no patience when other people speak.

- *Restlessness.* Individuals affected by ADHD have trouble focusing or completing projects, even in their hobbies.
- *Inattention.* Students with ADHD show inattention or lack of concentration in class or when reading.
- *Lack of problem-solving skills.* Persons with ADHD have trouble finishing simple tasks, particularly those that require problem-solving skills.
- *Lack of social skills.* Individuals with ADHD tend to interact with others in an awkward manner at school, in the workplace, or during social events.
- *Forgetfulness.* People with ADHD tend to routinely lose personal items, such as schoolwork, pens, books, purses, or cell phones.
- *Panic.* Lastly, persons diagnosed with ADHD often display uncontrollable anxiety, fear, and excessive nervousness.

What Are the Risk Factors for ADHD?
- *Family and genetics.* ADHD is linked to genetics. Carriers of LPHN3 and CDHI3 gene polymorphic variants have an increased risk of ADHD. In studies of twins, having one twin with ADHD increased the risk of the other twin having ADHD by 70–80%. Children with a parent with ADHD have a 57% greater chance of having it as well.
- *Alcohol consumption during pregnancy.* Alcohol consumption during pregnancy increases the risk of giving birth to a child with ADHD. Dopamine is an important neurotransmitter that fosters communication between the neurons in the brain. Alcohol reduces dopamine production in the fetal brain, which increases the risk of ADHD during childhood. Any amount of alcohol consumption during pregnancy is harmful to the fetus. Unfortunately, this concept is still not widely accepted.

- *Premature infants.* A preterm baby has a higher risk of ADHD. Babies that are severely underweight or overweight at birth have an elevated risk of ADHD. Insufficient blood perfusion in certain regions of the brain is common in children with ADHD. Those regions of the brain that are not adequately supplied with oxygen and nutrients are often the same regions that control behavior and attention.
- *Abused children.* About 30% of ADHD adults are physically or sexually abused during childhood. Whether childhood abuse leads to ADHD or deviated behavior associated with ADHD increases a child's chance of being abused is still an open question.

What Is the Association between Omega-3 Fatty Acids and ADHD?

- Omega-3 fatty acids are essential nutrients that support development and neurotransmission in the central nervous system.
- Omega-3 fatty acids are the major components of phospholipids that form the bilayer structure of cellular membranes in neurons. They regulate membrane fluidity, which is crucial for the activity and functions of membrane proteins embedded in cell membranes. Omega-3 fatty acid deficiency increases the rigidity of the cell membrane, affects communication between the neurons, and causes developmental disorders and ADHD.

Meta-analysis

- *Omega-3 fatty acids.* A meta-analysis of 25 research papers conducted with 1,994 ADHD patients on the relationship between omega-3 fatty acids and ADHD confirmed that the blood level of omega-3 fatty acids was lower in ADHD patients compared to healthy controls. Supplementation with omega-3 fatty acids was found to significantly alleviate inattention and hyperactive behavior in ADHD patients.

Recommendation
- *Prevention.* For children at risk of attention-deficit/hyperactivity disorder, take daily 1 g omega-3 fatty acids (27).
- *Treatment.* For children with attention-deficit/hyperactivity disorder, take daily 2 g omega-3 fatty acids (27).

42

AUTISM SPECTRUM DISORDER

Autism spectrum disorder—characterized by difficulties with social interactions and emotional expression, problems with verbal or non-verbal communication, and repetitive behaviors—is a disease caused by developmental disorders of the brain during childhood. The root cause of autism spectrum disorder is still unknown. The disease often starts in children aged 2–3. According to the data from the Centers for Disease Control and Prevention, 1 in every 68 children in the US has autism. The most recent data from the questionnaire survey conducted by the US Department of Health and Human Services' National Center for Health Statistics reveal that 1 in every 45 children aged 3–17 has autism. Based on this statistical data, about 1.2 million children have autism in the US. This number is indeed alarming! The incidence of autism has increased tenfold in the past 40 years in the US. Both environmental and genetic factors potentially contribute to the cause of autism. However, within a 40-year time span, our genes have not changed in any significant manner; therefore, the rapid rise in the incidence rate of autism is most likely related to the environment.

What Are the Symptoms of Autism Spectrum Disorder?

- *Unresponsiveness.* Children with autism are typically unresponsive when called, even at 12 months old.
- *Lack of confidence.* Individuals with autism avoid eye contact with other people and prefer being alone.
- *Lack of empathy.* Individuals with autism will not follow another's gaze or look at the same objects that others find interesting.
- *Repetitive behaviors.* Persons with autism exhibit common repetitive behaviors, including rocking, jumping, and twirling.
- *Lack of sympathy.* People diagnosed with autism are unable to feel others' pain, sorrow, and sadness.
- *Routine life.* Furthermore, individuals with autism keep a strict daily routine. For example, perhaps a person with autism has to have cereal first and then eggs every morning.
- *Inability to point out objects of interest.* A person with autism is incapable of using his fingers to point at an object that interests him.
- *Attention only to parts, not the whole.* A child with autism pays attention only to a small part of a toy instead of the toy as a whole.
- *Poor people skills.* Lastly, individuals with autism show no interest in getting to know others.

What Are the Risk Factors for Autism Spectrum Disorder?

- *Parents' age and genetics.* Both parents' ages at the child's conception, particularly the father's age, increase the risk of autism in children. Fathers who are 35 years of age can pass on mutated genes to offspring. A 36-year-old father has twice as many gene mutations as a 20-year-old father. For example, the CUL3 gene encodes a protein that influences the size of a person's head and body. CUL3 gene mutations may increase the risk of autism.

- *Fetal hypoxia.* Excessive bleeding and hypertension during pregnancy, as well as labor dystocia and cesarean section during childbirth, can result in fetal hypoxia, which increases the incidence rate of autism in children. Women who wait two to five years before getting pregnant again with a second child reduce the risk of autism.

- *Gestational diabetes.* Gestational diabetes increases the risk of autism. A high blood glucose level in the uterus of women with gestational diabetes can damage the placenta and cause fetal hypoxia, chronic inflammation, and gene mutations, all of which raise the risk of autism. However, women with type 2 diabetes have no increased risk of giving birth to children with autism compared to women without diabetes.

- *Psychoactive drugs.* Risperidone and aripiprazole are drugs approved by the FDA to treat autism. In addition to these two drugs, physicians prescribe psychoactive drugs to nearly 50% of all children with autism. Common side effects of psychoactive drugs include epilepsy, anxiety, bipolar disorder, depression, panic attacks, and ADHD. All of these symptoms are prevalent in children with autism.

- *Aluminum.* On average, a child receives at least 18 vaccinations from birth through their teenage years in the US. Vaccines contain aluminum as an adjuvant, which can boost the body's immune response to produce antibodies. Aluminum is a known neurotoxin. Scientists question whether aluminum in vaccines has caused the sharp rise in the incidence of autism in children in the past 40 years in the US.

What Is the Association between Vitamin D and Autism Spectrum Disorder?

- Children with autism often have low blood levels of vitamin D compared to healthy children. Infants with low blood levels of vitamin D at birth have an increased risk of autism during childhood.

- Supplementation with vitamin D significantly alleviated the symptoms of children with autism. The suggested dose is 4,000 IU of vitamin D3 daily for at least three months.
- Vitamin D prevents autism by decreasing the production of inflammatory cytokines, reducing oxidative damage to the neurons, and improving the antioxidant capacity of the brain.

Meta-analysis

- *Vitamin D.* A meta-analysis of 11 research papers explored the association between vitamin D and autism in 870 autistic patients and 782 healthy controls. Analysis confirmed that the blood level of vitamin D in autistic patients was significantly lower compared to healthy controls.

Recommendation

- *Prevention.* For pregnant women and breastfeeding women whose children may be at risk of autism, take daily 1,000 IU vitamin D3 (11).
- *Prevention.* For newborn babies at risk of autism, take daily 400 IU vitamin D3 (11).
- *Treatment.* For children with autism, take daily 2,000 IU vitamin D3 (11).

43

AUTOIMMUNE
THYROID DISEASE

Autoimmune thyroid disease—characterized by autoimmune antibodies attacking thyroid hormone–producing cells in the thyroid gland, mistaking them as foreign—is an autoimmune disease. The autoimmune antibodies attack the thyroid gland and reduce the blood level of thyroid hormones, leading to hypothyroidism. The root cause of autoimmune thyroid disease is still largely unknown. Both genetics and environment potentially contribute to the disease. Among all age groups, middle-aged women are the group at highest risk. An estimated 1.5 million autoimmune thyroid disease cases occur in the US every year.

Autoimmune thyroid disease can be divided into three major types—namely, Graves' disease, Hashimoto's disease, and postpartum thyroiditis.

- *Graves' disease.* Patients with Graves' disease produce too much thyroid hormone, which causes hyperthyroidism manifested by symptoms that include attention deficit, heat intolerance, frequent bowel movements, sweating, increased appetite, weight loss, anxiety, and an enlarged goiter.
- *Hashimoto's disease.* Patients with Hashimoto's disease produce insufficient amounts of thyroid hormone, leading to hypothyroidism. It is the most common type of autoimmune thyroid disease. Its symptoms include malaise, hair loss, weight gain, cold intolerance, constipation, dry skin, menorrhagia, and attention deficit.
- *Postpartum thyroiditis.* This type occurs within the first year after giving birth. Its symptoms, similar to hyperthyroidism, include anxiety, irritability, fatigue, unexplained weight loss, and insomnia. About 5–10% of new mothers are afflicted with postpartum thyroiditis.

What Are the Risk Factors for Autoimmune Thyroid Disease?
- *Systemic sclerosis.* Systemic sclerosis increases the risk of autoimmune thyroid disease. Systemic sclerosis—characterized by chronic degenerative disorders in the body, including the skin, joints, organs, and blood vessels—is a rare autoimmune disease. About 40% of patients with systemic sclerosis are also afflicted with autoimmune thyroid disease, and almost 100% of systemic sclerosis patients with papillary thyroid cancer have autoimmune thyroid disease.
- *Type 1 diabetes.* Type 1 diabetes is an autoimmune disease. About 30% of type 1 diabetes patients are afflicted with autoimmune thyroid disease. A type 1 diabetes patient's uncontrollable blood glucose level could have been caused by autoimmune thyroid disease. In addition to autoimmune thyroid disease, type 1 diabetes patients are also likely to suffer from celiac disease and Addison's disease.
- *Iodine overdose.* High blood iodine levels may increase the risk of autoimmune thyroid disease. On the one hand, iodized salt

seems to have resolved the iodine deficiency problem. On the other hand, iodine overdose caused by overconsumption of iodized salt has become a global public health concern. High blood iodine levels enhance the production of cytokines and chemokines, both of which guide immune cells to enter the thyroid gland, cause injuries to the thyroid hormone–producing cells, and increase the risk of autoimmune thyroid disease.

- *Family and genetics.* Autoimmune thyroid diseases such as Graves' disease and Hashimoto's disease are linked to polymorphic gene variants. More than 20 genes have been identified to be associated with autoimmune thyroid disease.
- *Environment.* Environmental factors—including polychlorinated biphenyl (PCB) and dioxin—are known risks factors for autoimmune thyroid disease.
- *Other factors.* Selenium deficiency and chronic hepatitis C are also known risk factors.

What Is the Association between Vitamin D and Autoimmune Thyroid Disease?

- Blood levels of vitamin D are often lower in patients with autoimmune thyroid disease compared to healthy individuals. About 92% of patients with Hashimoto's disease have low blood levels of vitamin D.
- Vitamin D enhances immune functions by inhibiting autoimmune antibody production and preventing the immune system from wrongly attacking tissues and organs.
- Vitamin D deficiency weakens the immune system and increases the incidence rate of autoimmune thyroid disease.

What Is the Association between Selenium and Autoimmune Thyroid Disease?

- Patients with autoimmune thyroid disease often have lower blood levels of selenium compared to healthy individuals. Selenium is a cofactor that supports enzymes involved in the synthesis of thyroid hormones. Supplementation with selenium was found to significantly reduce autoimmune antibody production in patients with autoimmune thyroid disease.

- Selenium is a cofactor that supports the activity of glutathione peroxidase, an enzyme that degrades hydrogen peroxide. Excessive hydrogen peroxide production can induce oxidative damage to thyroid hormone–producing cells and increase the risk of autoimmune thyroid disease.

Meta-analysis

- *Vitamin D.* A meta-analysis of 20 research papers explored the relationship between vitamin D and autoimmune thyroid disease in 3,603 individuals, including 1,782 autoimmune thyroid disease patients and 1,821 healthy controls. Analysis confirmed that the blood levels of vitamin D were lower in autoimmune thyroid disease patients compared to healthy controls.
- *Selenium.* Nine research papers investigated the efficacy of selenium supplementation in the treatment of autoimmune thyroid disease in 787 autoimmune thyroid disease patients. Supplementation with selenium was found to significantly lower the blood level of autoimmune antibodies and improve the moods and emotional well-being of patients with autoimmune thyroid disease.

Recommendation

- *Prevention.* For people at risk of autoimmune thyroid disease, take daily 800 IU vitamin D3 (11) and 50 mcg selenium (26).
- *Treatment.* For autoimmune thyroid disease patients, take daily 2,000 IU vitamin D3 (11) and 100 mcg selenium (26).

44

BLADDER CANCER

Bladder cancer often begins with the uncontrollable growth of the cells in the inner layer of the urinary bladder. The urinary bladder is a bag-like organ located inside the pelvis. Its main function is to collect urine, which is then discharged through the urethra. If the uncontrollable growth of the cells is restricted to the inner layer of the urinary bladder, the cancer is less invasive and treatable. On the other hand, if the malignant cells spread to the entire bladder wall, the cancer is invasive and difficult to treat. An estimated 560,000 bladder cancer cases occur in the US every year. Among them, 150,000 patients die of bladder cancer.

What Are the Symptoms of Bladder Cancer?
- Bloody urine (often an early sign of bladder cancer)
- Frequent urination or discomfort during urination
- Difficulty urinating or weak and slow urine flow
- Foot edema

- Bone aches all over the body
- Fatigue, loss of appetite, and weight loss

What Are the Risk Factors for Bladder Cancer?

- *Smoking.* Cigarette smoke contains harmful chemicals that are known carcinogens. For example, aromatic amines are known to cause bladder cancer.
- *Working environment.* Some industrial chemicals, such as benzidines and naphthylamines in dye factories and chemicals used in rubber, leather, and paint manufacturing, are causative agents for bladder cancer.
- *Drugs.* Long-term use of type 2 diabetes medications, such as pioglitazone and cyclophosphamide, increases the risk of bladder cancer.
- *Arsenic.* Drinking arsenic-contaminated water can lead to bladder cancer. Arsenic can induce gene mutations and tumor transformation of bladder cells into cancerous cells, causing bladder cancer.
- *Dehydration.* Insufficient daily water intake increases the incidence of bladder cancer. Adequate consumption of water can cleanse the urinary bladder by shortening the time that toxins stay in the bladder. People who don't drink enough water have an increased risk of bladder cancer.

What Is the Association between Vitamin A and Bladder Cancer?

- Blood levels of vitamin A are lower in patients with bladder cancer compared to healthy individuals. Vitamin A has antioxidant properties. It neutralizes free radicals and prevents them from causing gene mutations and oxidative damage to chromosomes.
- Vitamin A enhances cell differentiation and inhibits cell proliferation. Cell proliferation allows cancerous cells to multiply and form a tumor mass in the body.

What Is the Association between Vitamin C and Bladder Cancer?

- Carcinogens, such as 3-hydroxy-2-amino-benzoic acid, are known to cause bladder cancer. Vitamin C can neutralize benzoic acid derivatives and decrease the risk of bladder cancer.
- Vitamin C has antioxidant and anti-inflammatory functions. It inhibits the proliferation and spread of cancerous cells. Blood levels of vitamin C are lower in patients with bladder cancer compared to healthy controls. Sufficient dietary intake of vitamin C was found to decrease the incidence of bladder cancer.
- High-dose IV vitamin C therapy can treat certain forms of cancers. High blood levels of vitamin C produce hydrogen peroxide, which can kill cancer cells in the body. (For details, see chapter 47, "Breast Cancer.")

What Is the Association between Vitamin D and Bladder Cancer?

- Vitamin D deficiency is linked to a twofold increased risk of bladder cancer and a sixfold increased risk of invasive and untreatable bladder cancer.
- Vitamin D possesses anticancer functions. It inhibits the proliferation of cancerous cells and prevents them from growing new blood vessels.

What Is the Association between Vitamin E and Bladder Cancer?

- Vitamin E scavenges free radicals in the cell membrane and protects the structural integrity of the cells. A low blood level of vitamin E is common in patients with bladder cancer compared to healthy individuals. Sufficient dietary intake of vitamin E was shown to curtail the incidence rate of bladder cancer.
- Vitamin E can boost immune functions, regulate gene expression, and inhibit the proliferation and growth of cancerous cells.

What Is the Association between Vitamin B9 and Bladder Cancer?

- Vitamin B9 participates in the methylation and repair of DNA in the cells. Vitamin B9 insufficiency can lead to inadequate methylation of DNA, which is a hallmark of cancer cells.
- Blood levels of vitamin B9 are lower in bladder cancer patients compared to healthy controls. Supplementation with B9 was found to reduce the incidence rate of bladder cancer.

What Is the Association between Selenium and Bladder Cancer?

- Selenium exhibits antioxidant properties by scavenging hydrogen peroxide and preventing oxidative damage to DNA and gene mutation.
- Selenium enhances immune functions by reducing systemic inflammation and preventing the proliferation of cancerous cells. Selenium-dependent enzymes can force cancerous cells to commit apoptosis, or programmed cell death.
- Lower blood levels of selenium are common in patients with bladder cancer. Sufficient dietary intake of selenium was found to decrease the incidence rate of bladder cancer.

What Is the Association between Zinc and Bladder Cancer?

- Free radical–induced oxidative damage is a causative factor for bladder cancer. Zinc-dependent enzymes possess strong antioxidant properties. They neutralize free radicals and prevent them from causing oxidative damage to DNA and from inducing gene mutation and tumor transformation.
- Zinc deficiency increases the risk of bladder cancer. Supplementation with zinc was shown to reduce the risk of bladder cancer.

Meta-analysis

- *Vitamin A.* A meta-analysis of 25 research papers explored the relationship between vitamin A and bladder cancer in 11,580 bladder cancer patients. Analysis confirmed that sufficient dietary intake of vitamin A significantly reduced the risk of bladder cancer.

- *Vitamin C and vitamin E.* Twenty research papers investigated the association between antioxidant vitamins and bladder cancer. The meta-analysis confirmed that sufficient dietary intake of vitamin C and vitamin E decreased the incidence rate of bladder cancer.
- *Vitamin D.* Seven research papers conducted with 62,141 people investigated vitamin D and bladder cancer. The meta-analysis confirmed that low blood levels of vitamin D significantly increased the risk of bladder cancer.
- *Vitamin B9.* A meta-analysis of 12 research papers evaluated the relationship between vitamin B9 and bladder cancer. Analysis confirmed that sufficient dietary intake of vitamin B9 curtailed the incidence rate of bladder cancer.
- *Selenium.* Seven research papers studied the relationship between selenium and bladder cancer in 17,339 people. The result confirmed that high blood levels of selenium decreased the incidence rate of bladder cancer by 39%.
- *Zinc.* A meta-analysis of six research papers investigated the association between zinc and bladder cancer. The result confirmed that blood levels of zinc were significantly lower in bladder cancer patients compared to healthy controls.

Recommendation

- *Prevention.* For people at risk of bladder cancer, take daily 2,000 IU vitamin A (1), 200 mg vitamin C (10), 800 IU vitamin D3 (11), 30 IU vitamin E (12), 400 mcg vitamin B9 (8), 50 mcg selenium (26), and 10 mg zinc (20).
- *Treatment.* For bladder cancer patients, take daily 5,000 IU vitamin A (1), 500 mg vitamin C (10), 2,000 IU vitamin D3 (11), 100 IU vitamin E (12), 800 mcg vitamin B9 (8), 100 mcg selenium (26), and 20 mg zinc (20).

45

BLOOD CANCERS

Blood cancers are a collective term for cancers that affect the blood, bone marrow, and lymphatic system. They often start with the uncontrollable growth of abnormal stem cells in the bone marrow. Under normal physiological conditions, stem cells in the bone marrow can develop into three major types of blood cells—namely, red blood cells, white blood cells, and platelets. When stem cells transform into cancerous cells, the bone marrow is unable to produce sufficient amounts of normal blood cells. These cancer cells lose the ability to perform the normal physiological functions of blood cells. In the US, an estimated 172,000 blood cancer cases occur every year. A new case of blood cancer is diagnosed every three minutes.

What Are the Three Major Types of Blood Cancers?
- *Leukemia.* Leukemia is caused by the uncontrollable growth of stem cells, producing a large quantity of abnormal white blood cells. Not only are these abnormal white blood cells unable to fight against infections, but they also adversely affect

the bone marrow's ability to produce other blood cells, such as red blood cells and platelets.

- *Lymphoma.* Normal lymphocytes play an important role in immune defense against bacterial or viral infections. Abnormal lymphocytes may transform into cancerous lymphoma cells and lose anti-infection functions. Cancerous lymphoma cells then accumulate at lymph nodes to form lymphoma, further compromising immune defense.
- *Myeloma.* Myeloma is caused by the uncontrollable growth of abnormal plasma cells in the bone marrow. Plasma cells are a type of white blood cell that produces antibodies. Cancerous plasma cells have lost their antibody-producing abilities, compromising the immune defense system.

What Are the Symptoms of Blood Cancers?
- *Leukemia.* Leukemia negatively affects the bone marrow's ability to produce red blood cells. Insufficient red blood cells lead to anemia, weakness, and fatigue. Patients with leukemia sweat easily and experience shortness of breath, even after performing only minor household chores.
- *Lymphoma.* The major symptom of lymphoma is an enlarged lymph node. Patients may not feel any pain at all. Other symptoms include weight loss, lack of appetite, and fever.
- *Myeloma.* Initially, there are no apparent symptoms associated with myeloma. As the disease progresses, patients may feel fatigue and back pain and experience frequent infections, shortness of breath, and chest pains.

What Are the Risk Factors for Blood Cancers?
- *Age and gender.* Childhood leukemia is the most common type of cancer in children. However, most blood cancers, particularly lymphoma, occur at age 60 and older. Men are more susceptible to blood cancers than women are.
- *Family and genetics.* Familial acute myeloid leukemia is associated with CEBPA gene polymorphic variants. CEBPA genes

encode for a transcription factor that supports the differentiation of white blood cells. Mutation of the CEBPA gene increases the risk of leukemia. On the other hand, lymphoma is not a hereditary disease, and parents with lymphoma will not pass the disease to children. Myeloma, caused by cancerous plasma cells, is also not a hereditary disease.

- *Immunodeficiency.* Immunodeficiency increases the risk of blood cancers. Antirejection medications after organ transplantation surgery, AIDS, and autoimmune disorders, including rheumatoid arthritis and lupus erythematosus, can lead to immunodeficiency.
- *Radiation.* Judging from the data obtained from nuclear bomb explosions in Japan and nuclear reactor accidents around the world, exposure to gamma radiation can cause blood cancers. Cancer patients receiving radiation therapy also have an increased risk of blood cancers.
- *Chemicals.* Exposure to benzene, herbicides, or pesticides at the workplace increases the risk of blood cancers. Benzene and its derivatives can damage the chromosomes of stem cells in the bone marrow, leading to gene mutations and blood cancers.
- *Chemotherapy.* Certain chemotherapeutic agents to treat blood cancers may cause second-time blood cancers in patients. For example, alkylating agents, such as melphalan and chlorambucil, are chemotherapeutic agents commonly used to treat blood cancers. These chemotherapeutic agents may cure blood cancers, but they can also inflict second-time blood cancers on patients. The symptoms of second-time blood cancers resemble those of benzene-induced leukemia.
- *Obesity.* Obesity increases the risk of leukemia. In addition to leukemia, obesity also elevates the risk of cancers in the esophagus, stomach, liver, kidney, pancreas, and colon. In obese people, the abovementioned organs lining the digestive tract are filled with fats known as visceral fats. Visceral fats release chemicals and hormones that promote the transformation

of normal cells to cancerous cells and activate the target of rapamycin (TOR) pathway, which facilitates the proliferation and survival of cancerous cells in the inflicted organs.

What Is the Association between Vitamin D and Blood Cancers?

- Low blood levels of vitamin D increase the risk of blood cancers. People who live at elevations of 2,000 feet or higher are less likely to be afflicted with blood cancers due to an increased production of vitamin D from the skin in mountainous regions where ultraviolet B is strong. On the other hand, people who live far away from the equator, where ultraviolet B is weak and the skin produces less vitamin D, have an elevated risk of blood cancers. The rate of leukemia in children is higher in the winter months compared to that in the summer months because blood levels of vitamin D are lower during winter.

- A low blood level of vitamin D also increases the mortality rate in patients with blood cancers. However, sufficient dietary intake of vitamin D alleviates the symptoms and severity of blood cancers. Vitamin D can strengthen the immune system and prevent the growth and proliferation of cancerous cells.

Meta-analysis

- *Vitamin D.* A meta-analysis of seven research papers explored the relationship between vitamin D and blood cancers in 2,643 blood cancer patients. Low blood levels of vitamin D were found to significantly increase the mortality rate of patients with blood cancers.

Recommendation

- *Prevention.* For people at risk of blood cancer, take daily 800 IU vitamin D3 (11).
- *Treatment.* For blood cancer patients, take daily 2,000 IU vitamin D3 (11).

46

BONE FRACTURES

A bone fracture is a condition in which the continuity of the bone is interrupted. Two major types of bone fractures include a fracture caused by strong exterior pressure and a fracture caused by pathological changes in the bones, such as in osteoporosis, called a "pathologic fracture." In this chapter, we are concerned with pathologic fractures. An estimated 9 million bone fractures occur due to osteoporosis every year worldwide.

What Are the Risk Factors for Bone Fractures?
- *Osteoporosis.* Low bone density and degeneration of bone structure in osteoporosis patients increases the incidence rate of bone fractures after accidental falls. The most common bone fractures in osteoporosis patients are fractures of vertebra, called "vertebral compression fractures." It is estimated that 1.5 million vertebral compression fractures occur in the US every year.

- *Bone-related diseases.* Bone-related diseases can weaken bone structure and increase chances of suffering a bone fracture. These bone diseases include osteomalacia, bone cancer, bone cysts, osteogenesis imperfecta, and Paget's disease of bone. Vitamin D deficiency causes osteomalacia, characterized by body pains, muscle weakness, and softening of the bones. Bone cancer is a malignant tumor of the bone, which can destroy the bone tissue and result in fragile bones. In bone cysts, the bones are porous and filled with liquid, which makes the bones break easily. Osteogenesis imperfecta is a hereditary bone disease characterized by deformed and fragile bones. Paget's disease of bone is an age-related bone degenerative disease characterized by deformed and degenerative vertebrae and a similarly affected head bone and pelvic bone.

What Is the Association between Calcium and Bone Fractures?
- Calcium binds phosphate to form calcium phosphate, which is deposited into the bone matrix through the mineralization process. Calcium deficiency due to insufficient dietary intake or pathological factors can lead to bone loss and weakened bones, and it can increase the incidence rate of bone fractures after accidental falls.

What Is the Association between Vitamin D and Bone Fractures?
- Vitamin D is an essential nutrient for supporting the balance of calcium and phosphate levels in the bloodstream. Vitamin D enhances the mineralization of calcium phosphate and increases bone density. Vitamin D deficiency decreases the mineralization of calcium phosphate and reduces bone density, thus elevating the risk of osteoporosis and bone fractures.

Meta-analysis
- *Vitamin D.* A meta-analysis of eight randomized controlled clinical trial papers investigated the relationship between calcium and vitamin D supplements and the incident rate

of bone fracture in 30,970 individuals, including 195 hip-fracture patients and 2,231 other bone-fracture patients. The data confirmed that long-term supplementation with calcium and vitamin D significantly reduced the risk of bone fracture by 15% and the risk of hip fracture by 30%. In this analysis, the daily doses of supplements were 1,000–1,200 mg of calcium and 400–800 IU of vitamin D for one to seven years.

Recommendation
- *Prevention.* For people at risk of bone fracture, take daily 500 mg calcium (14) and 800 IU vitamin D3 (11).
- *Treatment.* For bone fracture patients, take daily 1,000 mg calcium (14) and 2,000 IU vitamin D3 (11).

47

BREAST CANCER

Breast cancer usually starts from an uncontrollable growth of abnormal cells in the milk ducts or the lobules that produce milk in the breast. A breast cancer that starts from the milk ducts is called ductal carcinoma, while a breast cancer that starts from the lobules is called lobular carcinoma. Either ductal or lobular carcinoma can grow to a mass and expand to other parts of the breast. Invasive breast cancer can spread through lymph nodes in the armpits and metastasize to other organs in the body. In the US, one in every eight women will suffer from breast cancer in her lifetime. It is estimated that this year alone, 250,000 women will be diagnosed with invasive breast cancer, and an additional 60,000 women will be diagnosed with noninvasive breast cancer.

What Are the Symptoms of Breast Cancer?
- A mass in the breast
- Change in breast shape

- Skin indentations in the breast
- Nipples secreting fluids

What Are the Risk Factors for Breast Cancer?

- *Age and gender.* The majority of breast cancer patients are women. The risk of breast cancer starts around age 40 and peaks at age 70. Men and younger women can also be afflicted with breast cancer, albeit at a lower incidence rate.
- *Alcohol.* Consumption of alcoholic beverages at two to three drinks per day increases the risk of breast cancer by 20%. Alcohol raises the blood level of estrogen, a female hormone that stimulates the growth and proliferation of cancer cells in the breast and increases the risk of breast cancer in post-menopausal women. Alcohol also lowers the blood level of folic acid, an essential nutrient that supports the synthesis and repair of DNA. The lack of folic acid increases errors in the synthesis of new DNA and destabilizes the structure of DNA, leading to gene mutation and tumor transformation.
- *Family and genetics.* Several gene polymorphic variants—such as BRCA1, BRCA2, p53, and PALB2—are associated with breast cancer. Among them, BRCA1 and BRCA2 are well-known genetic risk factors for breast cancer. About 8–10% of Ashkenazi Jews are carriers of the BRCA1 gene, while about 1% of Asians or Africans carry either the BRCA1 or BRCA2 gene.
- *Menstruation.* Women who began menstruation at age 12 or younger have a 20% increased risk of breast cancer. High blood levels of estrogen stimulate the growth and proliferation of cancerous cells in the breast.
- *Contraceptives.* The use of oral contraceptives increases the risk of breast cancer by 20–30%. The association between the risk of breast cancer and other birth control devices, such as the IUD or birth control patches, is not as clear. However, all contraceptive medications alter the blood levels of female sex hormones, and they will inevitably affect women's health.

In addition, women who receive estrogen replacement therapy for more than two years have an increased risk of breast cancer.

- *Smoking.* Lipophilic carcinogens, such as nitrosamines and aromatic amines in cigarette smoke, can enter the bloodstream and travel to fat tissues in the breast. These toxic chemicals can cause gene mutations and the transformation of breast cells to malignant cells. The p53 gene encodes a protein that supports the cell cycle and acts as a tumor suppressor. Women smokers were found to have more p53 mutated genes compared to nonsmoking women. Mutations in the p53 gene lead to unabated cell growth and increase the incidence rate of breast cancer.
- *Overweight/obesity.* Premenopausal women who are overweight experience a 20–40% decreased risk of breast cancer. However, postmenopausal women who are overweight experience a 30–60% increased risk of breast cancer. Obesity is a chronic inflammatory condition that stimulates the production of insulin and insulin-like growth factor and promotes the growth and proliferation of cancerous cells in the breast, particularly in postmenopausal women.
- *Lack of exercise.* Regular exercise decreases the risk of breast cancer by 10–20%. Exercise controls body weight, increases insulin sensitivity, and lowers estrogen levels, thus reducing the risk of breast cancer, particularly in postmenopausal women. On the other hand, a lack of exercise elevates the blood level of insulin and causes insulin resistance. Insulin resistance is associated with the growth and proliferation of cancer cells in the breast.

How Is Breast Cancer Diagnosed?
- *Breast exam.* Physicians perform breast exams to detect any masses or unusual shape changes in the breasts.
- *Mammogram.* The American Medical Association recommends that women aged 50 and older receive an X-ray mammogram every other year, rather than every year, to avoid

excessive radiation exposure. Nevertheless, women in the high-risk group for breast cancer may still require annual X-ray mammograms.

- *Breast ultrasound.* There is no risk of radiation exposure in a breast ultrasound.
- *Breast MRI.* Breast MRI scans provide valuable information regarding actual tumor size and shape and accurate staging for breast cancer without the risk of radiation exposure.

What Is the Association between Vitamin B6 and Breast Cancer?

- B vitamins—such as vitamins B6, B9, and B12—are involved in one-carbon metabolism, a biochemical pathway that supports the synthesis and methylation of DNA, and the maintenance of the structural integrity of chromosomes. Vitamin B6 deficiency leads to insufficient methylation of DNA, a salient characteristic of cancer cells. Insufficient gene methylation negatively affects the expression of tumor suppressor genes and increases the risk of tumor transformation.
- Sufficient dietary intake of vitamin B6 was found to decrease the risk of ER-positive breast cancer.

What Is the Association between Vitamin C and Breast Cancer?

- Taking a vitamin C supplement benefits cancer patients. It alleviates the symptoms associated with cancers—such as pain, vomiting, and fatigue—thus improving quality of life in cancer patients.
- Vitamin C can neutralize free radicals and prevent oxidative damage–induced gene mutation and tumor transformation. Oxidative damage is a major causative factor of breast cancer.
- High-dose IV vitamin C therapy may be a safe and effective treatment for certain types of cancers. As the name clearly implies, a megadose of vitamin C is injected as an intravenous infusion into a vein, which increases the cellular concentration of vitamin C in the body. High concentrations of vitamin C produce hydrogen peroxide, a strong oxidant that

can kill cancer cells. Hydrogen peroxide is converted to water and oxygen by catalase, an enzyme prevalent in normal cells. Cancer cells, on the other hand, are known to contain fewer catalase enzymes, and they cannot degrade hydrogen peroxide. High concentrations of hydrogen peroxide therefore can selectively kill cancer cells in the body. In other words, high-dose IV vitamin C therapy is a targeted therapy that kills cancer cells but spares normal cells. Although the treatment has not been approved by the FDA, physicians in the US and abroad often recommend high-dose IV vitamin C therapy to treat patients with advanced stages of cancer, particularly patients who are at late stages of the disease and refuse any further chemotherapy.

What Is the Association between Vitamin D and Breast Cancer?

- A low blood level of vitamin D is common in patients with breast cancer. Women with vitamin D deficiency have a higher risk of breast cancer compared to women with normal blood levels of vitamin D.
- High blood levels of vitamin D are associated with lower blood levels of estrogen, thus preventing the growth and proliferation of cancer cells in the breast.
- Sufficient dietary intake of vitamin D alleviates the debilitating symptoms of breast cancer and improves the survival rate of patients.

What Is the Association between Vitamin E and Breast Cancer?

- Vitamin E neutralizes free radicals and prevents free radical–induced lipid peroxidation of cell membranes. The destruction of cell membranes damages the integrity of cell organelles, such as the mitochondria and nucleus, and increases the risk of gene mutation and tumor transformation.
- Vitamin E has anticancer properties. It stimulates the expression of p53 tumor suppressor genes, activates heat shock

proteins, and inhibits the formation of new blood vessels in cancerous lesions in the breasts.

- The anticancer properties of vitamin E also include inhibiting the growth and proliferation of cancer cells, forcing cancer cells to commit apoptosis (cell death), and preventing the metastasis of cancer cells.

What Is the Association between Vitamin B9 and Breast Cancer?

- Sufficient blood levels of vitamin B9 decrease the risk of death in patients with breast cancer by 50%.
- A low blood level of vitamin B9 is common among patients with breast cancer. A normal blood level of vitamin B9 was found to significantly curtail the risk of breast cancer.
- Vitamin B9 is an essential nutrient that supports the synthesis and repair of DNA. Vitamin B9 deficiency increases errors in the synthesis and repair of DNA and decreases the structural stability of chromosomes, leading to gene mutation and tumor transformation.
- Sufficient dietary intake of vitamin B9 decreases the risk of ER-positive and PR-positive breast cancers.

Can Supplementation with Vitamin D Prevent Breast Cancer?

- Clinical studies have shown that supplementation with vitamin D3 at a daily dose of 1,100 IU together with calcium at a daily dose of 1,450 mg for four years decreased the risk of cancers, including breast cancer, by 70% in postmenopausal women.

What Is the Association between Selenium and Breast Cancer?

- Selenium-dependent enzymes can degrade carcinogens as well as heavy metals and other toxic chemicals.
- The anticancer properties of selenium-dependent enzymes include blocking the proliferation of cancer cells, encouraging cancer cells to commit apoptosis, and inhibiting the migration of cancer cells to neighboring cells.

What Is the Association between Omega-3 Fatty Acids and Breast Cancer?

- Supplementation with omega-3 fatty acids increases the efficacy of chemotherapy and reduces its side effects. Consumption of fish or supplementation with omega-3 fatty acids improves the survival rate of patients with breast cancer.
- Omega-3 fatty acids exhibit anticancer properties by inhibiting the formation of new blood vessels and the metastasis of cancer cells.
- Supplementation with omega-3 fatty acids reduces the production of inflammatory cytokines and alleviates the inflammation of breast tissues.

Meta-analysis

- *Vitamin B6.* A meta-analysis of 14 research papers studied the relationship between vitamin B6 and breast cancer in 14,260 breast cancer patients. Analysis confirmed that high blood levels of vitamin B6 reduced the risk of breast cancer, particularly in postmenopausal women.
- *Vitamin C.* Ten research articles explored the association between vitamin C and mortality rate in 17,696 breast cancer patients, including 1,558 cases of cancer death and 2,791 cases of all-cause mortality. The data confirmed that sufficient dietary intake of vitamin C significantly curtailed the risk of death in women with breast cancer. In addition, increasing dietary intake of vitamin C by 100 mg daily was found to reduce the risk of cancer mortality by 17% and the risk of all-cause mortality by 12%.
- *Vitamins C and E.* Forty research papers investigated the relationship between antioxidant vitamins and breast cancer. The meta-analysis confirmed that high blood levels of vitamin C and vitamin E reduced the risk of breast cancer.
- *Vitamin D.* A meta-analysis of 30 research articles studied the relationship between vitamin D and breast cancer in 6,092 breast cancer patients. Analysis confirmed that low blood

levels of vitamin D meant a decreased survival rate in women with breast cancer.

- *Vitamin B9.* Sixteen research papers investigated the association between vitamin B9 and breast cancer in 744,068 people, including 26,205 breast cancer patients. Analysis confirmed that dietary intake of vitamin B9 at a daily dose of 153–400 mcg reduced the risk of breast cancer.

- *Selenium.* A meta-analysis of 16 research papers explored the relationship between selenium and breast cancer. Analysis revealed that breast cancer patients had low blood levels of selenium compared to healthy women.

- *Omega-3 fatty acids.* Seventeen research papers evaluated the relationship between omega-3 fatty acids and breast cancer in 16,178 breast cancer patients and 527,392 healthy controls. Analysis confirmed that supplementation with omega-3 fatty acids reduced the risk of breast cancer by 14%.

Recommendation

- *Prevention.* For women at risk of breast cancer, take daily 2 mg vitamin B6 (6), 200 mg vitamin C (10), 800 IU vitamin D3 (11), 30 IU vitamin E (12), 400 mcg vitamin B9 (8), 50 mcg selenium (26), and 1 g omega-3 fatty acids (27).

- *Treatment.* For women with breast cancer, take daily 10 mg vitamin B6 (6), 500 mg vitamin C (10), 2,000 IU vitamin D3 (11), 100 IU vitamin E (12), 800 mcg vitamin B9 (8), 100 mcg selenium (26), and 2 g omega-3 fatty acids (27).

48

CARDIOVASCULAR DISEASE

Cardiovascular disease is a group of related diseases and conditions caused by pathological changes in the heart and vascular system and functional alterations in the cardiovascular system. Atherosclerosis and blood clots are the two major contributing factors of cardiovascular disease, which lead to the narrowing of the arterial wall and the reduction of blood flow. Heart attack and stroke are in part caused by blood clots occluding the blood flow to the heart and brain, respectively. In the US, 84 million people suffer from cardiovascular disease, and of those, 2,200 die from the disease every day. Every 40 seconds, someone in the US dies from cardiovascular disease.

What Are the Major Types of Heart-Related Diseases?
- *Heart attack.* A blood clot blocks the blood flow to the heart and stops the heartbeat due to lack of oxygen and nutrients.

- *Heart failure.* The heart is unable to pump out sufficient amounts of blood for body's needs, often due to an enlarged heart.
- *Atrial fibrillation.* The fibrosis of heart muscle causes an irregular heartbeat.

What Are the Symptoms of a Heart Attack?
- Chest pain, chest discomfort, or pressure inside the chest
- Shortness of breath
- Cold feet and hands
- Numbness and pain in the feet and hands
- Pain and discomfort in the neck, mandible, throat, stomach, or back

The warning signs of a heart attack differ between men and women. Men complain about chest pain, while women experience shortness of breath, nausea, or vomiting.

What Are the Risk Factors for Cardiovascular Disease?
- *Hypertension.* Hypertension is the major risk factor for cardiovascular diseases, including coronary artery disease and stroke. About 50% of ischemic stroke and cerebral hemorrhagic stroke are caused by hypertension. Hypertension exerts extra pressure on the arterial wall, injuring the blood vessels and causing endothelial dysfunction, which leads to atherosclerosis and blood clot formation. Aging raises blood pressure, particularly systolic pressure. Systolic pressure is indicative of one's biological age, the higher the systolic pressure, the older one's biological age. High systolic pressure is also a warning sign of cardiovascular disease. Biological age, not chronological age, is associated with hypertension and cardiovascular disease.
- *Hypercholesterolemia.* Cholesterol in the bloodstream is mainly stored in low-density lipoproteins (LDL) and high-density lipoproteins (HDL). LDL is often called "bad" cholesterol, while HDL is called "good" cholesterol. Hypercholesterolemia

means a high LDL level and a low HDL level in the bloodstream, increasing the risk of cardiovascular disease.

- *High triglycerides.* High blood levels of triglycerides are associated with atherosclerosis and blood clot formation and increased incidence rates of stroke, heart attack, and coronary artery disease. Individuals with high blood levels of triglycerides often suffer from hypertension, diabetes, and metabolic syndrome, all of which are risk factors for cardiovascular disease. High triglycerides increase the risk of cardiovascular disease.

- *Smoking.* Cigarette smoke contains harmful chemicals that enter the bloodstream and travel to the brain, heart, lungs, liver, pancreas, digestive tract, and the like and cause injuries to these organs and tissues. Toxic chemicals from cigarette smoke can also directly injure arterial vessels, leading to atherosclerosis and blood clot formation, thus increasing the risk of cardiovascular disease.

- *Lack of exercise.* Regular exercise like running, jogging, or swimming can strengthen muscles and bones in the body. Regular exercise increases insulin sensitivity, raising the efficiency of energy production and lowering the blood glucose level. Regular exercise can also reduce the risk of heart attack, coronary artery disease, stroke, and diabetes. On the other hand, lack of exercise brings on weight gain, hypertension, and diabetes, increasing the risk of cardiovascular disease.

- *Diabetes.* High blood glucose is a major symptom of diabetes. High blood glucose induces the production of superoxide anion radicals and hydroxyl radicals. Both radicals can cause oxidative damage to LDL and generate oxidized LDL. Oxidized LDL embedded in endothelial cells can cause plaque and blood clot formation in the arterial wall.

- *Salty food.* Habitual consumption of salty food can lead to hypertension. In response to the ingestion of salty food, the kidneys decrease the excretion of water and reabsorb discharged water in order to dilute high sodium concentrations in the bloodstream. This excessive amount of water in the bloodstream exerts extra pressure on the arterial wall and causes hypertension, a major risk factor for cardiovascular disease.

- *Aging.* A healthy cardiovascular system allows oxygenated blood from the lungs to enter the heart and travel via the vascular system to various organs and tissues. Aging causes the deterioration of the heart and vascular system, including the hardening of the arterial wall, endothelial dysfunction, and failure to control systolic pressure in the left ventricle of the heart—all of which adversely affect the delivery of oxygenated blood to various organs and tissues and exacerbate the risk of cardiovascular disease.

- *Family and genetics.* The cardiovascular system consists of the heart and vascular system. More than 40 gene polymorphic variants have been associated with cardiovascular disease. Environmental factors that influence gene expression at epigenetic levels—such as smoking, exercise, and diet—also play an important role in the pathology of cardiovascular disease.

What Is the Association between Vitamin C and Cardiovascular Disease?

- Vitamin C can lower LDL levels and blood pressure. A low blood level of vitamin C is common in patients with cardiovascular disease compared to healthy individuals. Supplementation with vitamin C improves endothelial functions and prevents cardiovascular disease.

- Vitamin C can neutralize free radicals and prevent free radical–induced damage to the heart and vascular system. Vitamin C inhibits the oxidation of LDL and reduces the risk of plaque and blood clot formation, thus decreasing the risk of cardiovascular disease.

What Is the Association between Vitamin D and Cardiovascular Disease?

- A lower blood level of vitamin D is associated with the risk of cardiovascular disease. Low blood levels of vitamin D are associated with an increased risk of sudden cardiac arrest in patients with cardiovascular disease.
- C reactive protein is a marker of inflammation. A high blood level of C reactive protein is indicative of systemic inflammation, such as in cardiovascular disease. Vitamin D inhibits the ability of the liver to produce C reactive protein and reduces the risk of cardiovascular disease.

What Is the Association between Vitamin E and Cardiovascular Disease?

- Vitamin E can inhibit free radical–induced oxidative damage to blood vessels and prevent endothelial dysfunction, atherosclerosis, and blood clot formation, all of which are risk factors for cardiovascular disease.
- Vitamin E can lower the blood level of C reactive protein and attenuate inflammation. A low blood level of vitamin E is common among patients with cardiovascular disease. Supplementation with vitamin E was shown to improve heart function and reduce the risk of cardiovascular disease.

What Is the Association between Magnesium and Cardiovascular Disease?

- The benefits of magnesium to cardiovascular functions include increasing vasodilatation, reducing blood pressure, alleviating inflammation, preventing platelet coagulation, enhancing homeostasis of blood insulin levels, and regulating fat metabolism.
- Cardiovascular disease patients had a lower blood level of magnesium compared to healthy individuals. Supplementation with magnesium was shown to reduce the risk of cardiovascular disease.

What Is the Association between Omega-3 Fatty Acids and Cardiovascular Disease?

- Omega-3 fatty acids have antioxidant properties. They block free radical–induced oxidative damage to the heart and vascular system. A low blood level of omega-3 fatty acids is common in patients with cardiovascular disease compared to healthy individuals. Supplementation with omega-3 fatty acids alleviates the symptoms of cardiovascular disease.
- Omega-3 fatty acids regulate the fluidity of cell membranes in endothelial cells of the heart and vascular system and maintain normal cardiovascular functions.

Meta-analysis

- *Vitamin C.* A meta-analysis of 44 clinical research reports evaluated the relationship between vitamin C and cardiovascular disease. The participants included patients with atherosclerosis, diabetes, and heart failure. Analysis confirmed that supplementation with vitamin C improved endothelial functions and alleviated the symptoms of cardiovascular disease, such as in atherosclerosis and heart failure.
- *Vitamin D.* Nineteen research papers explored the relationship between vitamin D and cardiovascular disease in 65,994 individuals, including 6,123 cardiovascular disease patients. The data confirmed that low blood levels of vitamin D had an increased risk of cardiovascular disease as well as an increased risk of all-cause mortality.
- *Vitamin D.* A meta-analysis of 10 clinical research papers investigated the relationship between vitamin D and C reactive proteins in 924 individuals. Analysis revealed that supplementation with vitamin D significantly lowered the blood's C reactive protein content. A high blood level of C reactive protein is a known risk factor for cardiovascular disease. The data confirmed that vitamin D curtailed the risk of cardiovascular disease.

- *Vitamin E.* A meta-analysis of 12 clinical research reports conducted with 246 participants in the vitamin E group and 249 participants in the placebo group explored the relationship between vitamin E and cardiovascular disease. The meta-analysis confirmed that supplementation with vitamin E reduced the blood level of C reactive protein and the risk of cardiovascular disease.
- *Magnesium.* Nineteen research papers studied the relationship between magnesium and cardiovascular disease in 532,979 people, including 19,926 cardiovascular disease patients, of whom 6,668 were stroke patients and 5,836 heart disease patients. The data revealed that sufficient dietary intake of magnesium reduced the risk of cardiovascular disease by 15%. Supplementation with magnesium at a daily dose of 150–400 mg was found to significantly reduce the risk of cardiovascular disease.
- *Omega-3 fatty acids.* A meta-analysis of 11 randomized controlled clinical trial studies evaluated the relationship between omega-3 fatty acids and cardiovascular disease in 15,348 cardiovascular disease patients. Analysis confirmed that supplementation with omega-3 fatty acids significantly improved survival rates in patients with cardiovascular disease compared to the placebo group.

Recommendation
- *Prevention.* For people at risk of cardiovascular disease, take daily 200 mg vitamin C (10), 800 IU vitamin D2 (11), 30 IU vitamin E (12), 100 mg magnesium (17), and 1 g omega-3 fatty acids (27).
- *Treatment.* For cardiovascular disease patients, take daily 500 mg vitamin C (10), 2,000 IU vitamin D3 (11), 100 IU vitamin E (12), 200 mg magnesium (17), and 2 g omega-3 fatty acids (27).

49

CATARACTS

Cataracts are caused by lens cloudiness, leading to diminished vision. The lenses in the eyes collect and focus images and then present the images to a light-sensitive membrane called the retina. The function of the lenses in the eyes resembles the lens in a camera. In healthy eyes, the lenses are transparent so that images presented to the retina are clear. In eyes with cataracts, the lenses are cloudy, and images become blurred when they reach the retina. Aging is a major risk factor for cataracts. About 25 million people aged 40 years and older have cataracts in the US. By age 75, 50% of people suffer from cataracts.

What Are the Causes of Cataracts?
- A lens consists mainly of water and proteins. When alpha crystalline proteins align properly, the lens is transparent. Aging accelerates structural alterations and derangement of alpha crystalline proteins, causing the lens to become opaque and leading to cataracts.

What Are the Major Types of Cataracts?

- *Nuclear sclerotic cataracts.* A cataract appears in the center of the lens. In the beginning, it seems like aggravated myopia. Thereafter, the color of the lens turns yellow and then brown. In severe cases, the vision weakens to an extent that patients can no longer distinguish different shades of color.
- *Cortical cataracts.* A cataract shows up in the periphery of the lens. The color of the lens in the periphery turns cloudy, and white, wedge-like opacities gradually migrate to the center of the lens. At this stage, patients generally avoid glaring lights.
- *Posterior subcapsular cataracts.* A cataract appears in the posterior region of the lens. The color of the lens in the posterior region turns cloudy. Patients have blurred vision that interferes with reading and driving.
- *Congenital cataracts.* A cataract develops when the fetus is still in the mother's womb. Infants whose mothers were infected with German measles during pregnancy could be afflicted with congenital cataracts in childhood.

What Are the Symptoms of Cataracts?

- Blurred or dim vision
- Night blindness, with vision worsening to the point that glares appear on objects at night or under dim light
- Color of the eyes turns yellow
- Double images appear in one eye (diplopia)
- Objects seem to change color, taking on dark hues

What Are the Risk Factors for Cataract?

- *Age.* Aging accelerates free radical–induced oxidative damage to the lenses and alters the structure of alpha crystalline proteins, leading to opacity of the lenses and cataracts. This is the main reason cataracts tend to occur in old age.
- *Diabetes.* High blood glucose stimulates the activity of aldose reductase, an enzyme that converts glucose to sorbitol, resulting in an increased sorbitol concentration in the eyes. The

accumulation of sorbitol increases intraocular pressure and induces damage to alpha crystalline proteins in the lenses, causing cataracts.

- *Obesity.* Fat tissues release leptin, a protein that informs the brain that the body has stored enough energy and can stop eating. Leptin resistance is common in obese individuals whose brains ignore the messages sent by leptin, bringing about the feeling of being hungry all the time, even right after having a meal. Leptin resistance triggers fat tissues to produce more leptin in obese people. The high amount of leptin enters the bloodstream and travels to the eyes, where leptin induces damage to alpha crystalline proteins in the lenses and causes cataracts.

- *Alcohol.* Moderate alcohol consumption may not hurt the eyes. However, heavy alcohol consumption can disrupt calcium homeostasis in the lenses. High concentrations of calcium in the lenses increase the risk of cataracts. In addition, excessive alcohol can also denature and alter the shapes of alpha crystalline proteins and lead to cataracts.

- *Smoking.* Cigarette smoke contains harmful chemicals that enter the bloodstream and travel to the eyes. These toxic chemicals induce a surge of free radical production, including superoxide anion radical and hydroxyl radical, and cause oxidative damage to alpha crystalline proteins in the lenses. Toxic chemicals from cigarette smoke can also deplete the zinc contents of the lenses. Zinc-dependent enzymes exhibit strong antioxidant properties. Insufficient zinc weakens the antioxidant capacity of the lenses, increasing the risk of cataracts.

- *Sun exposure.* People who do not wear sunglasses outdoors have a higher risk of cataracts. Ultraviolet rays from sun exposure induce a surge of free radical production in the lenses, which can cause oxidative damage to alpha crystalline proteins in them and lead to cataracts.

What Is the Association between Vitamin A and Cataracts?

- Vitamin A exerts antioxidant functions by protecting the cornea and maintaining normal vision. A low blood level of vitamin A is common among patients with cataracts compared to healthy individuals. Vitamin A deficiency could lead to cataracts and even blindness.
- Sufficient dietary intake of vitamin A curtailed the risk of cataracts. Supplementation with vitamin A prevented cataracts in older individuals.

What Is the Association between Vitamin C and Cataracts?

- Vitamin C, a strong antioxidant, can quench free radicals and reduce oxidative damage to alpha crystalline proteins in the lenses.
- A low blood level of vitamin C is common in patients with cataracts. Sufficient dietary intake of vitamin C reduced the risk of cataracts by 64%.

What Is the Association between Vitamin E and Cataracts?

- Lipid-soluble vitamin E stored in the lenses can neutralize free radicals produced by sun exposure and prevent oxidative damage to alpha crystalline proteins.
- Vitamin E can activate vitamin C and glutathione and increase antioxidant capacity in the eyes.
- Sufficient dietary intake of vitamin E reduced the risk of cataracts. Supplementation with vitamin E was found to prevent cataracts in older people.

Meta-analysis

- *Vitamin A.* A meta-analysis of 22 research papers studied the relationship between vitamin A and cataracts. Analysis revealed that sufficient dietary intake of vitamin A and beta-carotene significantly decreased the risk of cataracts.
- *Vitamin C.* Twenty research papers explored the relationship between vitamin C and cataracts. Sufficient dietary intake of

vitamin C curtailed the risk of cataracts. A high blood level of vitamin C meant a decreased risk of cataracts, as confirmed in this meta-analysis.

- *Vitamin E.* A meta-analysis of eight research papers investigated the relationship between vitamin E and cataracts in 15,021 people, including 2,258 cataract patients. Analysis confirmed that sufficient dietary intake of vitamin E reduced the risk of cataracts. Increasing daily intake of vitamin E by 7 IU was found to significantly curtail the risk of cataracts.

Recommendation

- *Prevention.* For people at risk of cataracts, take daily 2,000 IU vitamin A (1), 200 mg vitamin C (10), and 30 IU vitamin E (12).
- *Treatment.* For cataract patients, take daily 5,000 IU vitamin A (1), 500 mg vitamin C (10), and 100 IU vitamin E (12).

50

CERVICAL CANCER

Cervical cancer is a disease in which malignant cells form in the cervix. The cervix, located between the uterus and vagina, is the entrance to the uterus. Cervical cancer usually starts with the transformation of epithelial cells to malignant cells in the cervix. It is estimated that 12,990 women will be diagnosed with cervical cancer; among them, 4,120 women will die from cervical cancer in the US this year. For the past 30 years, the incidence rate of cervical cancer has reduced by 50%, mostly due to early detection of the cancer by Pap smears. The success rate of treatment is rather high for patients with early stages of cervical cancer.

What Are the Symptoms of Cervical Cancer?
- *Vaginal bleeding.* Bleeding between periods, during sexual intercourse, or after menopause
- *Abnormal vaginal secretions.* Secretion of smelly light-red fluid from the vagina
- *Pelvic pain.* Pelvic pain during sexual intercourse

What Are the Risk Factors for Cervical Cancer?

- *Herpes simplex virus.* About 50% of women with invasive cervical cancer are infected by herpes simplex virus-2, a virus that specifically infects the reproductive organs of both sexes. Herpes simplex virus-2 infection alone cannot cause cervical cancer. However, a herpes simplex virus infection together with a human papillomavirus (HPV) infection increases the risk of cervical cancer.

- *Human papillomavirus (HPV).* Analyses of viral genomes have identified more than 200 different types of HPV. About 30 of these types can infect reproductive organs such as the cervix, vagina, outer labia, and penis, as well as the anus, but only four of these types of HPV—namely, types 16, 18, 31, and 45—are associated with invasive cervical cancer. HPV type 16 is responsible for about 50% of all invasive cervical cancers in the US and Europe. Another 25–30% of invasive cervical cancers are caused by types 18, 31, and 45. Overall, HPV infections are involved in 99.7% cases of cervical squamous cell carcinoma worldwide.

- *Smoking.* Women who smoke cigarettes have an increased risk of HPV infection and cervical cancer. Cigarette smoke contains nicotine and benzopyrene, carcinogens that can trigger the insertion of HPV genes into the chromosomes of cervical cells and lead to the transformation of cervical cells to malignant cells. Other toxic chemicals from cigarette smoke can also stimulate cell proliferation, inhibit apoptosis, and enhance new blood vessel formation in malignant lesions. HPV infection may increase the risk of noninvasive cervical cancer converting to invasive cervical cancer in women smokers.

What Is the Association between Vitamin A and Cervical Cancer?

- Vitamin A regulates normal cell growth and differentiation and inhibits the metastasis of cancerous cells in the cervix. Vitamin A deficiency increases the risk of cervical cancer.

- A low blood level of vitamin A is common in patients with cervical cancer compared to healthy women. Sufficient dietary intake of vitamin A reduces the risk of cervical cancer.

What Is the Association between Vitamin B12 and Cervical Cancer?

- Vitamin B12 supports the methylation and synthesis of DNA. Vitamin B12 deficiency leads to insufficient methylation of DNA, a characteristic of malignant cells in cervical cancer.
- A low blood level of vitamin B12 is common among patients with cervical cancer compared to healthy women. Sufficient dietary intake of vitamin B12 reduces the risk of cervical cancer.

What Is the Association between Vitamin C and Cervical Cancer?

- Water-soluble vitamin C can quench free radicals in both the cytoplasm and nucleus and prevent free radical–induced oxidative damage to mitochondria and DNA, thus reducing the risk of tumor transformation.
- High-dose IV vitamin C therapy is a safe and effective treatment for certain types of advanced cancers. (See chapter 47, "Breast Cancer," for details.)

What Is the Association between Vitamin E and Cervical Cancer?

- Lipid-soluble vitamin E can scavenge free radicals in the cell membrane and maintain the structural integrity of the cell and its organelles, such as the nucleus and mitochondria. Oxidative damage to cell membranes leads to the destruction of cellular integrity and increases the risk of tumorigenesis.
- Women with cervical cancer have low blood levels of vitamin E compared to healthy women. Sufficient dietary intake of vitamin E curtailed the risk of cervical cancer.

Meta-analysis
- *Vitamin A.* A meta-analysis of 11 research articles evaluated the relationship between vitamin A and cervical cancer. Analysis confirmed that higher blood levels of vitamin A decreased the risk of cervical cancer.
- *Vitamin B12, vitamin C, and vitamin E.* Twenty-two research papers conducted with 10,073 people investigated the relationship between vitamin B12/antioxidant vitamins and cervical cancer. The result has shown that sufficient dietary intake of these vitamins reduced the risk of cervical cancer. Vitamin B12, vitamin E, and vitamin C reduced the risk of cervical cancer by 65%, 44%, and 33%, respectively.

Recommendation
- *Prevention.* For women at risk of cervical cancer, take daily 2,000 IU vitamin A (1), 100 mcg vitamin B12 (9), and 200 mg vitamin C (10).
- *Treatment.* For cervical cancer patients, take daily 5,000 IU vitamin A (1), 400 mcg vitamin B12 (9), and 500 mg vitamin C (10).

51

CERVICAL INTRAEPITHELIAL NEOPLASIA

Cervical intraepithelial neoplasia, also known as cervical dysplasia, is characterized by the uncontrollable growth of squamous cells on the surface of the cervix. Cervical intraepithelial neoplasia is not a cancer but a potentially premalignant transformation, often eliminated by the immune system. The majority of cases of cervical intraepithelial neoplasia spontaneously regress, and only about 10% might progress to cervical cancer. Cervical intraepithelial neoplasia is caused by a human papillomavirus (HPV) infection through sexual intercourse. Cervical intraepithelial neoplasia is symptomless and detected primarily during Pap smear examinations. In the US, each year about 50,000 women are afflicted with cervical intraepithelial neoplasia, predominantly at ages 25–35.

What Are the Risk Factors for Cervical Intraepithelial Neoplasia?

- *Human papillomavirus (HPV).* Human papillomavirus infections are the major cause of cervical intraepithelial neoplasia. The majority of HPV infections are cured spontaneously, without the need for any medical intervention. However, some infections lead to cervical intraepithelial neoplasia and progress to cervical cancer. There are more than 200 different types of HPV. Types 16 and 18 are responsible for more than 90% of all cases of cervical intraepithelial neoplasia. The two genes in HPV, E6 and E7, enable the virus to invade the human uterus. The E6 gene disarms the antitumor function of the host, while the E7 gene transforms epithelial cells to premalignant cells in the cervix.
- *HIV.* HIV infections increase the risk of cervical intraepithelial neoplasia. Lack of CD4 T cells and a high blood level of HIV-RNA are common in HIV patients, and both of these are known risk factors for cervical intraepithelial neoplasia. HIV patients are also more susceptible to HPV infections.
- *Environmental factors.* Cigarette smoking, sexually transmitted infections, and use of oral contraceptives are risk factors for cervical intraepithelial neoplasia. The mechanisms by which these factors induce tumor transformation in cervical intraepithelial neoplasia are similar to the mechanisms by which these factors induce cervical cancer.

What Is the Association between Vitamin C and Cervical Intraepithelial Neoplasia?

- Free radical–induced oxidative damage to the cervical tissue is a known causative factor for cervical intraepithelial neoplasia. Vitamin C can neutralize free radicals and prevent oxidative damage to the cervical tissue and tumor transformation.
- A low blood level of vitamin C is common in patients with cervical intraepithelial neoplasia compared to healthy women. Sufficient dietary intake of vitamin C reduces the risk of cervical intraepithelial neoplasia.

Meta-analysis

- *Vitamin C.* A meta-analysis of 12 research papers studied the relationship between vitamin C and cervical intraepithelial neoplasia. Analysis confirmed that sufficient dietary intake of vitamin C reduced the risk of cervical intraepithelial neoplasia. Increasing daily dietary intake of vitamin C by 50 mg was found to significantly reduce the risk of cervical intraepithelial neoplasia.

Recommendation

- *Prevention.* For women at risk of cervical intraepithelial neoplasia, take daily 200 mg vitamin C (10).
- *Treatment.* For cervical intraepithelial neoplasia patients, take daily 500 mg vitamin C (10).

52

CHRONIC KIDNEY DISEASE

Chronic kidney disease is caused by progressive deterioration and loss of kidney function. The deterioration of kidney function decreases the glomerular filtration rate and hinders waste excretion from the kidneys. Accumulation of waste in the bloodstream can lead to hypertension, anemia, diabetes, and bone loss. Hypertension and diabetes are two major causative factors of chronic kidney disease. If untreated, chronic kidney disease leads to kidney failure. Kidney failure patients require long-term hemodialysis or kidney transplants. In the US, 26 million people are afflicted with chronic kidney disease.

The American Kidney Foundation recommends that chronic kidney disease be divided into five stages, based primarily on glomerular filtration rate. The normal glomerular filtration rate is 90 (though having a glomerular filtration rate of 90 does not necessarily mean you have normal kidney function). These five different stages of chronic kidney disease are as follows:

- *Stage 1.* Kidney is damaged, but glomerular filtration rate is still 90 or higher.
- *Stage 2.* Glomerular filtration rate is 60–89. Injured kidney affects renal functions.
- *Stage 3.* Glomerular filtration rate is 30–59. Symptoms appear, including anemia and bone problems.
- *Stage 4.* Glomerular filtration rate drops to 15–29. Patient requires hemodialysis.
- *Stage 5.* Glomerular filtration rate is below 15. Kidney failure patient requires long-term hemodialysis or kidney transplant.

What Are the Symptoms of Chronic Kidney Disease?
- Frequent urination at night but producing little urine each time; foamy, dark, or bloody urine
- Edema in face, hands, legs, or ankles
- Fatigue and frailty due to anemia (injured kidney cannot support the production of new red blood cells, causing anemia)
- Skin itching, nausea, and vomiting (induced by waste buildup in the bloodstream)
- Shortness of breath (caused by pulmonary edema and anemia)
- Body chills even on hot summer days (body unable to adapt to ambient temperature due to anemia)

What Are the Risk Factors for Chronic Kidney Disease?
- *Diabetes.* High blood glucose causes damage to kidney cells, resulting in metabolic disorders and mitochondrial malfunction. Mitochondrial malfunction results in the loss of energy production and deterioration of renal functions, leading to chronic kidney disease. Diabetes-related chronic kidney disease is the major cause of kidney failure.

- *Hypertension.* Hypertension causes damage to the arterial vessels and further aggravates the symptoms of chronic kidney disease.
- *Smoking.* Cigarette smoke contains harmful chemicals that enter the bloodstream and travel to the kidneys. These toxic chemicals cause oxidative damage to the kidneys and induce insulin resistance in renal cells, thus increasing the risk of chronic kidney disease.
- *Obesity.* Obesity fattens glomerular cells and reduces the glomerular filtration rate. A decrease in glomerular filtration rate is a sign of chronic kidney disease.
- *High triglycerides.* High blood levels of triglycerides are associated with atherosclerosis, which is a contributing factor to chronic kidney disease. In addition, a low glomerular filtration rate in chronic kidney disease further elevates blood levels of triglycerides.
- *Age.* Aging accelerates renal fibrosis, glomerulosclerosis, tubular atrophy, atherosclerosis, and renal dysfunction, thus increasing the risk of chronic kidney disease.

What Is the Association between Vitamin B9 and Chronic Kidney Disease?

- A high blood level of homocysteine means an increased risk of cardiovascular disease in patients with chronic kidney disease. Vitamin B9 lowers blood levels of homocysteine.
- Blood levels of homocysteine are high in patients with chronic kidney disease compared to healthy individuals. Supplementation with vitamin B9 was found to reduce the blood level of homocysteine and alleviate the symptoms of chronic kidney disease.

What Is the Association between Vitamin D and Chronic Kidney Disease?

- Vitamin D deficiency is common in patients with chronic kidney disease. The kidney is the organ where the active form of vitamin D is produced in the body. Chronic kidney disease decreases the production of the active form of vitamin D and causes vitamin D deficiency. Supplementation with vitamin D enhances the production of the active form of vitamin D and increases the survival rate of patients with chronic kidney disease.

- Vitamin D regulates the renin-angiotensin system, controls blood pressure, and alleviates the symptoms of chronic kidney disease. Vitamin D deficiency exacerbates the symptoms of chronic kidney disease.

Meta-analysis

- *Vitamin B9.* A meta-analysis of seven randomized controlled trials evaluated the relationship between vitamin B9 and chronic kidney disease in 3,886 chronic kidney disease patients. The data have shown that sufficient dietary intake of vitamin B9 resulted in a 15% reduction in the risk of cardiovascular disease in patients with chronic kidney disease.
- *Vitamin D.* Twenty research papers studied vitamin D supplementation and chronic kidney disease. The meta-analysis confirmed that supplementation with vitamin D reduced the incidence rate of death from cardiovascular disease and all-cause mortality in patients with chronic kidney disease.

Recommendation

- *Prevention.* For people at risk of chronic kidney disease, take daily 800 IU vitamin D3 (11) and 400 mcg vitamin B9 (8).
- *Treatment.* For chronic kidney disease patients, take daily 2,000 IU vitamin D3 (11) and 800 mcg vitamin B9 (8).

53

CHRONIC OBSTRUCTIVE PULMONARY DISEASE

Chronic obstructive pulmonary disease, characterized by progressive deterioration of lung function and difficulty breathing, is a type of chronic pulmonary disease. Pathological changes in and hardening of the trachea, bronchi, and alveoli result in a loss of lung function. In severe cases, patients are barely able to walk and have difficulty climbing stairs. In the US, about 6.8% of people are afflicted with chronic obstructive pulmonary disease, of which half do not even know that they have the disease. About 700,000 chronic obstructive pulmonary disease patients are hospitalized and in need of inpatient care each year. Chronic obstructive pulmonary disease can be divided into chronic bronchitis and emphysema. Most chronic obstructive pulmonary disease patients have the symptoms of both chronic bronchitis and emphysema.

What Are the Symptoms of Chronic Obstructive Pulmonary Disease?

- Cough with white, yellow, or green phlegm
- Shortness of breath, where even mild physical activity leads to breathing difficulties
- Fatigue and weight loss
- Frequent respiratory infections
- Tight chest
- Edema in legs, ankles, and feet

What Are the Risk Factors for Chronic Obstructive Pulmonary Disease?

- *Smoking.* Harmful chemicals from cigarette smoke enter the bloodstream and travel to the lungs, where they cause a wide array of damage to the structure and function of the lungs, including (1) inducing alveoli to produce protease, an enzyme that degrades proteins in alveoli and destroys the structure of lung tissue, causing emphysema; (2) activating fibrogenic growth factors in the bronchi (fibrogenic growth factors alter the structure of the bronchi, narrowing the bronchi in smokers); (3) reducing nitric oxide production (lack of nitric oxide induces pulmonary hypertension); and (4) forming metaplasia in goblet cells, manifested by excessive secretion of mucus from lung tissue. Emphysema, narrowing of the bronchi, pulmonary hypertension, and excessive secretion of mucus induced by harmful chemicals in cigarette smoke lead to chronic obstructive pulmonary disease. Elderly people who smoked previously or are still smoking have a great risk of chronic obstructive pulmonary disease.
- *Indoor air pollution.* Biomass fuels, such as coal and natural gas for heating and cooking purposes at home, increase indoor air pollution and the risk of chronic obstructive pulmonary disease if the conditions persist 25 years or longer.
- *Outdoor air pollution.* Air pollution causes respiratory diseases and conditions, such as pneumonia, asthma, pulmonary

embolism, and chronic obstructive pulmonary disease. Air pollution also increases the incidence of and mortality from respiratory diseases. Particulate matter in the air, such as PM10, enter the respiratory tract and travel to the lungs, where macrophages engulf the PM10 particles. A macrophage dies when more than 60% of its cell volume is occupied by PM10 particles and the like. The death of macrophages releases a tidal surge of free radicals, protease, and inflammatory cytokines, causing acute and chronic pulmonary inflammation.

- *Workplace pollution.* Toxic organic and inorganic chemicals can be found in workplaces such as machinery plants, fertilizer factories, chlorinated dye factories, explosives manufacturing plants, rubber factories, plastic factories, refrigeration plants, oil refineries, agriculture farms, textile factories, leather factories, food processing plants, and beauty salons. Chronic exposure to toxic organic and inorganic chemicals increases the risk of chronic obstructive pulmonary disease.

- *Forced vital capacity (FVC).* Forced vital capacity is a measurement used clinically in the diagnosis of obstructive and restrictive lung function. A lower FVC value means an increased risk of chronic obstructive pulmonary disease. A number of factors cause low FVC values, including abnormal lung development and frequent lower respiratory tract infections during childhood, tuberculosis infection, and malnutrition.

- *Family and genetics.* Heavy smokers have a high incidence rate of chronic obstructive pulmonary disease. The question is why some smokers suffer from chronic obstructive pulmonary disease while other smokers do not. The answer is in genetics. As mentioned above, toxic chemicals from cigarette smoke can induce pulmonary inflammation and release protease, an enzyme that degrades proteins and destroys lung tissues. Alveoli contain the SERPINA1 gene that encodes serine protease inhibitors, proteins that block protease activity. Smokers with normal SERPINA1 genes are less likely to suffer from chronic obstructive pulmonary disease. On the other hand, smokers with mutated SERPINA1 genes are more likely to suffer from chronic obstructive pulmonary disease.

- *Age.* Aging diminishes pulmonary function and induces chronic pulmonary inflammation, both of which are risk factors for emphysema. Aging also accelerates the deterioration of the cardiovascular and musculoskeletal systems, which further weakens pulmonary function and increases the risk of chronic obstructive pulmonary disease.

What Is the Association between Vitamin D and Chronic Obstructive Pulmonary Disease?

- Blood levels of vitamin D affect forced vital capacity (FVC) and lung function. High blood levels of vitamin D are correlated with higher FVC values and normal lung function.
- Vitamin D deficiency is common in patients with chronic obstructive pulmonary disease. Lower blood levels of vitamin D exacerbate the symptoms of chronic obstructive pulmonary disease.

How Does Vitamin D Affect Chronic Obstructive Pulmonary Disease?

- Vitamin D strengthens immune defenses and reduces viral and bacterial infections. Infections aggravate the symptoms of chronic obstructive pulmonary disease.
- Vitamin D deficiency causes chronic bronchitis and increases the risk of chronic obstructive pulmonary disease.
- Vitamin D strengthens the muscles in the bronchi. Vitamin D deficiency weakens the muscles in the bronchi, resulting in the narrowing of the bronchi.

Meta-analysis

- *Vitamin D.* A meta-analysis of 18 research papers investigated vitamin D and chronic obstructive pulmonary disease. Analysis confirmed that vitamin D deficiency aggravated the symptoms of chronic obstructive pulmonary disease. Sufficient dietary intake and/or supplementation with vitamin D to maintain blood levels of vitamin D at 30–40 ng/ml was found to significantly alleviate the symptoms of chronic obstructive pulmonary disease.

Recommendation
- *Prevention.* For people at risk of chronic obstructive pulmonary disease, take daily 800 IU vitamin D3 (11).
- *Treatment.* For chronic obstructive pulmonary disease patients, take daily 2,000 IU vitamin D3 (11).

54

CHRONIC PANCREATITIS

Chronic pancreatitis, characterized by irreversible morphologic changes to pancreatic tissues and impairment of food digestion, is a type of pancreatic inflammatory disease. Structural damage to the pancreas caused by chronic inflammation affects the secretion of pancreatic digestive enzymes that support food digestion in the small intestines. Digestive disorders and malnutrition are common in patients with chronic pancreatitis. In the US, 200,000 people are afflicted with chronic pancreatitis. The average incidence age is 30 to 40 years old. Men have a higher incidence rate compared to women.

What Are the Symptoms of Chronic Pancreatitis?
- Upper abdominal pain that spreads to the back
- Sudden abdominal pain brought on by a high-protein or high-fat diet

- Lack of appetite
- Nausea and vomiting
- Weight loss
- Diarrhea
- Oily, clay-colored feces

What Are the Risk Factors for Chronic Pancreatitis?

- *Alcohol.* Alcohol enters the bloodstream and travels to the pancreas, causing a hypoxic condition under which mitochondria in the pancreatic tissue can no longer produce energy. Low energy production limits the ability of pancreatic cells to perform normal physiological functions, such as the secretion of insulin. Aldehyde, a toxic byproduct of alcohol metabolism, induces a surge of free radical production, leading to oxidative damage and inflammation. Heavy alcohol consumption is a major causative factor for chronic pancreatitis.
- *Smoking.* Nicotine in cigarette smoke can stimulate the release of calcium from pancreatic tissue. Excessive intracellular calcium causes injuries to insulin-producing pancreatic cells. Furthermore, cigarette smoking can exacerbate alcohol-induced chronic pancreatitis.
- *Pancreatic duct obstruction.* Alcohol consumption also promotes the formation of stones in the digestive juices secreted by the pancreas. These stones rubbing against the surface of the pancreatic duct lead to inflammation, ulcers, and pancreatic duct obstruction. Pancreatic duct obstruction is a risk factor for chronic pancreatitis.
- *Family and genetics.* Hereditary pancreatitis is a genetically related pancreatic disease. Hereditary pancreatitis, although rare, can evolve into chronic pancreatitis and even pancreatic cancer.

What Is the Association between Antioxidant and Chronic Pancreatitis?

- Consumption of a diet high in protein or fat can lead to sudden abdominal pain in patients with chronic pancreatitis. Antioxidant supplements consisting of selenium, vitamin A, vitamin C, and vitamin E can alleviate the symptoms of chronic pancreatitis.
- Free radical–induced oxidative damage is a major causative factor for chronic pancreatitis. Alcohol consumption, cigarette smoking, and toxic petrochemicals can generate free radicals and initiate oxidative damage to pancreatic cells. Antioxidants—such as vitamin A, vitamin C, and vitamin E—neutralize free radicals, prevent oxidative damage, and alleviate abdominal pain in patients with chronic pancreatitis.

Meta-analysis

- *Antioxidants.* A meta-analysis of nine randomized controlled trials investigated the relationship between antioxidants and abdominal pain in 390 chronic pancreatitis patients. Analysis confirmed that supplementation with antioxidants significantly reduced abdominal pain in patients with chronic pancreatitis. Only a combination of antioxidants—which included selenium, vitamin A, vitamin C, and vitamin E—was found to be effective in alleviating abdominal pain in patients with chronic pancreatitis. Supplementing with only selenium, vitamin A, vitamin C, or vitamin E alone, however, was ineffective.

Recommendation

- *Prevention.* For people at risk of chronic pancreatitis, take daily 50 mcg selenium (26), 2,000 IU vitamin A (1), 200 mg vitamin C (10), and 30 IU vitamin E (12).
- *Treatment.* For chronic pancreatitis patients, take daily 100 mcg selenium (26), 5,000 IU vitamin A (1), 500 mg vitamin C (10), and 100 IU vitamin E (12).

55

COGNITIVE IMPAIRMENT

Cognitive functions—such as memory, attention, consciousness, and problem-solving abilities—are necessary for daily activities. Aging may lead to a decline in cognitive functions. Pathological changes in the brain cause the progression from cognitive decline to cognitive impairment. Dementia is a severe form of cognitive impairment, and it can lead to Alzheimer's disease. Although cognitively impaired patients experience the deterioration of memory, language, thought processes, and judgment, they are still able to perform daily life activities. In the US, 16 million people suffer from cognitive impairment.

What Are the Symptoms of Cognitive Impairment?
- Individuals with cognitive impairment tend to forget appointments with physicians or friends.

- Conversations with cognitively impaired persons are often interrupted because they tend to forget words and lose their train of thought.
- For cognitively impaired individuals, places previously visited may seem unfamiliar and strange.
- Persons with cognitive impairment are unable to manage their own expenses, receipts, or bank accounts.

What Are the Risk Factors for the Progression of Cognitive Impairment to Dementia and Alzheimer's Disease?

- *Family and genetics.* Genes are associated with pathological changes in cognitive impairment, dementia, and Alzheimer's disease. A multitude of gene polymorphic variants are linked to cognitive impairment, dementia, and Alzheimer's disease. Among them, ApoE and BDNF gene polymorphic variants are known to cause Alzheimer's disease.
- *Hippocampal atrophy.* The hippocampus is an area where short-term memory, long-term memory, and spatial orientation are stored in the brain. Hippocampal atrophy leads to permanent memory loss. Cognitively impaired patients with hippocampal atrophy are likely to suffer from dementia and Alzheimer's disease.
- *Age.* Forgetfulness, attention deficit, and loss of problem-solving skills are age-associated symptoms of cognitive impairment. If untreated, cognitive impairment may progress to dementia and Alzheimer's disease. Aging exerts an uneven effect on the brain—that is, some areas of the brain are severely affected, while other areas are less affected. For instance, the hippocampus, where the memory is stored, can be severely affected by aging, increasing the risk of dementia and Alzheimer's disease.
- *Depression.* Depression is common in elderly people. Symptoms of depression often start from age 60 to 65. Depression increases the risk of cognitive impairment and Alzheimer's disease. Depressed people have higher blood levels of glucocorticoid, an early sign of hippocampal atrophy.

- *Diabetes.* Type 2 diabetes is associated with cardiovascular disease. Cardiovascular disease symptoms, including ministroke, regional cerebral ischemia, and infarction, are risk factors for cognitive impairment.
- *White matter disease.* White matter disease, characterized by pathological changes in the capillaries in the white matter of the brain, is common in type 2 diabetes patients with cognitive impairment. White matter disease causes amyloid deposition in the brain, a prelude to Alzheimer's disease.
- *Hypertension.* High diastolic pressure at age 40–50 is associated with an increased risk of cognitive impairment at age 70. Elderly people whose blood pressure remains high during sleep have an elevated risk of cognitive impairment. Patients with diabetes with high diastolic pressure are particularly at risk of cognitive impairment. Hypertension can also lead to vascular dementia and lead to Alzheimer's disease.

What Is the Association between Vitamin D and Cognitive Impairment?

- Studies have shown that elderly people with blood levels of vitamin D at 12 ng/ml or lower performed twice as poorly in cognitive tests as elderly people with blood levels of vitamin D at 26 ng/ml or higher. Poor performances in cognitive and physical strength tests are signs of cognitive impairment. People with blood levels of vitamin D at 40 ng/ml or higher have a low risk of cognitive impairment.
- Vitamin D is considered a neurosteroid. It has anti-inflammatory properties. Vitamin D deficiency causes inflammation and morphologic changes in the structure of the brain, increasing the risk of cognitive impairment.

What Is the Association between Omega-3 Fatty Acids and Cognitive Impairment?

- Sufficient dietary intake of omega-3 fatty acids decreases the risk of cognitive impairment in elderly people. Supplementation with omega-3 fatty acids improves memory and alleviates the symptoms of cognitive impairment.

- Omega-3 fatty acids have anti-inflammatory and antioxidant functions. Omega-3 fatty acids regulate the membrane fluidity in the cell membrane of the neurons and control the traffic of substances being transported in and out of the neurons.

Meta-analysis

- *Vitamin D.* A meta-analysis of seven research papers investigated vitamin D and cognitive impairment in 7,688 people. Analysis confirmed that those with low blood levels of vitamin D had an increased risk of cognitive impairment.
- *Omega-3 fatty acids.* Six randomized controlled trials investigated the relationship between omega-3 fatty acids and cognitive impairment in elderly people. The daily doses of omega-3 fatty acids were 400–1,800 mg for 40 months. The meta-analysis confirmed that supplementation with omega-3 fatty acids lowered the incidence rate of cognitive impairment in elderly individuals compared to the placebo control.
- *Omega-3 fatty acids.* A meta-analysis of 15 research papers studied the relationship between omega-3 fatty acids and memory decline. The doses of omega-3 fatty acid supplements were 1–2 g daily for four to six months, and the participants were all 18 years old or older. Analysis confirmed that supplementation with omega-3 fatty acids significantly improved memory and prevented memory decline.

Recommendation

- *Prevention.* For people at risk of cognitive impairment, take daily 800 IU vitamin D3 (11) and 1 g omega-3 fatty acids (27).
- *Treatment.* For cognitively impaired patients, take daily 2,000 IU vitamin D3 (11) and 2 g omega-3 fatty acids (27).

56

COLORECTAL CANCER

Colorectal cancer is a cancer that originates in the colon or rectum. In the early stages, abnormal cells form polyps in the outer layer of the colon or rectum. Most polyps are benign, and only a few are cancerous adenomas. Polyps can readily be surgically removed during a colonoscopy. If untreated, cancerous adenoma may lead to colorectal cancer. In the US, one in every 20 people suffers from colorectal cancers. It is estimated that this year alone, 95,270 people will be afflicted by colon cancer and 39,220 people by rectal cancer in the US.

What Are the Symptoms of Colorectal Cancer?
- Frequent bleeding when defecating
- Constipation or thin, ribbon-like stools
- Stools that are dark in color
- Abdominal pain, weakness, fatigue, and low energy
- Weight loss

What Are the Risk Factors for Colorectal Cancer?

- *Age.* About 90% of those diagnosed with colorectal cancer are over the age of 50. Each chromosome in the cell has a special methylation region. Proper methylation turns on the expression of tumor suppressor genes, which suppress the growth and proliferation of tumor cells. However, overmethylation turns off the expression of tumor suppressor genes. The absence of tumor suppressor genes leads to uncontrollable growth and proliferation of tumor cells. Aging causes overmethylation of genes in the chromosomes, which turns off the expression of tumor suppression genes, thus increasing the risk of colorectal cancer.

- *Obesity.* Obesity causes chronic systemic inflammation, which includes inflammation of the colon and rectum. Men who are obese have a 30–70% increased risk of colorectal cancer. Obesity also increases the risk of colorectal cancer in women, although the risk is not as high as in men. Fat tissue releases hormones and other chemicals that alter the anatomical structure of the colon and rectum. Obesity also stimulates the overgrowth of harmful gut flora, which stimulates polyp formation and increases the risk of colorectal cancer.

- *Family and genetics.* Any immediate family member suffering from colorectal cancer increases your risk of the disease. Familial adenomatous polyposis, a hereditary disease, is associated with adenomas in the colon and rectum.

- *Diet.* Habitual consumption of red meats—such as beef and processed meats, including sausages, hot dogs, and ham—increases the risk of colorectal cancer. Barbecuing meats at high temperatures produces nitrosamines, carcinogens that are known to cause colorectal cancer.

- *Sedentary lifestyle.* Lack of physical activity increases the risk of colorectal cancer. Exercise shortens the retention time of foods in the gastrointestinal tract, enhances immune functions, and increases insulin sensitivity, all of which may reduce polyp formation in the colon or rectum.

- *Smoking.* Cigarette smoke contains toxic chemicals that enter the bloodstream, travel to the colon or rectum, and induce epigenetic modifications. The latter affects DNA methylation and gene expression in the colon or rectum, leading to colorectal cancer.
- *Alcohol.* Alcohol stimulates the growth and proliferation of mucous cells in the colon and rectum and activates nitrosamine carcinogens. The latter can transform epithelial cells in the colon or rectum to adenomas and increase the risk of colorectal cancer.
- *Inflammatory bowel disease.* Patients with inflammatory bowel diseases, including ulcerative colitis and Crohn's disease, have an increased risk of colorectal cancer.
- *Type 2 diabetes.* Chronic insulin therapy and high HbA1c values increase the incidence rate of colorectal cancer in patients with type 2 diabetes.

What Is the Association between Vitamin B2 and Colorectal Cancer?

- Vitamin B2 converts oxidized glutathione to reduced glutathione. Glutathione is the mother of all antioxidants in the cell. Low blood levels of vitamin B2 and glutathione are common in patients with colorectal cancer.
- Vitamin B2 enhances one-carbon metabolism. Vitamin B2 deficiency may lead to disorders in one-carbon metabolism, causing insufficient methylation of DNA, which is a hallmark of cancerous cells.

What Is the Association between Vitamin B6 and Colorectal Cancer?

- Vitamin B6 has anticancer properties. It participates in the methylation and synthesis of DNA, reduces inflammatory reactions, and inhibits the growth of new blood vessels. Cancer needs new blood vessels to grow and migrate to neighboring areas.

- Insufficient blood levels of vitamin B6 are associated with systematic inflammation, which is a risk factor for colorectal cancer. Sufficient dietary intake of vitamin B6 was found to decrease the risk of colorectal cancer by 30–50%.

What Is the Association between Vitamin B9 and Colorectal Cancer?

- Vitamin B9 deficiency may increase errors in the synthesis of new DNA by, for instance, using uracil instead of thymine. New DNA containing uracil is unstable and is prone to breakage, leading to gene mutation and cancer formation.
- Sufficient dietary intake of vitamin B9 was shown to decrease the risk of colorectal cancer by 30%. This protecting effect of vitamin B9 against colorectal cancer was diminished in those who excessively consumed alcohol.

What Is the Association between Vitamin B12 and Colorectal Cancer?

- Vitamin B12 supports one-carbon metabolism, which facilitates the synthesis and methylation of DNA. Insufficient methylation is common in the genes of cancerous cells. Vitamin B12 deficiency may lead to insufficient methylation of DNA in the epithelial cells of the colon and rectum and increase the risk of colorectal cancer.

What Is the Association between Vitamin D and Colorectal Cancer?

- Vitamin D has anticancer properties. It enhances the differentiation of the epithelial cells in the colon and rectum to prevent them from transforming into cancerous cells and inhibits the formation of new blood vessels in cancerous lesions.
- Patients with colorectal cancer often have low blood levels of vitamin D compared to healthy individuals. Studies have shown that higher blood levels of vitamin D lowered the risk of colorectal cancer. In addition, maintaining high blood

levels of vitamin D reduced the risk of mortality in patients with colorectal cancer.

What Is the Association between Calcium and Colorectal Cancer?

- Sufficient dietary intake of calcium, such as from drinking milk, may prevent colorectal cancer. Calcium decreases bacterial-induced inflammation and tumorigenesis in the gastrointestinal tract, thus reducing the risk of colorectal cancer.
- Supplementation with calcium may reduce the risk as well as the recurrence of colorectal cancer.

What Is the Association between Magnesium and Colorectal Cancer?

- Sufficient dietary intake of magnesium was shown to decrease the risk of colorectal cancer by 22%.
- Magnesium has anticancer properties. It may reduce oxidative damage, increase insulin sensitivity, and prevent tumor transformation in the epithelial cells of the colon or rectum.

What Is the Association between Selenium and Colorectal Cancer?

- Selenium-dependent enzymes may induce apoptosis and autophagy in cancerous cells. Autophagy is a normal cellular phenomenon in which a cell undergoes a self-destruction process in order to ensure the survival of neighboring cells. However, cancerous cells often undergo autophagy to elude destruction by the host defense system.
- Selenium-dependent enzymes can degrade hydrogen peroxide and prevent it from damaging DNA, leading to gene mutation and tumorigenesis.

What Is the Association between Zinc and Colorectal Cancer?

- Zinc-dependent enzymes may prevent tumor transformation in the body. They inhibit oxidative damage, promote the synthesis and repair of DNA, and regulate the cell cycle to prevent tumorigenesis.

- Zinc deficiency increases the risk of colorectal cancer. Sufficient dietary intake of zinc was found to reduce the risk of colorectal cancer.

Meta-analysis
- *Vitamin B2.* A meta-analysis of eight research papers studied the relationship between vitamin B2 and colorectal cancer in 7,750 colorectal cancer patients. Sufficient dietary intake of vitamin B2 was found to significantly lower the risk of colorectal cancer.
- *Vitamin B6.* Thirteen research papers explored the relationship between vitamin B6 and colorectal cancer. The meta-analysis has shown that higher blood levels of vitamin B6 decreased the risk of colorectal cancer.
- *Vitamin B9.* A meta-analysis of 13 clinical reports conducted with 725,134 participants, including 5,720 colorectal cancer patients, investigated the relationship between vitamin B9 and colorectal cancer. Analysis confirmed that sufficient dietary intake of vitamin B9 decreased the risk of colorectal cancer. Increasing daily intake of vitamin B9 by 100 mcg was shown to significantly reduce the risk of colorectal cancer.
- *Vitamin B12.* A meta-analysis of 17 clinical studies investigated the association between vitamin B12 and colorectal cancer in 10,601 participants. The data have shown that sufficient dietary intake of vitamin B12 decreased the risk of colorectal cancer. Increasing daily intake of vitamin B12 by 4–5 mcg significantly reduced the risk of colorectal cancer.
- *Vitamin D.* Four clinical research reports explored the relationship between vitamin D and the survival of colorectal cancer patients in 2,575 cases. Maintaining blood levels of vitamin D at 40 ng/ml or higher was shown to significantly decrease mortality in patients with colorectal cancer.
- *Calcium.* A meta-analysis of eight research papers examined the relationship between calcium supplements and colorectal cancer in 11,005 people. Daily doses of calcium supplements

ranged from 333 to 2,229 mg. Analysis revealed that supplementation with calcium decreased the risk of colorectal cancer by 23%.

- *Calcium.* A meta-analysis of four randomized controlled trials conducted with 2,984 colorectal cancer patients evaluated the relationship between calcium supplements and the recurrence of colorectal cancer. Daily doses of calcium supplements ranged from 1,200 to 2,000 mg for 36–60 months. Analysis confirmed that calcium supplementation significantly reduced the recurrence of colorectal cancer.

- *Magnesium.* A meta-analysis of eight observational studies that included 338,979 participants and 8,000 colorectal cancer patients examined the association between magnesium intake and colorectal cancer. Analysis confirmed that increasing daily intake of magnesium by 50 mg decreased the risk of colon cancer by 5% and rectal cancer by 7%.

- *Magnesium.* Thirteen research papers evaluated the relationship between magnesium intake and colorectal cancer in 1,236,004 participants. Sufficient dietary intake of magnesium was shown to decrease the risk of colorectal cancer by 22%. This protecting effect of magnesium was more robust in women compared to men.

- *Selenium.* A meta-analysis of seven research papers explored the association between selenium and colorectal cancer. Analysis has shown that higher blood levels of selenium reduced the risk of colorectal cancer by 33%.

- *Zinc.* A meta-analysis of 19 research articles conducted with 400,000 people studied the relationship between zinc intake and colorectal cancer. Analysis has shown that high dietary intake of zinc decreased the risk of colorectal cancer by 18%.

Recommendation
- *Prevention.* For people at risk of colorectal cancer, take daily 2 mg vitamin B2 (3), 2 mg vitamin B6 (6), 100 mcg vitamin B12 (9), 800 IU vitamin D3 (11), 400 mcg vitamin B9 (8),

500 mg calcium (14), 100 mg magnesium (17), 50 mcg selenium (26), and 10 mg zinc (20).

- *Treatment.* For colorectal cancer patients, take daily 10 mg vitamin B2 (3), 10 mg vitamin B6 (6), 400 mcg vitamin B12 (9), 2,000 IU vitamin D3 (11), 800 mcg vitamin B9 (8), 1,000 mg calcium (14), 200 mg magnesium (17), 100 mcg selenium (26), and 20 mg zinc (20).

57

CORONARY ARTERY DISEASE

Coronary artery disease is caused by plaques in the coronary arteries, which reduce the blood flow and cause a hypoxic condition in the heart. The accumulation of plaques in the coronary arteries can also lead to atherosclerosis. Coronary artery disease increases the risk of heart failure, heart attack, and atrial fibrillation. Coronary artery disease is the leading cause of death in terms of heart-related diseases in both men and women in the US. About 15 million adult Americans suffer from coronary artery disease.

What Are the Symptoms of Coronary Artery Disease?
- *Chest pain.* Angina is the most prominent sign of coronary artery disease. Angina brings on chest pain, and it can spread from the chest to the shoulders, arms, neck, and back.

- *Difficulty breathing.* Inadequate blood flow into the lungs leads to pulmonary edema and difficulty breathing.
- *Heart attack.* In severe cases, coronary artery disease can lead to heart attack.
- *Heart failure.* Chronic ischemia in cardiac muscles can cause the enlargement of the heart and heart failure.
- *Dizziness.* Atrial fibrillation or arrhythmia can lead to dizziness.

What Are the Risk Factors for Coronary Artery Disease?

- *Smoking.* Cigarette smoke contains harmful chemicals that enter the bloodstream and travel to the heart. These toxic chemicals can induce inflammation and blood clot formation in the heart. These smoke-related chemicals can also induce the oxidation of LDL. Oxidized LDL becomes embedded in the coronary arteries, leading to plaque formation and atherosclerosis.
- *Diabetes.* High blood glucose causes systemic inflammation and endothelial dysfunction in the coronary arteries. Leucocytes and oxidized LDL build up on the injured endothelial layer of the coronary arteries and form plaques and blood clots, increasing the risk of coronary artery disease.
- *Obesity.* Fat tissues release hormones and other chemicals that can lead to insulin resistance. Obesity also raises blood levels of LDL and triglycerides. Excessive fats, such as LDL and triglycerides, in the bloodstream can lead to endothelial dysfunction and plaque formation.
- *High triglycerides.* High blood levels of triglycerides increase the risk of plaque formation and atherosclerosis. Genomic studies revealed that certain gene mutations were common in individuals with high blood levels of triglycerides and coronary artery disease, suggesting that high blood levels of triglycerides increase the risk of coronary artery disease.
- *Hypertension.* Hypertension can lead to endothelial dysfunction, plaque formation, and atherosclerosis. Hypertension also enlarges the atrium, which increases the risk of coronary artery disease.

- *Hypercholesterolemia.* High blood levels of LDL elevate the risk of coronary artery disease. Oxidized LDL can become embedded in the endothelial layer of blood vessels, leading to plaque formation. Leucocytes, fat, and cholesterol are deposited onto ruptured plaques and form blood clots, causing atherosclerosis and coronary artery disease.

What Is the Association between Vitamin B9 and Coronary Artery Disease?

- Vitamin B9 is an essential nutrient that supports the endothelial cell layer in blood vessels. In addition, vitamin B9 can reduce blood levels of homocysteine. High blood levels of homocysteine increase the risk of coronary artery disease and other cardiovascular diseases.
- Insufficient blood levels of vitamin B9 are common in patients with coronary artery disease. Sufficient dietary intake of vitamin B9 was shown to alleviate the symptoms of coronary artery disease.

What Is the Association between Omega-3 Fatty Acids and Coronary Artery Disease?

- Omega-3 fatty acids, through modification of lipid composition and contents in the bloodstream, may inhibit plaque formation in the arterial wall. Omega-3 fatty acid supplementation was found to reduce blood pressure, increase anti-inflammatory functions, and prevent atrial fibrillation in patients with coronary artery disease.
- A lower blood level of omega-3 fatty acids is common in patients with coronary artery disease. Supplementation with omega-3 fatty acids significantly improved the survival rate of patients with coronary artery disease.

Meta-analysis

- *Vitamin B9.* A meta-analysis of six randomized controlled trials studied the relationship between vitamin B9 and coronary artery disease in 377 coronary artery disease patients, including 191 patients in the vitamin B9 group and 186 patients in the placebo group. The studies were each two to three months in duration. Analysis has shown that patients in the vitamin B9 group had higher elasticity of coronary arteries and lower blood levels of homocysteine compared to the placebo group. The data revealed that intake of vitamin B9 at a dose of 5 mg daily for four weeks alleviated the symptoms of coronary artery disease.

- *Omega-3 fatty acids.* A meta-analysis of 14 randomized controlled trials explored the association between omega-3 fatty acids and coronary artery disease in 32,656 coronary artery disease patients, including 16,338 patients in the omega-3 fatty acid group and 16,318 patients in the placebo group. Analysis confirmed that patients in the omega-3 fatty acid group had a significantly increased survival rate compared to the placebo group.

Recommendation

- *Prevention.* For people at risk of coronary artery disease, take daily 400 mcg vitamin B9 (8) and 1 g omega-3 fatty acids (27).
- *Treatment.* For coronary disease patients, take daily 5 mg vitamin B9 (8) and 2 g omega-3 fatty acids (27) for one month, and after that, take daily 800 mcg vitamin B9 (8) and 2 g omega-3 fatty acids (27).

58

DEPRESSION

Depression is a common mood disorder characterized by persistent melancholy, apathy, and listlessness. The disease affects patients' daily activities, such as eating, bathing, dressing, thinking, and sleeping. In severe cases, a depressed person may have suicidal thoughts or attempt suicide. Depression can happen in any age group. It often starts at age 32 and peaks at ages 49–54. In the US, 15 million people suffer from depression, representing 6.7% of the adult population. Women have a higher incidence rate of depression compared to men.

What Are the Symptoms of Depression?
- Feeling persistently sad, anxious, and empty
- Feeling pessimistic and irritable
- Feeling guilty, helpless, and impotent
- Showing low interest in past hobbies or activities
- Feeling fatigued, weak, and tired
- Talking and walking slower than before

- Feeling impatient and restless
- Having difficulty concentrating or making decisions
- Being unable to sleep at night and feeling tired and sleepy during the day
- Experiencing overall discomfort, including headaches and abdominal pain; medications seem useless
- Having suicidal thoughts or attempting suicide

What Are the Risk Factors for Depression?

- *Family and genetics.* About 50% of depression is related to genes, and the other 50% is attributed to environmental factors. Having a parent or sibling with depression increases your risk of depression two- to threefold, but genomic research thus far has not found any "depression gene." Depression is likely caused not by a single gene mutation but by an interplay of many different genes. Inheriting a particular gene from a parent who has depression doesn't mean that one will inevitably suffer from depression. How gene mutation leads to depression is still an open question.
- *Neurotransmitters.* Neurotransmitters support communication between neurons in the brain. Three major neurotransmitters are serotonin, norepinephrine, and dopamine. Serotonin regulates a multitude of physiological functions, including sleep, anger, eating, sexual desire, and emotion. Norepinephrine helps the body to cope with stress and dangerous situations. Dopamine controls pleasure and satisfaction. Depressed people have low levels of neurotransmitters in their brains. Insufficient neurotransmitters lead to mood disorders and depression.
- *Gender.* Women are twice as likely to suffer from depression compared to men. The higher incidence rate of depression in women is linked to female hormones. Premenstrual dysphoric disorder—characterized by severe depression, irritability, and premenstrual anxiety—is a psychiatric syndrome. Postpartum depression within one year after giving birth is common

in new mothers. Hormonal fluctuation causes depression in premenopausal women. Men also suffer from depression, but they often try to hide it by drinking alcoholic beverages. Depressed men are more irritable and have low thresholds to cope with stress. More depressed women attempt suicide than men, but more depressed men die from suicide than women.

- *Age.* Although depression affects all age groups, adolescent youth are among the highest at risk. A depressed mother, disrupted family life, neglect, and mental and/or physical abuse, all cause depression in adolescent youth. Depressed adolescents are vulnerable to alcohol and drug abuse, exacerbating emotional and psychological problems. Depression is often associated with illnesses—such as Alzheimer's disease, Parkinson's disease, or cancer—in elderly people. The loss of one's life partner can also lead to depression. In the US, elderly people aged 85 and older have the highest suicide rate among all age groups.
- *Diseases.* Severe or chronic diseases can bring about a sense of despair and lead to depression. Chronic diseases—such as hypothyroidism, fibromyalgia, arthritis, stroke, heart failure, heart attack, insomnia, Alzheimer's disease, or Parkinson's disease—adversely affect the mood and increase the risk of depression. Medications also increase the risk of depression.

What Are the Complications Associated with Depression?
- Obesity
- Alcohol and substance abuse
- Anxiety, panic, and social phobia
- Family conflict, relationship stress, and problems in school and at work
- Suicidal thoughts or attempts
- Self-mutilation

What Is the Association between Vitamin B9 and Depression?

- Vitamin B9 supports one-carbon metabolism, a biochemical pathway involved in the synthesis and repair of DNA and regulation of gene expression in the neurons.
- Vitamin B9 deficiency raises the blood level of homocysteine. High blood levels of homocysteine increase the risk of depression. Depressed patients have low blood levels of vitamin B9 compared to healthy individuals.

What Is the Association between Vitamin B12 and Depression?

- Depressed patients, particularly women, have lower blood levels of vitamin B12. Supplementation with vitamin B12 may alleviate the symptoms of depression.
- Vitamin B12 protects the structural integrity of myelin shields on the outer layers of the nerve fibers and supports the production of new red blood cells. Vitamin B12 deficiency can lead to irritability, personality changes, depression, cognitive impairment, and psychosis.

What Is the Association between Vitamin D and Depression?

- Vitamin D receptors are ubiquitously present in the neurons, implying that vitamin D plays an important role in neuron-to-neuron communications in the brain.
- Vitamin D regulates the production of neurotransmitters, such as dopamine and serotonin. Vitamin D deficiency reduces dopamine and serotonin levels in the brain, leading to depression.
- According to historical records dating back 2,000 years ago, physicians knew that sun exposure could treat patients with depression. Upon sun exposure, the skin produces vitamin D. High blood levels of vitamin D decrease the risk of depression, and vitamin D deficiency is associated with depression.

What Is the Association between Omega-3 Fatty Acids and Depression?

- Depressed patients have low blood levels of omega-3 fatty acids compared to healthy individuals. Supplementation with omega-3 fatty acids mitigates the symptoms of depression, such as feeling guilty, depressed, and helpless and suffering from insomnia.
- Omega-3 fatty acids alleviate the symptoms of depression by controlling inflammatory and oxidative damage and regulating the membrane fluidity of neurons for optimal neuron-to-neuron communications.

Meta-analysis

- *Vitamin B9.* A meta-analysis of three randomized controlled trials evaluated the association between vitamin B9 and depression in 247 depressed patients. The degree and extent of depression during the 10-week studies was assessed using the Hamilton Depression Scale. The results confirmed that sufficient dietary intake of vitamin B9 significantly reduced the symptoms of depression as measured by the Hamilton Depression Scale.
- *Vitamin B12.* Twelve research papers explored the relationship between vitamin B12 and depression in 8,242 people. The meta-analysis revealed that women with low blood levels of vitamin B12 had an increased risk of depression. The correlation, however, was less robust in men.
- *Vitamin D.* A meta-analysis of 15 randomized controlled trials investigated the relationship between vitamin D and depression. The result has shown that supplementation with vitamin D at a daily dose of 800 IU significantly decreased the symptoms of depression. The efficacy of vitamin D supplementation was found to be similar to that of antidepressant drugs.
- *Omega-3 fatty acids.* Eight randomized controlled trials investigated the relationship between omega-3 fatty acids and

depression in 367 depressed women, including 182 patients in the omega-3 fatty acid group and 185 patients in the placebo group. The meta-analysis has shown that supplementation with omega-3 fatty acids significantly curtailed the symptoms of depressed women.

Recommendation
- *Prevention.* For people at risk of depression, take daily 100 mcg vitamin B12 (9), 800 IU vitamin D3 (11), 400 mcg vitamin B9 (8), and 1 g omega-3 fatty acids (27).
- *Treatment.* For depression patients, take daily 400 mcg vitamin B12 (9), 2,000 IU vitamin D3 (11), 800 mcg vitamin B9 (8), and 2 g omega-3 fatty acids (27).

59

TYPE 1 DIABETES

Type 1 diabetes is an autoimmune disease characterized by the immune system attacking the pancreas, mistaking it as foreign. The cause is still unknown. The attack by the immune system diminishes the production of insulin from insulin-producing cells in the pancreas.

Like a key, insulin opens the door and allows glucose to get into the cell. The body utilizes glucose to produce energy. Low blood levels of insulin in patients with type 1 diabetes prevent glucose from entering into the cell, leading to the accumulation of glucose in the bloodstream and lack of energy production in the body. If untreated, high blood glucose can cause damage to the eyes, kidneys, neurons, and heart and even end in death. In the US, about 1.25 million people are afflicted with type 1 diabetes.

Insulin Therapy for Type 1 Diabetes
Insulin therapy is an effective treatment for type 1 diabetes. It provides a spare key that allows glucose to get into the cell.

What Are the Symptoms of Type 1 Diabetes?
- Fatigue and weakness
- Thirst and frequent urination
- Nausea and vomiting
- Frequent abdominal pain
- Blurred vision
- Slower wound healing
- Moodiness and irritability

How Is Type 1 Diabetes Diagnosed?
- *Glycated hemoglobin (HbA1c).* Glucose reacts chemically with hemoglobin in red blood cells to form an adduct called HbA1c. The amount of HbA1c correlates with the amount of glucose in the bloodstream. The higher the blood glucose level, the higher the HbA1c level. A 5% HbA1c value means that 5 out of 100 hemoglobin molecules are glycated by glucose in the bloodstream. An HbA1c value over 6.5% is indicative of diabetes, between 5.7–6.4% is prediabetes, and below 5.7% is normal.
- *Fasting blood glucose test.* The blood glucose test is taken after fasting overnight. A blood glucose level below 100 mg/dl is normal, between 101–125 mg/dl is prediabetes, and over 126 mg/dl is diabetes.
- *Autoantibodies.* The presence of glutamic acid decarboxylase antibodies (GAD65) or islet cell antibodies (ICA) in the bloodstream is indicative of type 1 diabetes. Detection of these autoantibodies in the blood is often used to diagnose type 1 diabetes.
- *Ketone bodies.* A high blood level of ketone bodies in the bloodstream is a marker of type 1 diabetes.

How to Differentiate Type 1 Diabetes from Type 2 Diabetes
- Diabetes is often diagnosed upon confirmation from test results of one's HbA1c value and fasting blood glucose levels. Additional blood tests for GAD65 or ICA autoantibodies are

needed for differentiating type 1 diabetes from type 2 diabetes. The presence of autoantibodies in the bloodstream usually confirms the incidence of type 1 diabetes.

What Are the Risk Factors for Type 1 Diabetes?

- *Family and genetics.* Type 1 diabetes is an autoimmune disease. A multitude of gene polymorphic variants are associated with type 1 diabetes; among them are HLA-DQA1, HLA-DQB1, and HLA-DRB1 genes, which all belong to the human leukocyte antigen complex. The major functions of the human leukocyte antigen complex include enhancing immune functions, discerning self from nonself, protecting organs and tissues, and attacking foreign invaders, such as bacteria and viruses. Mutations in these genes lead to immune disorders and the inability of the immune system to discern self from nonself. In type 1 diabetes, immune cells attack insulin-producing beta cells, mistaking them as foreign, causing the death of beta cells.
- *Geography.* People who live far away from the equator have a higher incidence rate of type 1 diabetes. The risk of type 1 diabetes is higher in the winter months compared to the summer months. Northern Europeans are prone to type 1 diabetes with a high incidence rate of 60 per 100,000 people. Contrary to that, the incidence rate of type 1 diabetes is only 0.1 per 100,000 people in China, India, and Venezuela.
- *Age and gender.* Although type 1 diabetes can affect any age group, children ages 4–7 and 10–14 are most susceptible. In general, autoimmune diseases are more common in women compared to men. However, in type 1 diabetes, men have a higher incidence rate than women.
- *Other autoimmune diseases.* Patients with rheumatoid arthritis, lupus erythematosus, ankylosing spondylitis, or autoimmune thyroid disease have an increased risk of type 1 diabetes.

What Is the Association between Vitamin D and Type 1 Diabetes?
- Newborn babies with sufficient dietary intake of vitamin D, particularly during the first year, have a reduced risk of type 1 diabetes. In addition, pregnant women with adequate dietary intake of vitamin D lower the risk of type 1 diabetes in their newborn babies.
- Vitamin D regulates the production of insulin from beta cells and controls blood glucose levels. Vitamin D deficiency increases the risk of type 1 diabetes. A lower blood level of vitamin D is common in patients with type 1 diabetes.

Meta-analysis
- *Vitamin D.* A meta-analysis of 10 research papers studied the relationship between vitamin D and type 1 diabetes. The result has shown that low blood levels of vitamin D were common in children with type 1 diabetes compared to healthy children. Analysis confirmed that vitamin D deficiency was prevalent in children with type 1 diabetes.

Recommendation
- *Prevention.* For new babies at risk of type 1 diabetes, take daily 400 IU vitamin D3 (11).
- *Prevention.* For adults at risk of type 1 diabetes, take daily 800 IU vitamin D3 (11).
- *Treatment.* For type 1 diabetes patients, take daily 2,000 IU vitamin D3 (11).

60

TYPE 2 DIABETES

Type 2 diabetes, a disease that interferes with glucose metabolism, affects mostly adults. Glucose is the major fuel for energy production in the body. Inability to metabolize glucose and convert it to energy causes a multitude of pathological changes and malfunctions in organs and tissues. In recent years, more children ages 8–10 are afflicted with type 2 diabetes, which coincides with the prevalence of childhood obesity. In the US, 20 million people suffer from type 2 diabetes, and an additional 87 million people are prediabetic.

What Are the Two Kinds of Type 2 Diabetes?
- *Insulin deficiency.* Insulin is required for glucose to enter into the cell. When beta cells in the pancreas cannot produce enough insulin, that insulin deficiency causes glucose to build up in the bloodstream, resulting in high blood glucose. This condition damages the cardiovascular and nervous systems, as well as the kidneys.

- *Insulin resistance.* Obese individuals release chemicals and hormones from fat tissues into the bloodstream, causing insulin resistance—characterized by a high blood level of insulin and lack of insulin elsewhere in the body. Despite enough insulin being produced by the pancreas, insulin is unable to open the door for glucose to get into the cell, leading to high blood glucose and causing damage to organs and tissues.

What Are the Causes of Type 2 Diabetes?

- *Family and genetics.* Genetics is linked to type 2 diabetes. Unfavorable conditions in the uterus, such as high blood glucose and hypercholesterolemia during pregnancy, cause epigenetic modifications in the genomes of infants, increasing the risk of type 2 diabetes in newborns.
- *Obesity.* Fat tissues in obese people release fatty acids, glycerol, hormones, and inflammatory cytokines into the bloodstream, leading to insulin resistance, which forces the pancreas to work harder to produce more insulin. Working extra shifts over a long period of time injures insulin-producing beta cells in the pancreas, causing type 2 diabetes. In addition, accumulation of fat in the abdomen rather than in the thighs or legs increases the risk of type 2 diabetes in obese people.
- *Diet.* High sugar consumption increases the risk of type 2 diabetes. Fructose from sugar is converted to fat in the liver. Excessive fat buildup in either subcutaneous or visceral regions causes obesity, a risk factor for type 2 diabetes.
- *Little physical exercise.* Exercise increases insulin sensitivity in the muscles and decreases the risk of insulin resistance. Exercise also enhances glucose metabolism in muscle cells and lowers the blood glucose level. Lack of physical exercise increases the risk of insulin resistance and type 2 diabetes.
- *Age.* Aging adversely affects the ability of beta cells to produce insulin and hampers the growth and proliferation of insulin-producing beta cells in the pancreas.

- *Hypertension.* High blood pressure is common among patients with type 2 diabetes. About 75% of type 2 diabetes patients suffer from hypertension. Likewise, hypertensive patients have a high incidence rate of type 2 diabetes. Hypertension can lead to insulin resistance and heighten the risk of type 2 diabetes.

How Is Type 2 Diabetes Diagnosed?
- Blood tests of one's HbA1c value and fasting blood glucose levels are used clinically for the diagnosis of type 2 diabetes. (See chapter 59, "Type 1 Diabetes," for details.)

What Is the Association between Vitamin D and Type 2 Diabetes?
- Vitamin D enhances a beta cell's ability to produce insulin and increases insulin sensitivity. Vitamin D deficiency can lead to insulin resistance and type 2 diabetes. A low blood level of vitamin D is common in patients with type 2 diabetes.
- Vitamin D regulates fat synthesis in the liver and prevents fatty liver disease. Vitamin D deficiency causes the accumulation of fat in the liver, increasing the risk of insulin resistance and type 2 diabetes.
- Vitamin D supplementation reduces insulin resistance and alleviates the symptoms of type 2 diabetes.

What Is the Association between Magnesium and Type 2 Diabetes?
- Magnesium enhances insulin sensitivity and lowers the risk of type 2 diabetes. Magnesium deficiency negatively affects insulin production in the pancreas. Insufficient dietary intake of magnesium causes insulin resistance in patients with type 2 diabetes.
- Supplementation with magnesium lowers the blood level of insulin, reduces insulin resistance, and alleviates the symptoms of type 2 diabetes.

Can Vitamin D Prevent Type 2 Diabetes?

- High blood levels of vitamin D decrease the risk of type 2 diabetes.
- People with high blood levels of vitamin D in their prime years are less likely to suffer from type 2 diabetes in old age.
- Supplementation with vitamin D at a daily dose of 2,000 IU may prevent type 2 diabetes in prediabetic individuals.

What Is the Association between Zinc and Type 2 Diabetes?

- Lower blood levels of zinc may cause microvascular complications in patients with type 2 diabetes. Severe microvascular complications can lead to kidney disease.
- Supplementation with zinc may prevent metabolic syndrome, increase insulin sensitivity, lower blood glucose levels, and enhance antioxidant functions.

What Is the Association between Chromium and Type 2 Diabetes?

- Chromium is an essential nutrient that supports insulin function and regulates blood glucose levels. Chromium has antioxidant and anti-inflammatory properties. Low blood levels of chromium are common in patients with type 2 diabetes.
- Chromium activates insulin receptor proteins and increases insulin sensitivity. Supplementation with chromium decreases blood glucose levels and alleviates the symptoms of type 2 diabetes.

What Is the Association between Omega-3 Fatty Acids and Type 2 Diabetes?

- Omega-3 fatty acids increase insulin sensitivity, facilitating cellular uptake of glucose and reducing blood glucose levels. Omega-3 fatty acids also prevent platelet aggregation and enhance the endothelial function of blood vessels.
- Supplementation with omega-3 fatty acids decreases the blood levels of triglycerides and HbA1c in patients with type 2 diabetes. The American Diabetes Association recommends that

patients with type 2 diabetes consume sufficient daily amounts of omega-3 fatty acids from foods or supplements.

Meta-analysis

- *Vitamin D.* A meta-analysis of six research papers studied the relationship between vitamin D and type 2 diabetes in 1,484 patients with diabetes. Analysis confirmed that lower blood levels of vitamin D aggravated the symptoms of type 2 diabetes.
- *Magnesium.* Fifteen research papers explored the association between magnesium intake and type 2 diabetes in 539,735 participants, including 25,252 type 2 diabetes patients. The meta-analysis has shown that increasing daily intake of magnesium by 100 mg decreased the risk of type 2 diabetes by 16%.
- *Zinc.* A meta-analysis of 14 research articles conducted with 3,978 people evaluated the relationship between zinc intake and type 2 diabetes. Analysis revealed that sufficient dietary intake of zinc prevented type 2 diabetes. Supplementation with zinc was found to significantly reduce HbA1c values as well as blood glucose levels in type 1 diabetes and type 2 diabetes, as well as in obese people.
- *Chromium.* Thirteen randomized controlled trials investigated the association between chromium supplements and type 2 diabetes. The doses of chromium supplements ranged from 42 to 1,000 mcg, and the duration of the studies was 30–120 days. The meta-analysis confirmed that supplementation with chromium lowered fasting blood glucose levels in type 2 diabetes patients as well as in prediabetic individuals.
- *Omega-3 fatty acids.* A meta-analysis of 20 randomized controlled trials explored the association between omega-3 fatty acid supplements and type 2 diabetes. Analysis has shown that omega-3 fatty acid supplementation significantly reduced triglyceride levels in patients with type 2 diabetes.
- *Omega-3 fatty acids.* Twenty-four research papers investigated the relationship between omega-3 fatty acids and type 2 diabetes

in 545,275 participants, including 245,092 type 2 diabetes patients. The meta-analysis confirmed that regular consumption of fish or supplementation with omega-3 fatty acids reduced the risk of type 2 diabetes.

Recommendation

- *Prevention.* For people at risk of type 2 diabetes, take daily 800 IU vitamin D3 (11), 100 mg magnesium (17), 10 mg zinc (20), 50 mg chromium (25), and 1 g omega-3 fatty acids (27).
- *Treatment.* For type 2 diabetes patients, take daily 2,000 IU vitamin D3 (11), 200 mg magnesium (17), 20 mg zinc (20), 200 mg chromium (25), and 2 g omega-3 fatty acids (27).

61

DRY EYES

Dry eye is a common eye disease caused by insufficient tear production or tears that dry out too quickly. Tears, a watery fluid secreted by the lachrymal glands, provide moisture and lubricate the surface of the eye and eyelid. If untreated, dry eyes can lead to pain and corneal abrasions. Dry eyes cause discomfort in reading or using computers. The risk of dry eyes is higher in old age, particularly for women. About 7% of Americans are afflicted with dry eyes, while about 33% of Asians suffer from the disease.

What Are the Symptoms of Dry Eyes?

- Itching and pain in the eyes
- Stabbing pain caused by mucous fluid secreted from the eyes
- Redness and light sensitivity of the white part of the eye (the sclera)
- Constant feeling of eye irritation
- Difficulty wearing contact lenses or driving at night
- Watery eyes

What Are the Causes of Dry Eyes?

- *Computers.* If you spend a lot of time looking at computers, you may be at risk of dry eye syndrome. You should try to blink the eyes at least 10 times for every 30 minutes of computer use. Good adherence to this habit can avoid dry eye syndrome.

- *Contact lenses.* Contact lenses block the normal supply of oxygen to the cornea. You may select lenses with higher gas permeability, such as silicone hydrogel contact lenses or rigid gas-permeable contact lenses, to reduce the problem of dry eyes.

- *LASIK.* Laser-assisted in-situ keratomileusis (LASIK) eye surgery, which allows one to avoid wearing glasses, is a common cornea refractive surgery to correct vision problems. Dry eye syndrome is a common side effect of LASIK surgery, affecting about 4% of all patients, and is often caused by accidentally damaging the trigeminal nerve during the surgical procedure. The issue of dry eyes could persist for months and even years after surgery.

- *Environmental factors.* Both indoor and outdoor air pollution can cause dry eye syndrome. Globally, 3 billion households burn coal, wood, charcoal, dried plant stalks, and animal waste for indoor cooking and heating. Exhaust from automobile gasoline and diesel fuels, pollutants released from industrial factors, and particulate matter from air pollution, such as PM2.5 and PM10, are all risk factors for dry eyes.

- *Smoking.* Cigarette smoke contains harmful chemicals that enter the bloodstream and the eyes and lead to eye injuries. These toxic and irritable chemicals damage the tear film, resulting in the loss of moisture control on the surface of the eyes. These smoke-related chemicals can also irritate the conjunctival mucosa of the eye, induce swelling and inflammation, decrease tear formation, and increase the incidence of dry eyes.

What Is the Association between Omega-3 Fatty Acids and Dry Eyes?

- Omega-3 fatty acids inhibit the production of inflammatory cytokines and enhance tear production in the eyes.
- Supplementation with omega-3 fatty acids appears to be effective for treating the problem of dry eyes.

Meta-analysis

- *Omega-3 fatty acids.* A meta-analysis of five randomized controlled trials studied the relationship between omega-3 fatty acid supplements and dry eyes in 790 participants for three months. Analysis has shown that supplementation with omega-3 fatty acids reduced the symptoms of dry eyes.

Recommendation

- *Prevention.* For people at risk of dry eyes, take daily 1 g omega-3 fatty acids (27).
- *Treatment.* For dry eye patients, take daily 2 g omega-3 fatty acids (27).

62

ECZEMA

Eczema, characterized by skin inflammation, is a group of common child-hood dermatitis problems. These skin diseases cause swollen blisters and dry, itchy skin. Lesions of eczema frequently occur on the forehead, cheeks, scalp, arms, knees, and feet. Eczema is linked to family and genetics. It can be divided into two types, atopic eczema and nonatopic eczema. Atopic eczema is related to IgE immunoglobulin, and nonatopic eczema is not related to IgE immunoglobulin. In the US, 32 million people are afflicted with eczema, including 18 million with moderate and severe forms of eczema. About 10.7% of children have eczema problems in the US.

What Are the Symptoms of Eczema?
- Dry, sensitive skin
- Swollen, inflamed skin
- Unbearable skin itching
- Darkened lesions on the skin
- Peeling, coarse skin

What Risk Factors Trigger or Exacerbate Eczema?

- *Family and genetics.* Atopic eczema is linked to FLG gene mutations. FLG genes encode filament aggregate protein, an important matrix protein in keratinocytes. FLG gene mutations alter the structure of the keratinocyte layer and weaken its antibacterial function. Hence an eczema patient's skin lacks this antibacterial function and becomes more susceptible to bacterial infections, such as infections by *Staphylococcus aureus* and yeast. Bacterial infection triggers the immune response to recruit leukocytes, lymphocytes, and macrophages, all of which release inflammatory cytokines into the infected skin, causing skin inflammation and eczema.
- *Environmental factors.* Environmental factors can trigger and exacerbate eczema. These include clothes made of wool and synthetic fibers, soaps, detergents, cosmetics, perfumes, dust, chemical solvents, high or low temperatures, and high or low levels of humidity.
- *Allergies.* Patients with allergies have a higher risk of eczema. Allergens that augment the risk of eczema include pollens, animal dander, dust mites, cigarette smoke, and molds.
- *Age.* Eczema affects any age group, although infants and children are among the highest risk group. About 65% of eczema patients have suffered from eczema since age one, and about 90% of eczema patients have been afflicted with eczema since age five. Symptoms of eczema often disappear with age; however, about 50% of eczema patients suffer from eczema their entire lives.

What Is the Association between Vitamin D and Eczema?

- Low blood levels of vitamin D are common in children and adults with eczema. Vitamin D regulates immune functions. Vitamin D deficiency exacerbates bacterial infections in the skin, leading to dermatitis and eczema.
- Supplementation with vitamin D improves the symptoms of eczema.

Meta-analysis

- *Vitamin D.* A meta-analysis of nine research articles studied the association between vitamin D and eczema. Analysis has shown that supplementation with vitamin D significantly alleviated the symptoms of eczema. These data confirmed that vitamin D supplements are effective in treating patients with eczema.

Recommendation

- *Prevention.* For people at risk of eczema, take daily 800 IU vitamin D3 (11).
- *Treatment.* For eczema patients in remission, take daily 1,000 IU vitamin D3 (11).
- *Treatment.* For eczema patients, take daily 2,000 IU vitamin D3 (11).

63

ENDOMETRIAL CANCER

Endometrial cancer is also known as uterine cancer and is characterized by the transformation of endometrial cells to malignant cells in the uterus. The uterus wall consists of two different layers, the inner endometrial layer and the outer muscle layer. The function of the outer muscle layer is in part to push the fetus from the uterus to the vagina during childbirth. Uterine cancer often initiates from the endometrial layer, causing endometrial cancer. Endometrial cancer is the most common cancer in women's reproductive systems. An estimated 60,050 new cases of endometrial cancer will occur, and 10,470 women will die from it, in the US this year.

What Are the Symptoms of Endometrial Cancer?
- Vaginal bleeding between menstrual cycles
- Vaginal bleeding after menopause

- Abnormal discharge from the vagina
- Pelvic pain
- Weight loss

What Are the Risk Factors for Endometrial Cancer?

- *Family and genetics.* About 10% of endometrial cancer cases are linked to genetics, and the other 90% are not genetically related. Hereditary endometrial cancer is mainly caused by PTEN gene mutations. PTEN genes encode tyrosine kinase, a protein that supports the expression of tumor suppressor genes. Mutations in the PTEN gene reduce the expression of tumor suppressor genes and increase the risk of endometrial cancer.
- *Oral contraceptives and contraceptive devices.* Women who use oral contraceptives reduce the risk of endometrial cancer by 50%. Such protective effects can last for 10–20 years. About 70–80% of endometrial cancer cases are associated with excessive estrogens that stimulate abnormal growth and proliferation of endometrial cells. Oral contraceptives contain progestin, a hormone that counters the action of estrogens, thus reducing the risk of endometrial cancer. Contraceptive devices can also lower the risk of endometrial cancer. However, both oral contraceptives and contraceptive devices increase the risk of breast cancer.
- *Obesity.* Women who are obese have a two- to fivefold increased risk of endometrial cancer. The fat tissues of obese women release fatty acids, hormones, and other substances that can stimulate the growth and proliferation of endometrial cells. Obese women tend to have elevated levels of estrogens that can stimulate abnormal growth and proliferation of endometrial cells, increasing the risk of endometrial cancer.
- *Diabetes.* Patients with diabetes have high blood insulin levels and insulin resistance, both of which are risk factors for endometrial cancer. Women with diabetes have a fourfold increased risk of endometrial cancer compared to healthy women. Proper body weight, regular exercise, and a nutrient-balanced

diet can reduce the risk of endometrial cancer in women with type 1 or type 2 diabetes.

- *Lack of exercise.* Lack of physical exercise increases the risk of endometrial cancer. Exercise controls body weight, increases insulin sensitivity, and prevents type 2 diabetes and endometrial cancer. Women who exercise regularly and eat nutrient-balanced diets curtail the risk of endometrial cancer by 60%.
- *Breast cancer.* Tamoxifen is a therapeutic agent for treating breast cancer. Tamoxifen elevates the risk of endometrial cancer in postmenopausal women with breast cancer. The incidence rate of endometrial cancer in women with tamoxifen-treated breast cancer was 0.3% compared to only 0.1% in women with non-tamoxifen-treated breast cancer.

What Is the Association between Vitamin A and Endometrial Cancer?

- Vitamin A keeps endometrial cells in a differentiated state and prevents the tumorigenesis of endometrial cells.
- Vitamin A regulates more than 500 genes in the body. Vitamin A deficiency causes morphological changes in endometrial cells and increases the risk of endometrial cancer.

What Is the Association between Vitamin C and Endometrial Cancer?

- Hypoxia-inducible factors allow solid tumors to grow and proliferate under hypoxic conditions. Vitamin C inhibits the ability of solid tumors to produce hypoxia-inducible factors and prevents the growth and proliferation of cancerous cells under hypoxic conditions.
- The anticancer properties of vitamin C also include stimulating immune functions, inhibiting the activation of carcinogens (such as nitrosamines), and preventing oxidative damage to organs and tissues.
- A high-dose intravenous injection of vitamin C is an effective therapeutic approach for the treatment of cancers. High

concentrations of vitamin C produce hydrogen peroxide, which can kill cancerous cells in the body. (See chapter 47, "Breast Cancer," for details.)

What Is the Association between Vitamin E and Endometrial Cancer?

- Vitamin E is a lipid-soluble antioxidant that quenches free radicals in the cell membrane and prevents the oxidative destruction of the cell and its organelles, such as the nucleus and mitochondria. Lipid peroxidation causes the structural instability of the nucleus and mitochondria, increasing the risk of tumor formation.

Meta-analysis

- *Antioxidants.* A meta-analysis of 17 research articles explored the association between antioxidant vitamins and endometrial cancer. Analysis has shown that sufficient dietary intake of antioxidant vitamins—including vitamin C, beta-carotene, and vitamin E—reduced the risk of endometrial cancer by 15%, 12%, and 9%, respectively.

Recommendation

- *Prevention.* For women at risk of endometrial cancer, take daily 2,000 IU vitamin A (1), 200 mg vitamin C (10), and 30 IU vitamin E (12).
- *Treatment.* For female endometrial cancer patients, take daily 5,000 IU vitamin A (1), 500 mg vitamin C (10), and 100 IU vitamin E (12).

64

ESOPHAGEAL CANCER

Esophageal cancer occurs when malignant cells form in the tissues of the esophagus. The esophagus is a 20–30 cm long tubular structure made of muscles in between the throat and stomach. Esophageal cancer often starts from the tumorigenesis of cells in the mucous layer of the esophagus and then spreads to the outer layer. In the US, 16,000 people will be afflicted with esophageal cancer this year.

What Are the Symptoms of Esophageal Cancer?
- Difficulty swallowing
- Feeling like something is stuck in the throat
- Lack of appetite
- Malnutrition
- Weight loss
- Hoarse and husky voice
- Nausea and vomiting
- Persistent coughing

What Are the Risk Factors for Esophageal Cancer?

- *Steaming-hot food.* Very hot foods—such as rice, soup, and tea—can cause injuries to mucous cells in the esophagus. Consumption of steaming-hot foods elevates the risk of esophageal cancer.
- *Acid reflux.* Acid reflux injures mucous cells in the esophagus and causes Barrett's esophagus with precancerous mucous cells, increasing the risk of esophageal cancer. Nevertheless, most patients with Barrett's esophagus never develop esophageal cancer.
- *Smoking.* Cigarette smoke contains more than 60 known carcinogens, some of which enter the bloodstream and travel to the esophagus. These carcinogens may induce DNA mutations and transform mucous cells to cancerous cells in the esophagus.
- *Alcohol.* Alcohol from alcoholic beverages can enter the blood circulation system, travel to the esophagus, and cause damage to mucous cells. Alcohol is also degraded into aldehyde in the body. Both alcohol and aldehyde affect the methylation of DNA and increase the risk of esophageal cancer.
- *Human papillomavirus (HPV).* People infected with HPV have an increased risk of esophageal cancer.
- *Obesity.* Obese people are more likely to have acid reflux and Barrett's esophagus. In addition, fat tissues in obese people stimulate the immune cells to produce inflammatory cytokines, which can injure the mucous layer of the esophagus and increase the risk of esophageal cancer.

What Is the Association between Vitamin C and Esophageal Cancer?

- Vitamin C can inhibit the formation of nitrosamines, carcinogens that cause esophageal cancer. Vitamin C can also mitigate acid reflux and decrease the risk of esophageal cancer.
- Sufficient dietary intake of vitamin C reduces the risk of esophageal cancer.

- High-dose IV vitamin C therapy is an effective treatment for certain types of cancers. High concentrations of vitamin C produce hydrogen peroxide, which can kill cancerous cells in the body. (See chapter 47, "Breast Cancer," for details.)

What Is the Association between Vitamin B9 and Esophageal Cancer?

- Vitamin B9 supports the synthesis and methylation of DNA and maintains the structural stability of DNA. Vitamin B9 deficiency may increase errors in the synthesis of new DNA, leading to gene mutation and tumorigenesis.
- Sufficient dietary intake of vitamin B9 lowers the risk of esophageal cancer.

Meta-analysis

- *Vitamin B9.* A meta-analysis of 16 research papers studied the association between vitamin B9 and esophageal cancer. Analysis confirmed that sufficient dietary intake of vitamin B9 significantly lowered the risk of esophageal cancer.
- *Vitamin C.* Fifteen research articles investigated the relationship between vitamin C intake and esophageal cancer in 3,955 esophageal cancer patients and 7,063 healthy individuals. The meta-analysis confirmed that sufficient dietary intake of vitamin C significantly reduced the risk of esophageal cancer. Increasing daily intake of vitamin C by 50 mg was found to reduce the risk of esophageal cancer by 13%.

Recommendation

- *Prevention.* For people at risk of esophageal cancer, take daily 200 mg vitamin C (10) and 400 mcg vitamin B9 (8).
- *Treatment.* For esophageal cancer patients, take daily 500 mg vitamin C (10), and 800 mcg vitamin B9 (8).

65

EXERCISE-INDUCED BRONCHOCONSTRICTION

Exercise-induced bronchoconstriction, also known as exercise-induced asthma, is caused by the narrowing of the bronchi after exercise, making it difficult to exhale air from the lungs and leading to asthma and its complications. Athletes who perform strenuous exercise inhale hot and/or cold air into the lungs, which triggers the constriction of the bronchi and causes exercise-induced bronchoconstriction. About 90% of asthma patients suffer from exercise-induced bronchoconstriction. It is estimated that 10% of the world population and 50% of all athletes have problems with exercise-induced bronchoconstriction.

What Are the Symptoms of Exercise-Induced Bronchoconstriction?
- Shortness of breath
- Difficulty breathing

- Coughing
- Asthma
- Tightening in the chest

What Are the Risk Factors for Exercise-Induced Bronchoconstriction?

- *Atopy.* Atopy refers to the genetic tendency to develop allergic rhinitis, asthma, and eczema. Atopic patients are prone to exercise-induced bronchoconstriction.
- *Strenuous exercise.* Strenuous exercise includes skiing, football, cross-country, hockey, swimming, and soccer. Athletes who perform these forms of strenuous exercise, particularly in cold weather, have an increased risk of exercise-induced bronchoconstriction.

What Is the Association between Vitamin C and Exercise-Induced Bronchoconstriction?

- Vitamin C supports lung function. Athletes who take vitamin C supplements right before exercise lower their risk of exercise-induced bronchoconstriction.
- Vitamin C inhibits the actions of bronchoconstrictors, such as histamines and prostaglandins.

Meta-analysis

- *Vitamin C.* A meta-analysis of three randomized controlled trials explored the relationship between vitamin C and exercise-induced bronchoconstriction in 40 participants. Analysis revealed that vitamin C supplementation at a dose of 0.5 to 2 g right before exercise reduced the risk of exercise-induced bronchoconstriction by 8.4%.

Recommendation

- *Prevention.* For people at risk of exercise-induced bronchoconstriction, take 500 mg vitamin C (10) before exercise.

66

FATTY LIVER DISEASE

The liver, located below the left side of the rib cage, is the second largest organ in the body. The liver has a multitude of important physiological functions, one of which is to convert nutrients to energy. During this conversion, fat is generated and stored in the liver. Fatty liver disease occurs when the amount of fat stored in the liver exceeds 5–10% of the weight of the liver. Obesity, hypercholesterolemia, and high blood triglyceride levels are risk factors for fatty liver disease. Anorexia and rapid weight loss can also cause fatty liver disease. In the US, about 20% of the population has fatty liver disease, which means 75 million to 100 million Americans suffer from this affliction. Fatty liver disease can affect any age group, but people aged 40–49 have the highest incident rate. Still, it is the most common liver-related disease in children aged 2–19.

Fatty liver disease can be divided into two types:

- *Alcoholic fatty liver disease.* Heavy consumption of alcohol can induce alcoholic fatty liver disease. Alcohol is converted into fat and stored in the liver. Alcoholic people are likely to suffer from alcoholic fatty liver disease.

- *Nonalcoholic fatty liver disease.* High consumption of fructose makes one susceptible to nonalcoholic fatty liver disease. Like alcohol, fructose is converted into fat and stored in the liver. Excessive consumption of sugary beverages increases the risk of nonalcoholic fatty liver disease.

What Are the Symptoms and Complications of Fatty Liver Disease?

- Fatty liver disease is symptomless. The enlarged liver is often discovered during a medical examination.
- The patient may feel fatigue and abdominal discomfort.
- Excessive fat accumulated in the liver can lead to chronic inflammation, cirrhosis, and liver cancer.
- Excessive fat in the liver induces insulin resistance in the liver and muscle tissues. Insulin resistance causes damage to insulin-producing beta cells in the pancreas.

What Are the Risk Factors for Fatty Liver Disease?

- *Family and genetics.* Genes are linked to fatty liver disease. PNPLA3 gene polymorphic variants, particularly 1148M mutations, are associated with the accumulation of fats in the liver and insulin resistance, leading to fatty liver disease. The PNPLA3 gene encodes a phospholipase enzyme that hydrolyzes phospholipids and regulates fat metabolism in the liver and adipocytes. The 1148M gene mutation inactivates a phospholipase enzyme, causing disorders in fat metabolism and the accumulation of fats in the liver and adipocytes. About 60% of fatty liver disease is caused by PNPLA3 gene mutations.
- *Alcohol.* Alcohol in the bloodstream enters the liver, where alcohol is converted to fat and stored, causing alcoholic fatty liver disease. Besides fatty liver disease, alcohol can induce hepatic inflammation, oxidative damage, fibrosis, and cirrhosis. Acetaldehyde, a metabolite of alcohol, is a carcinogen that

can damage DNA and increase the incidence of tumorigenesis. Heavy consumption of alcohol can lead to alcoholic fatty liver disease and liver cancer.

- *Sugar.* Sucrose is the most common form of sugar found on food labels and consists of glucose and fructose. In the human digestive tract, sucrose is converted into glucose and fructose, both of which are then absorbed by the intestines and enter the bloodstream. Glucose gets into the brain, heart, liver, muscle, and all other organs and tissues in the body, where it is used as fuel to produce energy. On the other hand, all fructose in the bloodstream ends up in the liver, where it is converted to fat, causing nonalcoholic fatty liver disease.

- *Smoking.* Chemicals in cigarette smoke enter the bloodstream and travel to the liver. These chemicals can induce the fibrosis of hepatic cells, decrease insulin sensitivity, and aggravate the symptoms of fatty liver disease. Obese people who smoke heighten their risk of fatty liver disease.

- *Metabolic syndrome.* Five contributing factors for metabolic syndrome include a thick waistline, high triglycerides, low HDL, hypertension, and high blood glucose. People with metabolic syndrome have at least three of those five contributing factors and have an elevated risk of fatty liver disease.

- *Obesity.* Fat in the liver is either made in the liver or transported into the liver. Alcohol and sugar increase the production of fat in the liver. On the other hand, fat tissues in obese people release fatty acids, which enter the bloodstream and travel to the liver, where fatty acids are converted to fats and stored in the liver, increasing the risk of fatty liver disease.

- *Type 2 diabetes.* Type 2 diabetes patients have a threefold increased risk of fatty liver disease compared to healthy individuals. Excessive fat in the liver affects insulin metabolism, leading to insulin resistance. Insulin resistance causes the liver to accumulate more fat. Type 2 diabetes patients who are obese have a high risk of fatty liver disease.

What Is the Association between Vitamin D and Fatty Liver Disease?

- Lower blood levels of vitamin D are common in patients with fatty liver disease compared to healthy individuals. Individuals with vitamin D deficiency are more susceptible to fatty liver disease. Sufficient dietary intake of vitamin D reduces the risk of fatty liver disease.
- Vitamin D alleviates the symptoms of fatty liver disease by preventing hepatic inflammation, cirrhosis, and fibrosis.

What Is the Association between Vitamin E and Fatty Liver Disease?

- Lower blood levels of vitamin E are common in patients with fatty liver disease compared to healthy individuals. Supplementation with vitamin E may assuage the symptoms of fatty liver disease.
- Vitamin E alleviates the symptoms of fatty liver disease by reducing the transport of fatty acids into the liver and curtailing hepatic inflammation and fibrosis.

What Is the Association between Omega-3 Fatty Acids and Fatty Liver Disease?

- Patients with fatty liver disease often have low blood levels of omega-3 fatty acids compared to healthy individuals. Supplementation with omega-3 fatty acids reduces the fat stored in the liver and inhibits de novo lipogenesis in the liver.
- Omega-3 fatty acids mitigate the symptoms of fatty liver disease by reducing hepatic inflammation, oxidative damage, fibrosis, and cirrhosis.

Meta-analysis

- *Vitamin D.* A meta-analysis of 33 research articles studied the relationship between vitamin D and fatty liver disease in 13,524 participants, including 5,896 nonalcoholic fatty liver disease patients and 7,628 healthy individuals. Analysis confirmed that patients with nonalcoholic fatty liver disease had low blood levels of vitamin D compared to healthy controls.

- *Vitamin E.* Five research papers investigated the association between vitamin E and fatty liver disease. The meta-analysis revealed that vitamin D reduced fatty liver index (a predictor of hepatic steatosis), mitigated hepatic inflammation, and alleviated the symptoms of fatty liver disease.
- *Omega-3 fatty acids.* A meta-analysis of nine research articles conducted with 355 fatty liver disease patients explored the relationship between omega-3 fatty acids and fatty liver disease. Supplementation with omega-3 fatty acids was found to significantly reduce the amount of fat stored in the liver.

Recommendation
- *Prevention.* For people at risk of fatty liver disease, take daily 800 IU vitamin D3 (11), 30 IU vitamin E (12), and 1 g omega-3 fatty acids (27).
- *Treatment.* For fatty liver disease patients, take daily 2,000 IU vitamin D3 (11), 100 IU vitamin E (12), and 2 g omega-3 fatty acids (27).

67

FIBROMYALGIA

Fibromyalgia is a common chronic disease characterized by pain in the muscles all over the body. Although its symptoms resemble those of arthritis, fibromyalgia is not an arthritic disease because it does not cause inflamed joints. Fibromyalgia patients feel pain and fatigue all the time. In the US, 10 million people are afflicted with fibromyalgia.

What Are the Causes of Fibromyalgia?
The cause of fibromyalgia is not clear at present. Physical or emotional stress, such as car accidents or chronic illnesses, can lead to fibromyalgia. Fibromyalgia might be related to how our genes regulate and cope with pain. Certain genes in the chromosomes of fibromyalgia patients are particularly sensitive to pain, which may invoke strong responses to pain. The existence of these genes has been confirmed, although the cause and effect are still not known.

How Is Fibromyalgia Diagnosed?

Fibromyalgia is often misdiagnosed by physicians. Symptoms of fibromyalgia, such as pain and fatigue, are also common in other diseases. Currently, no blood test is available for fibromyalgia. Some physicians tell patients with fibromyalgia that the pain is all in their heads and there is nothing they can do about it.

Physicians commonly follow the handbook of the American College of Rheumatology to diagnose fibromyalgia.

What Are the Symptoms of Fibromyalgia?

- Muscle stiffness all over the body, even after taking a walk
- Muscle stiffness after standing or sitting still for a while
- Chronic muscle pain and cramps all over the body
- Poor-quality sleep and feeling tired and sleepy during the day
- Gastrointestinal discomfort, such as frequent nausea, vomiting, abdominal pain, constipation, and diarrhea
- Morning stiffness
- Frequent migraines
- Numbness in the face, hands, and feet
- Anxiety and depression

What Are the Risk Factors for Fibromyalgia?

- *Gender and age.* Nine out of 10 fibromyalgia patients are women, particularly perimenopausal women. Women at the ages of 20–50 are the highest risk group for fibromyalgia.
- *Rheumatic disease.* Rheumatic diseases—including rheumatoid arthritis, osteoarthritis, lupus erythematosus, and ankylosing spondylitis—increase the risk of fibromyalgia.
- *Family and genetics.* Fibromyalgia is linked to genetics. If your parent or sibling has suffered from fibromyalgia, it increases your risk of the disease. Fibromyalgia is associated with functional somatic disorders, involving the interplay of multiple genes, although the exact mechanism is not clear at present.

What Is the Association between Vitamin D and Fibromyalgia?
- Fibromyalgia patients have low blood levels of vitamin D compared to healthy individuals. Taking 2,000 IU of vitamin D3 daily for eight weeks was shown to significantly assuage the symptoms of fibromyalgia.

Meta-analysis
- *Vitamin D.* A meta-analysis of 12 research articles studied the association between vitamin D and fibromyalgia in 1,854 fibromyalgia patients. Analysis confirmed that fibromyalgia patients had lower blood levels of vitamin D compared to healthy controls.

Recommendation
- *Prevention.* For people at risk of fibromyalgia, take daily 800 IU vitamin D3 (11).
- *Treatment.* For fibromyalgia patients, take daily 2,000 IU vitamin D3 (11).

68

GESTATIONAL DIABETES

When a woman without diabetes develops diabetes during pregnancy, it is called gestational diabetes. In the US, about 7–18% of pregnant women are afflicted with gestational diabetes. The cause of the disease is still unknown. Gestational diabetes occurs at a late stage of pregnancy and is characterized by insulin resistance and high blood glucose. If untreated, gestational diabetes can affect the health of both mother and infant. The mother has an increased risk of type 2 diabetes after childbirth, and the infant is at risk of obesity during childhood.

What Are the Symptoms of Gestational Diabetes?
- Gestational diabetes is symptomless. It is often discovered during routine blood glucose tests at weeks 24–28 of pregnancy. A high blood glucose level is indicative of gestational diabetes.

What Are the Risk Factors for Gestational Diabetes?

- *Age.* Women who are pregnant at age 25 and older have an increased risk of gestational diabetes.
- *Obesity.* Women who are obese during pregnancy have an increased risk of gestational diabetes. The relationship between body weight and increased risk of gestational diabetes as follows: overweight creates a twofold increase, obesity a fourfold increase, and severe obesity an eightfold increase.
- *Prediabetes.* Women with prediabetes also have an increased risk of gestational diabetes. Prediabetic individuals have blood glucose levels between 101 and 125 mg/dl.
- *Polycystic ovary syndrome.* Women with polycystic ovary syndrome have abnormal ovulation, irregular menstruation, and high blood glucose, increasing the risk of gestational diabetes.

What Is the Association between Vitamin D and Gestational Diabetes?

- Vitamin D can mitigate insulin resistance, increase cellular insulin sensitivity, and regulate beta cells in the pancreas that produce insulin.
- Pregnant women with gestational diabetes often have low blood levels of vitamin D. Vitamin D supplementation lowers blood glucose levels and increases glucose tolerance in women with gestational diabetes.

What Is the Association between Selenium and Gestational Diabetes?

- Selenium-dependent enzymes support immune response. They can mitigate inflammatory reactions during pregnancy.
- Pregnant women with gestational diabetes have low blood levels of selenium. Supplementation with selenium during pregnancy lowers the risk of gestational diabetes.

Meta-analysis

- *Vitamin D.* A meta-analysis of 20 research articles conducted with 16,515 people studied the relationship between vitamin D and gestational diabetes. Analysis revealed that pregnant women with low blood levels of vitamin D had a heightened risk of gestational diabetes.
- *Selenium.* Six research papers investigated the association between selenium and gestational diabetes in 147 patients with gestational diabetes and 360 healthy women. The meta-analysis confirmed that women with gestational diabetes had low blood levels of selenium compared to healthy women.

Recommendation

- *Prevention.* For women at risk of gestational diabetes, take daily 2,000 IU vitamin D3 (11) and 100 mcg selenium (26).

69

GLAUCOMA

Glaucoma is caused by the blockage of draining space between the cornea and iris in the front of the eyeball, affecting the discharge of fluid from the eyes. The buildup of fluid increases eyeball pressure and injures the optic nerve over time, causing glaucoma. If untreated, glaucoma may lead to blindness. In the US, 4 million people are afflicted with glaucoma, although about 50% of them do not even know it. Globally, 60 million people suffer from glaucoma.

Glaucoma can be divided into three main types:

- *Open-angle glaucoma.* Open-angle glaucoma induces damage to the optic nerve behind the eyeball and diminishes vision. This kind of glaucoma is caused by the blockage of fluid discharge from the eyes, resulting in increasing eyeball pressure and, in severe cases, leading to blindness. Open-angle glaucoma is the most common form of glaucoma.

- *Closed-angle glaucoma.* Closed-angle glaucoma is caused by a sudden blockage of fluid discharge and a rapid increase in eyeball pressure, although the incidence of this type of glaucoma is rather rare.
- *Congenital glaucoma.* Congenital glaucoma is linked to family and genetics. A hereditary eye developmental disorder of the fetus in the mother's womb causes high eyeball pressure and damage to the optic nerve. Children with congenital glaucoma often have larger eyeballs and opaque corneas and are sensitive to light.

What Are the Symptoms of Glaucoma?
- *Open-angle glaucoma.* Open-angle glaucoma is often symptomless. People could have had open-angle glaucoma for years without knowing it. Open-angle glaucoma is often discovered during an eye examination; by then, the condition could already be serious. Open-angle glaucoma can lead to permanent loss of eyesight.
- *Closed-angle glaucoma.* Symptoms of closed-angle glaucoma include blurred vision, sensitivity to light, narrowed peripheral vision, pain in the eyes due to a damaged optic nerve, bleeding, swollen eyelids, nausea, vomiting, and, in severe cases, blindness.

What Are the Risk Factors for Glaucoma?
- *Age.* The older the person, the higher his risk of glaucoma. Individuals aged 60 have a sixfold increased risk of glaucoma compared to those aged 20.
- *Family and genetics.* All three major types of glaucoma are related to genetics. CAV1/CAV2 and TMCO1 gene mutations are associated with open-angle glaucoma, PLEKHA7 and COL11A1 gene mutations are linked to closed-angle glaucoma, and CYP1B1 gene mutations are related to congenital glaucoma.

- *Eye injuries.* Eye injuries, particularly damage incurred in the fluid discharge passage in the front of the eyeball, increase the risk of glaucoma. People whose cornea thickness near the center is less than 0.5 mm have an increased risk of glaucoma.
- *Hypertension.* Sodium ion transport disorders are common in hypertension and glaucoma patients. Hypertension causes the kidneys to retain excessive sodium ions, while glaucoma causes the eyes to retain excessive sodium ions. Hypertension exerts extra pressure on the eyes of glaucoma patients and exacerbates the symptoms of glaucoma.
- *Diabetes.* Diabetes increases the risk of glaucoma. About 5% of patients with diabetes have glaucoma, while only 2% of people without diabetes suffer from it. Diabetes brings on damage to the microvascular structure in the optic nerve and increases the risk of open-angle glaucoma.

What Is the Association between Vitamin B9 and Glaucoma?
- Vitamin B9 reduces the blood level of homocysteine. High blood levels of homocysteine are associated with glaucoma.
- Sufficient dietary intake of vitamin B9 lowers the risk of glaucoma.

Meta-analysis
- *Vitamin B9.* A meta-analysis of five clinical research reports investigated vitamin B9 and glaucoma. Analysis has shown that glaucoma patients had low blood levels of vitamin B9 and high blood levels of homocysteine compared to healthy controls.

Recommendation
- *Prevention.* For people at risk of glaucoma, take daily 400 mcg vitamin B9 (8).
- *Treatment.* For glaucoma patients, take daily 800 mcg vitamin B9 (8).

70

GLIOMA

Glioma is a form of brain cancer caused by abnormal growth and tumor-igenesis of glial cells in the brain. About 80% of all invasive brain cancers are glioma, and glioblastoma is the most common form of glioma. Glioma is a fast-growing and aggressive cancer, and it can easily spread to other regions in the brain, as well as other organs in the body. In the US, an estimated 10,400 people will be afflicted with glioma this year.

Glial cells consist of three different types of cells—namely, astrocyte, oligodendrocyte, and ependymal cells, all of which can transform into cancerous cells. This means that glioma can be divided into three major types:

- *Astrocytoma.* Astrocytoma is caused by the transformation of astrocytes into cancerous cells; glioblastoma is a type of astrocytoma.
- *Oligodendroglioma.* Oligodendroglioma originates from cancerous oligodendrocytes.

- *Ependymoma.* Ependymoma is formed by the tumorigenesis of ependymal cells.

What Are the Symptoms of Glioma?
- Headaches and dizziness
- Personality changes
- Lack of strength in the face, hands, and feet
- Difficulty speaking
- Nausea and vomiting
- Waddling
- Vision and memory decline
- Incontinence
- Irritability
- Convulsions and spasming

What Are the Risk Factors for Glioma?
- *Age.* Glioma can affect any age group. It is the second-most common cancer in children aged 0–19 (blood cancers are the first). In adults, the average age at which one is afflicted with glioma is 59.
- *Family and genetics.* Genes are linked to glioma. Mutations of EGRF and PDGF genes and tumor suppressor genes—such as PTEN, RB1, and TP53—have been associated with the formation and growth of glioma.
- *Radiation.* Cancer patients who receive radiation therapy have an increased risk of glioma. Radiation therapy, particularly via X-ray, induces a surge of free radicals that can kill cancerous cells but also damage the DNA of normal brain cells, increasing the risk of glioma.

What Is the Association between Vitamin A and Glioma?
- Glioma patients have lower blood levels of vitamin A compared to healthy individuals. Vitamin A inhibits the growth and proliferation of glioma cells.

- Vitamin A supports the growth and development of the brain from childhood to adulthood and prevents free radical–induced DNA damage to the neurons. Sufficient dietary intake of vitamin A reduces the risk of glioma.

What Is the Association between Vitamin C and Glioma?

- Vitamin C has anticancer properties. It induces apoptosis of glioma cells and prevents the transformation of glial cells to cancerous cells.
- Glioma patients have lower blood levels of vitamin C. Supplementation with vitamin C reduces the incidence rate of glioma in its high-risk group.
- High-dose IV vitamin C therapy has been shown to be effective for treating cancers. High concentrations of vitamin C produce hydrogen peroxide, which can kill cancerous cells in the body. (See chapter 47, "Breast Cancer," for details.)

Meta-analysis

- *Vitamin A.* A meta-analysis of seven research articles studied the relationship between vitamin A and glioma in 1,841 glioma patients and 4,123 healthy individuals. The result has shown that sufficient dietary intake of vitamin A lowered the risk of glioma.
- *Vitamin C.* Fifteen research papers investigated the association between vitamin C and glioma in 3,409 glioma patients. The meta-analysis confirmed that sufficient dietary intake of vitamin C reduced the risk of glioma.

Recommendation

- *Prevention.* For people at risk of glioma, take daily 2,000 IU vitamin A (1) and 200 mg vitamin C (10).
- *Treatment.* For glioma patients, take daily 5,000 IU vitamin A (1) and 500 mg vitamin C (10).

71

GOUT

Gout is an inflammatory arthritic disease characterized by sudden swelling and acute pain in the joints of the hands and feet, particularly in the big toes. Gout is caused by a high content of uric acid in the bloodstream, which induces the formation of knife-sharp uric acid crystals in the joints of the big toes. Rubbing of these uric acid crystals against the cells or tissues causes swollen, inflamed tissues and acute pain. Excessive uric acid crystals in the kidneys can also lead to the formation of kidney stones. In the US, 6 million men and 2 million women are afflicted with gout.

What Are the Symptoms of Gout?
- Swelling and acute pain in the big toes, also known as "podagra"
- Mostly nighttime episodes that can persist for hours
- Swollen big toe, painful to touch (even by only bed linens)
- Red, swollen, and painful joints in the hands, feet, knees, and ankles
- Chronic inflammatory arthritis

What Are the Risk Factors for Gout?

- *Age and gender.* Men with high blood levels of uric acid have an elevated risk of gout compared to women. The average age of men afflicted is 30–50 years old. Postmenopausal women have a higher risk of gout compared to premenopausal women.
- *Family and genetics.* Genetics is related to gout. The ABCG2 gene encodes a membrane protein that supports the transport and excretion of uric acid from the blood. Mutation of the ABCG2 gene raises the uric acid contents of the blood and increases the risk of gout.
- *Diet.* Habitual consumption of purine-rich foods increases the risk of gout. Purine-rich foods include animals' internal organs, such as the liver and kidneys, and animal meats, such as pheasant, wild rabbit, venison, anchovies, herring, mackerel, trout, shellfish, and crabs. Alcoholic beverages, particularly beer, raise the blood level of uric acid.
- *Obesity.* Obesity increases the risk of gout twofold. Obese people tend to suffer from gout at least 11 years earlier than nonobese people.
- *Hypertension.* High blood levels of uric acid are common in hypertensive patients, who have a twofold increased risk of gout compared to healthy individuals. Hypertensive patients who are on diuretic medications further increase their risk of gout.
- *Diabetes.* High blood glucose and insulin resistance are risk factors for gout.
- *Kidney disease.* Kidney disease decreases the excretion of uric acid and elevates the blood level of uric acid. Kidney stones made of uric acid crystals can injure the cells and tissues in the kidneys and increase the risk of gout. In addition, gout exacerbates the symptoms of kidney disease.

What Is the Association between Vitamin C and Gout?
- A high blood level of uric acid can lead to gout. Vitamin C lowers the blood level of uric acid and enhances the kidneys' ability to excrete excess uric acid.
- Sufficient dietary intake of vitamin C reduces the risk of gout. Supplementation with vitamin C decreases the incidence rate of gout.

Meta-analysis
- *Vitamin C.* A meta-analysis of 13 randomized controlled trials conducted with 2,082 people studied the relationship between vitamin C and gout. Analysis revealed that vitamin C supplementation at a daily dose of 500 mg significantly lowered blood levels of uric acid as well as the risk of gout.

Recommendation
- *Prevention.* For people at risk of gout, take daily 200 mg vitamin C (10).
- *Treatment.* For gout patients, take daily 500 mg vitamin C (10).

72

GRAVES' DISEASE

Graves' disease is an autoimmune disorder characterized by excessive production of thyroid hormones, causing hyperthyroidism. The pituitary gland in the brain produces thyroid-stimulating hormones that regulate thyroid function. Graves' disease patients produce an autoantibody that resembles the thyroid-stimulating hormone. The synergistic effect of the thyroid-stimulating hormone and autoantibody brings on the overproduction of thyroid hormones in the thyroid gland, leading to hyperthyroidism. In the US, 3 million people are afflicted with Graves' disease. The incidence rate is five times higher in women compared to men.

What Are the Symptoms of Graves' Disease?
- Anxiety and irritability
- Chest pain
- Hypertension
- Insomnia

- Fatigue
- Palpitations and an irregular heartbeat
- Heat intolerance, sweating easily, and clammy skin
- An enlarged thyroid gland or goiter
- Exophthalmoses (abnormal protrusion of the eyeball or eyeballs)
- Weight loss despite a good appetite

What Are the Risk Factors for Graves' Disease?

- *Age and gender.* The average age of onset of Graves' disease is 40 or younger. Women have a seven to eight times higher incidence rate compared to men.
- *Family and genetics.* Gene mutations are linked to the cause of Graves' disease. Human leukocyte antigen, or HLA, complex, is responsible for differentiating self from nonself as part of the host's immune defense system. Mutation of HLA genes leads to Graves' disease, in which the immune cells attack thyroid hormone–producing cells in the thyroid gland, mistaking them as foreign.
- *Other autoimmune diseases.* Patients with autoimmune diseases such as type 1 diabetes or rheumatoid arthritis have an increased risk of Graves' disease.

What Is the Association between Vitamin D and Graves' Disease?

- Graves' disease patients have lower blood levels of vitamin D compared to healthy individuals.
- Radioactive iodine therapy is a therapeutic modality for treating Graves' disease. This treatment is effective only if the patient's blood level of vitamin D is higher than 20 ng/ml. Studies have shown that supplementation with vitamin D can significantly improve the effectiveness of radioactive iodine therapy for treating Graves' disease.

Meta-analysis

- *Vitamin D.* A meta-analysis of 26 research articles investigated the association between vitamin D and Graves' disease in 1,748 Graves' disease patients and 1,448 healthy individuals. The result has shown that Graves' disease patients had lower blood levels of vitamin D compared to healthy controls.

Recommendation

- *Prevention.* For people at risk of Graves' disease, take daily 800 IU vitamin D3 (11).
- *Treatment.* For Graves' disease patients, take daily 2,000 IU vitamin D3 (11).

73

HEART ATTACK

The heart needs oxygen and nutrients to maintain the heartbeat and perform its vital functions. A heart attack is caused by the sudden blockage of blood flow into the heart by blood clots, leading to the death of heart muscle cells. Blood clots formed elsewhere in the body enter the bloodstream, travel to the heart, and block the blood flow, resulting in cardiac hypoxia and heart attack. Atherosclerosis, diabetes, heart failure, and obesity are risk factors for blood clot formation and heart attack. In the US, each year 740,000 people suffer from heart attacks, among whom 530,000 are first-time heart attack patients and 210,000 are second-time heart attack patients. Every 43 seconds, someone suffers a heart attack in the US.

What Are the Alarming Signs of Heart Attack?

Many well-known signs of a heart attack, such as chest pain or tightening, are common in men, but women tend to have other alarming signs.

Alarming signs of heart attack in men include
- Chest pain or tightening
- Pain or discomfort in the arms, back, neck, and abdomen
- Shortness of breath
- Cold sweat
- Nausea and vomiting
- Dizziness and confusion

Alarming signs of heart attack in women include
- Shortness of breath
- Nausea and vomiting
- Back pain
- Jaw pain

What Are the Risk Factors for Heart Attack?

- *Smoking.* Cigarette smoke contains toxic chemicals that enter the bloodstream and travel to the heart. These chemicals lead to injuries to the endothelial cells of the blood vessels and induce endothelial dysfunction. Chemicals from the smoke can also increase inflammation, blood clot formation, and oxidation of LDL, leading to atherosclerosis and plaque formation, both of which are risk factors for heart attack.
- *Hypertension.* High blood pressure can lead to damage to the heart and vascular system. Leukocytes, triglycerides, and cholesterol adhere to the damaged arterial wall, causing atherosclerosis and plaque formation.
- *High triglycerides.* People with high blood triglyceride levels are at risk of heart attack. Triglycerides, together with cholesterol and oxidized LDL, participate in the formation of plaque and blood clots in damaged arterial walls.
- *Hypercholesterolemia.* Hypercholesterolemia or high LDL increases the risk of heart attack. Oxidized LDLs enter the endothelial layer of the blood vessel, where macrophages engulf oxidized LDLs to form enlarged foam cells. The death

of foam cells releases cellular debris, including cholesterol and fats, in the endothelial layer and initiates plaque formation and atherosclerosis.

- *Diabetes.* A high blood glucose level is a major risk factor for atherosclerosis and blood clot formation. Insulin resistance also increases the risk of heart attack.
- *Lack of exercise.* Lack of physical activity can lead to diabetes and hypertension, both of which are known risk factors for heart attack. The benefits of regular physical exercise to the heart include improving endothelial functions and preventing plaque and blood clot formation.
- *Obesity.* Obesity induces hypertension, high LDL, high triglyceride levels, diabetes, inflammation, and blood clot formation, increasing the risk of heart attack.
- *Stress.* Excessive daily stress leads to overproduction of white blood cells. Under normal conditions, white blood cells fight against infections and accelerate wound healing. However, excessive white blood cells produced under stress may stick to the arterial wall and exacerbate plaque formation and atherosclerosis. Persistent stress is a risk factor for heart attack.

What Is the Association between Vitamin E and Heart Attack?
- Vitamin E can quench free radicals and prevent oxidative stress–induced damage to the heart. Vitamin E deficiency weakens the antioxidant defense of endothelial cells against free radicals, increasing the risk of plaque and blood clot formation.
- Vitamin E enhances the blood flow in coronary arteries of the heart and prevents oxidative damage to blood vessels and blood clot formation.

What Is the Association between Magnesium and Heart Attack?
- Magnesium ions enhance vasodilatation, alleviate inflammation, and inhibit platelet aggregation.

- Magnesium is an essential element that supports normal electrical physiological functions of the heart. Magnesium deficiency brings on an irregular heartbeat.

Meta-analysis
- *Vitamin E.* A meta-analysis of 16 research articles studied the relationship between vitamin E and heart attack. The doses of vitamin E ranged from 33 to 800 IU daily for 0.5 to 9.4 years. Analysis confirmed that supplementation with vitamin E alone reduced the risk of heart attack. However, this protective effect of vitamin E against heart attack was abolished when vitamin E was taken together with other antioxidants.
- *Magnesium.* Sixteen research papers investigated the association between magnesium and heart attack in 313,041 participants, including 11,995 cardiovascular disease patients, 7,534 hypoxic heart attack patients, and 2,686 patients who died from hypoxic heart attack. The result has shown that increasing daily intake of magnesium by 200 mg decreased hypoxic heart attack by 22% and other cardiovascular diseases by 11%.

Recommendation
- *Prevention.* For people at risk of heart attack, take daily 30 IU vitamin E (12) and 100 mg magnesium (17).
- *Treatment.* For heart attack patients, take daily 100 IU vitamin E (12) and 200 mg magnesium (17).

74

HEART FAILURE

Heart failure is caused by enlarged cardiac muscles in the left ventricle and stiffness of the ventricular walls, making the heart unable to contract and relax properly. Contraction pumps the blood out of the heart, while relaxation allows the blood to return to the heart. Enlarged and hardened ventricles weaken the heart, and the weakened heart has to work harder to supply blood to the rest of the body. Exhaustive contraction and relaxation cycles further enlarge cardiac muscles, leading to heart failure. In the US, 5 million people are afflicted with heart failure.

Heart failure can be divided into four types:

- *Left-side heart failure.* Shortness of breath and pulmonary edema
- *Right-side heart failure.* Abdominal and leg edema
- *Contracting-stage heart failure.* Weakness in left ventricular contraction
- *Relaxing-stage heart failure.* Weakness in left ventricular relaxation

What Are the Symptoms of Heart Failure?
- Shortness of breath
- Fatigue
- Coughing
- Leg, ankle, and foot edema
- Nausea, vomiting, and lack of appetite
- Memory decline and feeling mentally foggy
- Fast and irregular heartbeat
- Abdominal edema

What Are the Risk Factors for Heart Failure?
- *Coronary artery disease.* Coronary artery disease reduces blood flow. Insufficient blood flow leads to enlarged ventricular muscles and heart failure.
- *Myocardial infarction.* Myocardial infarction diminishes blood flow, causing hypoxia and the death of cardiac muscle cells. Atherosclerosis and blood clots are common risk factors for myocardial infarction and heart failure. Myocardial infarction patients have an increased risk of heart failure compared to healthy individuals.
- *Hypertension.* Hypertension is associated with enlarged ventricles, systolic and diastolic pressure disorders, irregular heartbeat, and heart failure. To cope with the extra pressure on the arterial wall, the hearts of hypertensive patients enlarge in size as well as thickness. An enlarged heart is unable to perform the normal contract-and-relax cycle, increasing the risk of heart failure.
- *Diabetes.* Diabetes increases the risk of heart failure and the incidence rate of death from heart failure. High blood glucose induces endothelial dysfunction, damages cardiac muscle cells, and alters gene expression, all of which are risk factors for heart failure and heart attack.
- *Alcohol.* Alcohol induces alcoholic cardiomyopathy, which is characterized by an enlarged muscle layer in the left ventricle, increasing the risk of heart failure.

- *Smoking.* Nicotine from cigarette smoke lowers oxygen content and increases blood pressure and heartbeat. Nicotine can also damage cardiac muscle cells and increase the risk of heart failure.
- *Obesity.* Fat tissues in obese people release fatty acids, inflammatory cytokines, and hormones into the bloodstream. These substances, particularly fatty acids, can build up in the heart and induce cardiac lipotoxicity, a condition that damages cardiac muscle cells and affects cardiac function. These obesity-related pathological changes increase the risk of heart failure.

What Is the Association between Vitamin B1 and Heart Failure?
- Vitamin B1 dilates blood vessels and improves cardiac function.
- Vitamin B1 deficiency can lead to an enlarged heart and irregular heartbeat. Sufficient dietary intake of vitamin B1 lowers both systolic and diastolic pressure.

What Is the Association between Omega-3 Fatty Acids and Heart Failure?
- A low blood level of omega-3 fatty acids is associated with increased pressure on the chamber wall of the atrium and decreased efficiency of heart contraction in the atrium.
- Supplementation with omega-3 fatty acids reduces the incidence rate of death from myocardial infarction in heart failure patients.

Meta-analysis
- *Vitamin B1.* A meta-analysis of nine clinical research reports explored the relationship between vitamin B1 and heart failure. Analysis confirmed that supplementation with vitamin B1 alleviated the symptoms of heart failure.
- *Omega-3 fatty acids.* Seven research articles investigated the association between omega-3 fatty acids and heart failure in 176,441 participants, including 5,480 heart failure patients.

The meta-analysis confirmed that supplementation with omega-3 fatty acids curtailed the risk of heart failure.

Recommendation
- *Prevention.* For people at risk of heart failure, take daily 5 mg vitamin B1 (2) and 1 g omega-3 fatty acids (27).
- *Treatment.* For heart failure patients, take daily 100 mg vitamin B1 (2) and 2 g omega-3 fatty acids (27).

75

HEMODIALYSIS

Hemodialysis is an extracorporeal process by which wastes, salt, and water in the bloodstream are removed via a man-made machine. Regular hemodialysis is required for kidney failure patients to carry out routine daily life activities. In the US, 300,000 kidney failure patients require hemodialysis every year.

What Are the Complications Associated with Hemodialysis?
- *Hypotension.* About 40% of patients experienced low blood pressure, or hypotension, during hemodialysis, which can be attributed to several possible factors, including hypovolemia and the overproduction of nitric oxide. Nitric oxide is the strongest vasodilator produced in the body. Extracorporeal circulation activates a nitric oxide–producing enzyme in red blood cells to produce too much nitric oxide, causing hypotension during hemodialysis. Symptoms of hypotension

during hemodialysis include shortness of breath, abdominal pain, and muscle spasms.

- *Anemia.* Anemia is common in hemodialysis patients. Kidney failure patients are unable to produce erythropoietin, a protein that supports the synthesis of new red blood cells in the bone marrow, leading to anemia. Improper diet as well as the loss of iron and vitamins during hemodialysis can exacerbate the symptoms of anemia in hemodialysis patients.

- *Bone disease.* One important function of the kidneys is to convert vitamin D from its inactive form to its active form. Patients in hemodialysis are unable to produce the active form of vitamin D. Vitamin D deficiency leads to a multitude of health problems, including bone diseases such as osteomalacia and osteoporosis, both of which are prevalent in hemodialysis patients.

- *Hypertension.* Hypertension is common in hemodialysis patients. As mentioned above, about 40% of hemodialysis patients develop hypotensive episodes during hemodialysis. A bolus injection of saline solution is an effective way of expanding the blood volume and restoring blood pressure. However, excessive water from this saline solution cannot be removed by the kidneys in hemodialysis patients. Accumulation of excessive water in the blood exerts the pressure on the arterial wall and brings on hypertension. Hemodialysis patients who require bolus injections of saline solution have a greater risk of hypertension.

What Is the Association between Vitamin C and Hemodialysis?

- Chronic inflammation is common in hemodialysis patients. Vitamin C can reduce chronic inflammation in hemodialysis patients.

- Vitamin C enhances the body's ability to produce more hemoglobin and red blood cells and alleviates the symptoms of anemia in hemodialysis patients.

What Is the Association between Vitamin D and Hemodialysis?

- Vitamin D deficiency is common in hemodialysis patients. Vitamin D regulates calcium and phosphorus metabolism and prevents osteoporosis in hemodialysis patients.
- Vitamin D controls blood glucose levels. Sufficient dietary intake of vitamin D lowers blood glucose levels in hemodialysis patients.

What Is the Association between Omega-3 Fatty Acids and Hemodialysis?

- Supplementation with omega-3 fatty acids reduces the effects of an inflammatory diet and atherosclerosis in hemodialysis patients.
- A low blood level of omega-3 fatty acids is common in hemodialysis patients. Omega-3 fatty acids lower blood levels of triglycerides and LDL in hemodialysis patients.

Meta-analysis

- *Vitamin C.* A meta-analysis of six clinical research articles explored the relationship between vitamin C and hemoglobin content in hemodialysis patients. Analysis confirmed that supplementation with vitamin C significantly raised hemoglobin levels and reduced the necessary dosage of erythropoietin medication in hemodialysis patients.
- *Vitamin D.* Seventeen clinical research papers examined the association between vitamin D and blood glucose control in 131 hemodialysis patients without diabetes aged 40–50. Supplementation with vitamin D was found to lower fasting glucose and parathyroid hormone levels in hemodialysis patients. However, no effect was observed on the fasting insulin level.
- *Omega-3 fatty acids.* A meta-analysis of 14 randomized controlled trials conducted with 678 hemodialysis patients evaluated the relationship between omega-3 fatty acids and hemodialysis patients. The result confirmed that

supplementation with omega-3 fatty acids lowered the blood levels of triglycerides and LDL in hemodialysis patients.

Recommendation

- *Treatment.* For hemodialysis patients, take daily 500 mg vitamin C (10), 2,000 IU vitamin D3 (11), and 2 g omega-3 fatty acids (27).

76

HEPATITIS C

Hepatitis C is an infectious disease caused by a viral infection in the liver. The hepatitis C virus is a blood-borne virus. Blood transfusion, hemodialysis, and shared needles in illicit drug users are the major routes of hepatitis C viral infections. About 20–30% of infected individuals may recover from hepatitis C without any medical intervention. However, for 70–80% of patients, the infection will become chronic and last for years. In severe cases, complications from hepatitis C can lead to death. Currently, there is no vaccine for the hepatitis C virus. In the US, 5 million people are infected with hepatitis C, among whom 40–85% are carriers. Globally, 200 million people are afflicted with hepatitis C infections.

What Are the Symptoms of Hepatitis C?
- Initial symptoms are so mild in people who are infected with hepatitis C virus that infected individuals often do not seek medication or treatment. These symptoms include fever,

fatigue, abdominal pain, lack of appetite, nausea, vomiting, and jaundice. It takes 4–12 weeks for these symptoms to appear.

- A hepatitis C virus infection may be symptomless. Nevertheless, it can lead to chronic liver diseases such as cirrhosis and liver cancer.

What Are the Risk Factors for Hepatitis C Infections?

- *Intravenous drug abusers.* Illicit drug users, particularly those who inject drugs intravenously, are among the highest-risk group of hepatitis C patients because they tend to share contaminated needles and syringes. In fact, antibodies against hepatitis C virus are found in 50–80% of all intravenous drug abusers.
- *Blood transfusion.* About 5–10% of hepatitis C infections are related to blood transfusion. Before 1990, blood donors were not being tested for hepatitis C viruses or their antibodies in the US. People who received blood transfusions or organ transplants before 1990 are at risk of having hepatitis C.
- *Hemodialysis.* Hemodialysis patients have a higher risk of hepatitis C. Dialysis devices and medications are often contaminated by hepatitis C viruses in hemodialysis clinics. About 10% of hemodialysis patients suffer from hepatitis C infections.
- *Health-care professionals.* Nurses and other health-care professionals who give intravenous injections to patients could accidentally pierce through their own skin with contaminated needles and become afflicted with hepatitis C infections.

What Is the Association between Vitamin D and Hepatitis C?

- Vitamin D deficiency is common in chronic hepatitis C patients. The liver is the organ where vitamin D is converted to 25(OH) vitamin D. Hepatitis C patients are unable to produce 25(OH)D, causing vitamin D deficiency.

- Vitamin D reduces hepatic fibrosis, alleviates inflammation, and improves hepatic functions.

Meta-analysis
- *Vitamin D.* A meta-analysis of 11 research articles examined the relationship between vitamin D and hepatitis C in 1,575 hepatitis C patients. The result revealed that 71%—or 1,117—of hepatitis C patients had lower blood levels of vitamin D compared to healthy controls.

Recommendation
- *Prevention.* For people at risk of hepatitis C, take daily 800 IU vitamin D3 (11).
- *Treatment.* For hepatitis C patients, take daily 2,000 IU vitamin D3 (11).

77

HYPERCHOLESTEROLEMIA (HIGH BLOOD CHOLESTEROL)

Hypercholesterolemia is a condition characterized by high cholesterol levels in the blood. Cholesterol is required for a multitude of cellular functions in the body. Most cholesterol is made in the body, while only a small quantity is needed from dietary intake. Animal-based foods contain cholesterol, and plant-based foods contain no cholesterol. In other words, cholesterol comes from meat, milk, eggs, and the like, but not from fruits or vegetables. Overconsumption of meats and other greasy animal-based foods can lead to hypercholesterolemia, which is a major risk factor for heart attack and stroke. In the US, 73 million people are afflicted with hypercholesterolemia, which is equivalent to about 31% of the population.

Cholesterol in the blood can be divided into two major types:

- *High-density lipoprotein (HDL)*. HDL removes cholesterol from the arterial wall and transports it via blood circulation to organs and tissues, preventing cholesterol from sticking to the arterial wall and causing atherosclerosis. For its role, HDL is called "good cholesterol."
- *Low-density lipoprotein (LDL)*. LDL, on the other hand, transports cholesterol from organs to the bloodstream, where LDL may stick to the arterial wall and lead to atherosclerosis. For its role, LDL is called "bad cholesterol." High blood cholesterol, or hypercholesterolemia, often refers to a high LDL level in the bloodstream.

What Are the Risk Factors for Hypercholesterolemia?
- *Diet*. Habitual consumption of animal-based foods containing high saturated fat levels can lead to hypercholesterolemia. Sugary beverages can also increase cholesterol and triglyceride levels in the bloodstream.
- *Obesity*. Hypercholesterolemia is common in obese people. Obesity stimulates the body to produce more cholesterol. Without eating any high-cholesterol foods, obese people could still have very high cholesterol levels in the bloodstream and be afflicted with hypercholesterolemia. Weight loss can lower cholesterol levels in the bloodstream and reduce the risk of hypercholesterolemia in obese people. Weight loss, not medication, is the best way to lower blood levels of cholesterol.
- *Lack of exercise*. Regular exercise can reduce cholesterol levels in the blood. Studies have shown that regular exercise increased "good" cholesterol (HDL) and decreased "bad" cholesterol (LDL) in the blood. Contrary to that, lack of physical activity was shown to increase LDL and decrease HDL.
- *Smoking*. Chemicals in cigarette smoke may affect cholesterol levels in the blood. Studies revealed that "bad" cholesterol was high and "good" cholesterol was low in smokers compared to nonsmokers.

- *Diabetes*. Hypercholesterolemia is common in type 2 diabetes patients. High blood glucose stimulates the body to produce more cholesterol. Type 2 diabetes is a risk factor for hypercholesterolemia.

How Is Hypercholesterolemia Diagnosed?
Testing blood cholesterol levels is the best way to detect hypercholesterolemia. Hypercholesterolemia is defined as when total cholesterol is more than 200 mg/dl and HDL is less than 40 mg/dl in the blood. Additional blood tests may be needed if hypercholesterolemia is diagnosed to avoid the potential risk of heart attack and stroke. Some reference values are shown here:

Total cholesterol levels in the blood
- *Normal*. Below 200 mg/dl
- *Too high*. Greater than 200 mg/dl

LDL levels in the blood
- *Normal*. 100 to 129 mg/dl
- *Too high*. 160 to 189 mg/dl

HDL levels in the blood
- *Normal*. 40 to 59 mg/dl
- *Too low*. Less than 40 mg/dl

Triglyceride levels in the blood
- *Normal*. Less than 150 mg/dl
- *Too high*. Greater than 200 mg/dl

What Is the Association between Vitamin C and Hypercholesterolemia?
- Vitamin C can quench free radicals and prevent oxidative damage to LDL; oxidized LDL tends to stick to the surface of the arterial wall and leads to atherosclerosis.

- Vitamin C also protects HDL in the blood from free radical–induced oxidative damage.

Meta-analysis
- *Vitamin C.* A meta-analysis of 13 randomized controlled trials evaluated the relationship between vitamin C and hypercholesterolemia in 1,890 hypercholesterolemia patients. The experimental group received 500 mg of vitamin C daily for 3–24 weeks. Analysis has shown that supplementation with vitamin C decreased LDL levels by 7.9 mg/dl and increased HDL levels by 1.1 mg/dl in patients with hypercholesterolemia. In addition, supplementation with vitamin C was found to lower triglyceride levels by 20.1 mg/dl in patients with hypercholesterolemia.

Recommendation
- *Prevention.* For people at risk of hypercholesterolemia, take daily 200 mg vitamin C (10).
- *Treatment.* For hypercholesterolemia patients, take daily 500 mg vitamin C (10).

78

HYPERTENSION (HIGH BLOOD PRESSURE)

Blood pressure is generated when the heart pumps the blood out to the rest of the body. Hypertension, or high blood pressure, is caused by the hardening of the arteries and makes it more difficult for the heart to pump the blood out to the rest of the body. Hypertension often is symptomless. Chronic hypertension is a risk factor for heart attack, stroke, kidney disease, and even blindness. In the US, 78 million people suffer from hypertension—almost one in three adults is afflicted with hypertension.

Hypertension can be divided into two types:

- *Essential hypertension.* Genetics and lifestyle are linked to essential hypertension. Lifestyle factors include high consumption of sweet and salty foods, smoking, and drinking alcoholic beverages. Almost 90–95% of hypertension is essential hypertension.

- *Secondary hypertension.* Secondary hypertension is caused by kidney disease and certain medications. About 5–10% of hypertension is secondary hypertension.

What Are Systolic and Diastolic Pressure?
- *Systolic pressure.* The pressure on arterial vessels when the heart contracts
- *Diastolic pressure.* The pressure on arterial vessels when the heart relaxes

When someone's blood pressure is 120/80 mmHg, it means systolic pressure is 120 mmHg and diastolic pressure is 80 mmHg, and it is called normal blood pressure. Hypertension is when blood pressure is 140/90 mmHg or higher. Hypertension is symptomless; people may have hypertension but not be aware of it. However, when blood pressure reaches 180/110 mmHg, symptoms like pain and discomfort appear.

What Are the Symptoms of Hypertension?
When blood pressure reaches 180/110 mmHg or higher, patients may experience the following symptoms:

- Unrelenting headache persisting for several days
- Upset stomach, nausea, and vomiting
- Lightheadedness and dizziness
- Nosebleeds
- Irregular heartbeat
- Shortness of breath

What Are the Risk Factors for Hypertension?
- *Age.* Aging can lead to hypertension. Aging is associated with chronic inflammation and oxidative stress, which hampers the

production of nitric oxide in the endothelial layer of arterial vessels. Nitric oxide is the strongest vasodilator in the body. Insufficient nitric oxide production causes vasoconstriction and hypertension.

- *Family and genetics.* Having a parent or sibling with hypertension increases your risk of the disease. If both parents have hypertension, it increases your risk two- to fourfold. About 50% of hypertension is linked to genetics, while the other 50% is caused by environmental factors. Recent genomic research has shown that 13 gene polymorphic variants are linked to systolic pressure and an additional 20 gene polymorphic variants are linked to diastolic pressure.

- *Obesity.* Obesity raises blood pressure by activating blood pressure mediators, including renin, angiotensinogen, and aldosterone. In addition, obesity automatically raises blood pressure to cope with the increasing demand for blood supply due to the body's size.

- *Lack of exercise.* Lack of regular physical exercise is the main culprit of many chronic diseases, including hypertension, type 2 diabetes, coronary artery disease, heart failure, depression, colorectal cancer, breast cancer, and endometrial cancer.

- *Smoking.* Cigarette smoke contains thousands of chemicals, some of which enter the bloodstream and injure the arterial wall, increasing the risk of hypertension. In addition, nicotine from cigarette smoke stimulates the sympathetic nervous system and raises blood pressure.

- *Alcohol.* Alcohol from alcoholic beverages induces hypertension by damaging pressure regulators, stimulating the sympathetic nervous system, and activating renin-angiotensin system functions. In addition, alcohol causes chronic inflammation, free radical–induced oxidative damage, and the hardening of the arterial wall, all of which are risk factors for hypertension.

- *High salt.* The kidneys are the major organs that regulate blood pressure in the body. When the blood level of sodium is too high, the kidneys reabsorb water and release it back into the bloodstream to dilute the sodium ion concentration. The excessive water in the bloodstream causes the expansion of blood volume, which exerts extra pressure on the arterial wall and induces hypertension. This is the reason habitual consumption of salty foods can lead to hypertension.

- *Stress.* Stress increases the risk of hypertension. To cope with stress, the body produces more corticoid and less prostaglandin. The former is a vasoconstrictor, and the latter is a vasodilator. Too much corticoid and not enough prostaglandin in the bloodstream lead to hypertension.
- *Diabetes.* Insulin resistance is common among patients with diabetes. Insulin in endothelial cells of the blood vessel can counter the action of vasoconstrictors. The lack of insulin in endothelial cells increases the risk of hypertension in patients with diabetes.

What Are the Complications Associated with Hypertension?

Uncontrolled hypertension can lead to cardiovascular diseases and other diseases, including the following:

- *Heart attack and stroke.* Hypertension induces atherosclerosis, and it can lead to heart attack and stroke.
- *Aneurysm.* Hypertension weakens the arterial vessel to form a blood-filled bulge in the arterial wall, called an aneurysm. The eruption of an aneurysm in the arterial wall can be a life-threatening event.
- *Blindness.* Hypertension thickens and narrows the arterial wall in the eyes, leading to blindness.
- *Cognitive decline.* Hypertensive patients are prone to cognitive and memory decline.

What Is the Association between Vitamin B9 and Hypertension?

- Vitamin B9 supports the endothelial function of blood vessels. Vitamin B9 deficiency can lead to endothelial dysfunction and hypertension.

- Vitamin B9 facilitates the conversion of homocysteine to methionine, thus reducing the blood level of homocysteine. An elevated blood level of homocysteine is associated with endothelial dysfunction and hypertension.

What Is the Association between Vitamin C and Hypertension?
- Vitamin C reduces blood pressure by enhancing the ability of endothelial cells to produce nitric oxide, the strongest vasodilator in the body. Vitamin C also enhances the elasticity of coronary arteries.
- Hypertensive patients have lower blood levels of vitamin C compared to healthy individuals. Supplementation with vitamin C lowers both systolic and diastolic pressure in hypertensive patients.

What Is the Association between Vitamin D and Hypertension?
- People with low blood levels of vitamin D have a higher risk of hypertension. Supplementation with vitamin D lowers blood pressure in hypertensive patients.
- Vitamin D receptors are ubiquitous in the cardiovascular system, including the heart and vessel systems. Vitamin D deficiency leads to cardiovascular diseases, including hypertension.

What Is the Association between Potassium and Hypertension?
- Habitual consumption of salty foods raises the blood level of sodium and brings on hypertension. Potassium ions counter the actions of sodium ions and bring down blood pressure. Sufficient dietary intake of potassium reduces the risk of hypertension.
- Potassium ions bring down blood pressure by decreasing the fluid content in the blood, reducing the pressure on the arterial wall, and decreasing the activity of angiotensin, a vasoconstrictor. Potassium ions also relax the smooth muscles of arteries, decrease peripheral vascular resistance, and lower blood pressure.

What Is the Association between Magnesium and Hypertension?
- A low blood level of magnesium is common in patients with hypertension. Supplementation with magnesium lowers both systolic and diastolic pressure.
- Magnesium ions lower blood pressure by increasing nitric oxide production, improving endothelial functions, and enhancing vasodilatation.

What Is the Association between Omega-3 Fatty Acids and Hypertension?
- Omega-3 fatty acids improve endothelial function and lessen vascular resistance and blood pressure.
- Omega-3 fatty acids regulate the membrane fluidity of cell membranes in blood vessels and cardiac cells and maintain the elasticity of the cardiovascular system.

Meta-analysis
- *Vitamin C.* A meta-analysis of 29 clinical research papers explored the relationship between vitamin C and hypertension. The average dose of vitamin C was 500 mg daily for eight weeks. Analysis has shown that supplementation with vitamin C lowered systolic pressure by 3.84 mmHg and diastolic pressure by 1.48 mmHg.
- *Vitamin D.* Eighteen research papers investigated the association between vitamin D and hypertension. The meta-analysis confirmed that vitamin D deficiency was correlated with hypertension. High blood levels of vitamin D were found to significantly reduce the risk of hypertension.
- *Vitamin B9.* A meta-analysis of 12 randomized controlled trials evaluated the relationship between vitamin B9 intake and hypertension. The dose of vitamin B9 was 5,000 mcg daily for 2–16 weeks. Analysis revealed that sufficient dietary intake of vitamin B9 significantly reduced the blood pressure of the participants.

- *Potassium.* Fifteen randomized controlled trials investigated the relationship between potassium intake and hypertension in 917 participants. The result has shown that supplementation with potassium lowered systolic pressure by 6.8 mmHg and diastolic pressure by 4.6 mmHg.
- *Magnesium.* A meta-analysis of 22 clinical research papers studied the association between magnesium intake and hypertension. The doses of magnesium supplements ranged from 120 to 973 mg daily for 3–24 weeks. Analysis has shown that supplementation with magnesium lowered systolic pressure by 3–4 mmHg and diastolic pressure by 2–3 mmHg.
- *Omega-3 fatty acids.* Seventy randomized controlled trials explored the relationship between omega-3 fatty acids and hypertension. The meta-analysis confirmed that supplementation with omega-3 fatty acids lowered both systolic and diastolic pressure in hypertensive patients. The effect of omega-3 fatty acids on lowering blood pressure was found to be more profound in hypertensive patients who did not take antihypertensive drugs.

Recommendation
- *Prevention.* For people at risk of hypertension, take daily 200 mg vitamin C (10), 800 IU vitamin D3 (11), 400 mcg vitamin B9 (8), 500 mg potassium (15), 100 mg magnesium (17), and 1 g omega-3 fatty acids (27).
- *Treatment.* For hypertension patients, take daily 500 mg vitamin C (10), 2,000 IU vitamin D3 (11), 800 mcg vitamin B9 (8), 1,000 mg potassium (15), 200 mg magnesium (17), and 2 g omega-3 fatty acids (27).

79

INFLAMMATORY BOWEL DISEASE

Inflammatory bowel disease, caused by an autoimmune disorder, is an inflammatory disease of the digestive tract. The digestive tract includes the mouth, esophagus, stomach, small intestines, large intestines, and anus. The main functions of the digestive tract are to digest foods, absorb nutrients from foods, and discharge wastes. Inflammatory bowel disease—in which the immune cells attack the cells and tissues of the digestive tract, mistaking them as foreign—induces chronic inflammation. Chronic inflammation causes malfunctions of the digestive tract. Patients with inflammatory bowel disease often suffer from chronic abdominal pain, diarrhea, and, in severe cases, loss of life. In the US, 1.4 million people are afflicted with inflammatory bowel disease.

Inflammatory bowel disease can be divided into two types:

- *Ulcerative colitis.* Ulcerative colitis—characterized by cellular inflammation, ulceration, and pus formation in the innermost layer of the colon—is an inflammatory disease of the colon. Inflammation and ulceration lead to abdominal pain and diarrhea. Ulcerative colitis is caused by the immune system sending a large amount of leukocytes and other immune cells to the colon to fight against foods, bacteria, or other substances in the colon, mistaking them for foreign invaders, resulting in an inflamed and ulcerated colon.

- *Crohn's disease.* Crohn's disease resembles ulcerative colitis. However, there are distinct differences between the two. Ulcerative colitis affects only the colon, while Crohn's disease affects the entire digestive tract, from the mouth to the anus. The junction between the small and large intestines is the most vulnerable region in Crohn's disease. Additionally, ulcerative colitis only injures the innermost layer of the colon, while Crohn's disease injures the entire wall of the digestive tract.

What Are the Risk Factors for Inflammatory Bowel Disease?

- *Age and gender.* Although inflammatory bowel disease can affect any age group, the incidence of the disease is most common at age 15–35. The average ages of individuals afflicted with ulcerative colitis and Crohn's disease are 34.9 and 29.5, respectively. Although the incidence rate of inflammatory bowel disease is similar between men and women, men at age 50–60 are more susceptible to inflammatory bowel disease compared to women.

- *Family and genetics.* Both parents suffering from inflammatory bowel disease increases your risk of the disease by 36%. NOD2/CARD15 gene polymorphic variants are linked to Crohn's disease. About 20% of Crohn's disease patients in the US and Europe carry NOD2/CARD15 gene variants.

- *Childhood infection.* Inflammatory bowel disease is considered an autoimmune disorder. Children who grew up in a not-so-clean environment were found to have a stronger immune system compared to children who grew up in a clean environment. Studies have shown that children who lived in a clean environment had a higher incidence of inflammatory bowel disease compared to children who lived in a not-so-clean environment. Bacterial infections early in life seemed to boost the immune system. For example, *Helicobacter pylori* infections are common during childhood. Individuals infected by *Helicobacter pylori* in childhood were found to be less likely to suffer from inflammatory bowel disease in adulthood.

- *Vaccination.* Measles viruses can live parasitically in the human digestive tract and bring on inflammatory bowel disease. People who received measles vaccinations in the 1960s have had an increased risk of inflammatory bowel disease, including ulcerative colitis and Crohn's disease.

- *Antibiotics.* Antibiotics alter bacterial flora living in the digestive tract. Frequent use of antibiotics during childhood increases the risk of inflammatory bowel disease.

- *Nonsteroidal anti-inflammatory drugs (NSAIDs).* NSAID medications, such as naproxen and ibuprofen, can induce ulcerative damage to the mucous cell layer of the stomach, small intestines, and large intestines. NSAIDs also inhibit cyclooxygenase enzymes that support the synthesis of prostaglandins, which are lipid mediators that regulate immune functions. Inhibition of prostaglandin production increases the risk of inflammatory bowel disease.

What Is the Association between Vitamin D and Inflammatory Bowel Disease?

- Inflammatory bowel disease patients have lower blood levels of vitamin D compared to healthy individuals. People who live far from the equator have a greater risk of inflammatory bowel disease. Maintaining high blood levels of vitamin D alleviates the symptoms of inflammatory bowel disease.

- Supplementation with vitamin D was found to mitigate the symptoms of Crohn's disease. The suggested daily dose of vitamin D3 is 5,000 IU for 24 weeks.
- Vitamin D deficiency increases the incidence of colon cancer in patients with Crohn's disease.

Meta-analysis
- *Vitamin D.* A meta-analysis of 14 research articles studied the relationship between vitamin D and inflammatory bowel disease in 1,891 participants, including 938 inflammatory bowel disease patients and 953 healthy individuals. Analysis has shown that patients with inflammatory bowel disease had lower blood levels of vitamin D compared to healthy controls.

Recommendation
- *Prevention.* For people at risk of inflammatory bowel disease, take daily 800 IU vitamin D3 (11).
- *Treatment.* For inflammatory bowel disease patients, including those with ulcerative colitis and Crohn's disease, take 5,000 IU vitamin D3 (11) for 6 months, and after that, take daily 2,000 IU vitamin D3 (11).

80

KASHIN-BECK DISEASE

Kashin-Beck disease is a chronic disease of the cartilage. The disease affects several millions of people living in 15 provinces in China from the northeastern to southwestern regions. Kashin-Beck disease is caused by selenium deficiency in the soil. Children and teenagers aged 5–15 are most vulnerable to the affliction.

What Are the Symptoms of Kashin-Beck Disease?
- Retarded bone growth due to the death of chondrocytes, causing shorter stature in children and teenagers
- Swelling in the joints, such as the shoulder blades, elbows, ankles, knees, fingers, and toes
- Shortened and hardened bones

Meta-analysis

- *Selenium.* A meta-analysis of 15 research papers explored the association between selenium supplements and Kashin-Beck disease in 2,359 children in affected regions in China. Analysis has shown that supplementation with selenium reduced the incidence rate of Kashin-Beck disease by 84% in affected regions in China.

Recommendation

- *Prevention.* For children in Kashin-Beck disease regions, take daily 50 mcg selenium (26).
- *Treatment.* For Kashin-Beck disease patients, take daily 100 mcg selenium (26).

81

LIVER CANCER

Liver cancer is caused by the transformation of hepatic cells to malignant cells in the liver. Infections by hepatitis B and hepatitis C viruses and heavy alcohol consumption are the major causative factors of liver cancer. In the US, it is estimated that about 39,230 people will be diagnosed with liver cancer this year. The five-year survival rate of liver cancer is only 17%. The incidence rate of liver cancer is much higher in Asia compared to North America and Europe because hepatitis B and hepatitis C infections are more prevalent in Asia.

What Are the Symptoms of Liver Cancer?
- Weight loss
- Liver enlargement (mass on the right side of the upper abdomen)
- Pancreas enlargement (mass on the left side of the upper abdomen)
- Fullness in the stomach after eating only a small portion of food

- Itching all over the body
- Jaundice
- Nausea and vomiting
- Fever

What Are the Risk Factors for Liver Cancer?

- *Hepatitis B.* Hepatitis B infections increase the risk of liver cancer. Hepatitis B viruses can insert viral DNA into the chromosomes in liver cells, trigger gene mutations, and lead to liver cancer. Taiwan distinguished itself in the fight against hepatitis B infections. Starting in 1980, the island carried out a nationwide mandatory program of hepatitis B vaccinations in children. Since then, the incidence rate of hepatitis B infection in Taiwan has dropped from 10% in 1980 to less than 1% at present.
- *Hepatitis C.* Hepatitis C infections lead to fibrosis, cirrhosis, and liver cancer. Hepatitis C viruses can insert viral RNA into the chromosomes of liver cells, direct the infected cells to make viral proteins, and force them to undergo cell division and proliferation to produce more viruses. The hepatitis C–infected liver cells can transform into cancerous cells and cause liver cancer.
- *Cirrhosis.* Alcoholic or nonalcoholic cirrhosis increases the risk of liver cancer. Patients with liver cancer often had cirrhotic problems. Cirrhosis is characterized by loss of regenerative functions, fibrosis, and death of liver cells; all these pathological changes are risk factors for liver cancer.
- *Obesity.* Obesity causes chronic inflammation and releases inflammatory cytokines in the liver, resulting in fatty liver disease, cirrhosis, and fibrosis, all of which increase the risk of liver cancer.
- *Diabetes.* Patients with diabetes who receive inpatient hospital care have a fourfold increased risk of liver cancer, which is attributed to high blood levels of insulin, insulin resistance,

fatty liver disease, liver fibrosis, cirrhosis, and chronic hepatitis infections common in severe type 2 diabetes patients.

What Is the Association between Omega-3 Fatty Acids and Liver Cancer?

- Omega-3 fatty acids may inhibit the transformation of hepatic cells to malignant cells.
- Omega-3 fatty acids force injured liver cells to commit apoptosis and thus prevent them from transforming into cancerous cells.

Meta-analysis

- *Omega-3 fatty acids.* A meta-analysis of nine research papers studied the association between omega-3 fatty acids and liver cancer. Analysis revealed that sufficient dietary intake of omega-3 fatty acids decreased the risk of liver cancer by 51%. In addition, regular consumption of fish was found to reduce the risk of liver cancer by 35%.

Recommendation

- *Prevention.* For people at risk of liver cancer, take daily 1 g omega-3 fatty acids (27).
- *Treatment.* For cirrhosis patients, take daily 2 g omega-3 fatty acids (27).
- *Treatment.* For liver cancer patients, take daily 2 g omega-3 fatty acids (27).

82

LUNG CANCER

Lung cancer is a form of cancer that begins in the lungs. It can metastasize and spread to other parts of the body. In the US, 117,000 people will suffer from lung cancer, and 140,000 of them will die from the disease this year. The number of people who die from lung cancer is greater than the combined number of people who die from colon cancer, prostate cancer, endometrial cancer, and breast cancer.

Lung cancer can be divided into three major types:

- *Non–small cell lung cancer.* Non–small cell lung cancer is the most common form of lung cancer; 85% of lung cancer belongs to this type.
- *Small cell lung cancer.* Small cell lung cancer is an invasive form of cancer that can readily spread to other parts of the body; 10–15% of lung cancer is of this type.
- *Lung carcinoid cancer.* Lung carcinoid cancer is also known as "neuroendocrine lung cancer." Less than 5% of lung cancer

belongs to this type; it grows slowly and rarely spreads to other parts of the body.

What Are the Symptoms of Lung Cancer?
- Persistent coughing, which gets worse and more serious
- Expectorated sputum that displays abnormal colors or contains blood
- Shortness of breath
- Pain in chest, shoulder blades, and back
- Recurrent pneumonia and bronchitis infections
- Hoarse voice
- Weight loss
- Headache

What Are the Risk Factors for Lung Cancer?
- *Smoking.* Cigarette smoking is the greatest risk factor for lung cancer. About 90% of lung cancer is attributed to cigarette smoking. Cigarette smoke contains 60 known carcinogens, including aromatic hydrocarbons, n-nitrosamines, and volatile organic hydrocarbons. These carcinogens from the smoke can injure chromosomes and induce gene mutations in pulmonary cells, increasing the risk of lung cancer. In addition to lung cancer, smoking is also associated with oral cancer, pharyngeal cancer, esophageal cancer, urinary bladder cancer, kidney cancer, endometrial cancer, stomach cancer, blood cancer, and liver cancer.
- *Radon.* Radon is a radioactive gas released naturally from igneous rocks. Radon gas, which is tasteless and odorless, can emit alpha radiation. Upon being inhaled into the lungs, alpha radiation from radon gas injures lung cells and causes DNA breakage and gene mutations of pulmonary cells. One of every 15 houses in the US has an unsafe level of radon gas.
- *Asbestos.* Asbestos in the air enters the lungs and causes injuries to the cells and tissues of the lungs. It accumulates in the pleural mesothelial layer of the lungs and induces mesothelioma.

Asbestos in alveoli cells affects cell division and induces abnormalities in the chromosomes of alveoli cells, leading to lung cancer.

- *Arsenic.* Arsenic, a known carcinogen, comes from contaminated drinking water. Drinking arsenic-contaminated water is one of the reasons some nonsmokers are afflicted with lung cancer.
- *Diesel.* Exhaust from diesel engines contains carcinogens. Workers who are exposed to exhaust from diesel engines—such as railroad workers, operators of heavy machinery, miners, and truck drivers—have an increased risk of lung cancer.

What Is the Association between Vitamin A and Lung Cancer?

- Vitamin A supports the methylation of DNA and controls gene expression in the cell. Insufficient DNA methylation is a salient characteristic of cancerous cells.
- Vitamin A enhances the lungs' ability to produce carcinogen-degrading enzymes that can detoxify airborne carcinogens and decrease the risk of lung cancer.
- Vitamin A deficiency increases the risk that epithelial cells in the trachea and bronchi will transform into cancerous cells.
- Toxic chemicals from cigarette smoke induce the lungs to produce free radicals, which can deplete vitamin A contents stored in pulmonary cells. Vitamin A deficiency increases the risk of lung cancer.

What Is the Association between Vitamin C and Lung Cancer?

- Vitamin C increases collagen production in the lungs. Collagens form a wall-like structure to block cancerous cells from migrating into neighboring cells. In addition, cancerous cells cannot migrate through an intact layer of hyaluronic acid located in the interstitial space between lung cells. To circumvent the situation, cancerous cells release enzymes that degrade the hyaluronic layer. Vitamin C inhibits a cancerous cell's ability to degrade the hyaluronic acid layer and prevents the migration of cancerous cells in the lungs.

- High-dose IV vitamin C therapy is an effective treatment for cancer, particularly in late-stage cancer patients. (See chapter 47, "Breast Cancer," for details.)

What Is the Association between Vitamin D and Lung Cancer?

- Vitamin D has anticancer properties. It inhibits a cancer cell's ability to produce cyclin protein, a protein that allows cancer cells to divide and proliferate. In addition, vascular endothelial growth factor is a protein that activates the formation of new blood vessels in cancerous lesions. Vitamin D inhibits the production of vascular endothelial growth factor and blocks the formation of new blood vessels in cancerous lesions in the lungs.
- Low blood levels of vitamin D increase the risk of lung cancer. Sufficient dietary intake of vitamin D was found to improve the survival rate of patients with lung cancer. Sun exposure and supplementation with vitamin D alleviate the symptoms of lung cancer.

What Is the Association between Vitamin E and Lung Cancer?

- Vitamin E activates transcriptional factors in the cytoplasm, enhances the cell nucleus's ability to produce more antioxidant enzymes and glutathione, and heightens cellular antioxidant capacity.
- Vitamin E inhibits the lungs' ability to produce carcinogenic nitrosamines. Vitamin E quenches free radicals and prevents free radical–induced lipid peroxidation of phospholipids in the cell membrane. Lipid peroxidation leads to the structural instability of the nucleus and mitochondria, increasing the risk of tumor formation.

Meta-analysis

- *Vitamin A.* A meta-analysis of 19 research articles studied the association between vitamin A and lung cancer in 10,261 participants. The result confirmed that sufficient dietary intake of vitamin A reduced the risk of lung cancer.
- *Vitamin C.* Twenty-one research papers investigated the relationship between vitamin C and lung cancer in 8,938 lung cancer patients. The meta-analysis confirmed that sufficient dietary intake of vitamin C reduced the risk of lung cancer. Increasing daily intake of vitamin C by 100 mg was found to decrease the risk of lung cancer by 7%.
- *Vitamin D.* A meta-analysis of 12 research articles conducted with 288,778 participants investigated the relationship between vitamin D and lung cancer. Analysis revealed that higher blood levels of vitamin D decreased the risk of lung cancer. In addition, supplementation with vitamin D was found to reduce the incidence of lung cancer.
- *Vitamin E.* Eleven research papers evaluated the relationship between vitamin E and lung cancer in 4,434 participants. The meta-analysis confirmed that sufficient dietary intake of vitamin E reduced the risk of lung cancer. Lung cancer patients had lower blood levels of vitamin E compared to healthy controls.

Recommendation

- *Prevention.* For people at risk of lung cancer, take daily 2,000 IU vitamin A (1), 200 mg vitamin C (10), 800 IU vitamin D3 (11), 30 IU vitamin E (12), and 400 mcg vitamin B9 (8).
- *Prevention.* For smokers at risk of lung cancer, take daily 2,000 IU vitamin A (1), 300 mg vitamin C (10), 1,000 IU vitamin D3 (11), 30 IU vitamin E (12), and 800 mcg vitamin B9 (8).
- *Treatment.* For lung cancer patients, take daily 5,000 IU vitamin A (1), 500 mg vitamin C (10), 2,000 IU vitamin D3 (11), 100 IU vitamin E (12), and 800 mcg vitamin B9 (8).

83

LUPUS ERYTHEMATOSUS

Lupus erythematosus is a collection of autoimmune diseases in which the immune system attacks various organs in the body, like the lungs, liver, kidneys, skin, joints, heart, and nervous system, mistaking them as foreign. These erroneous attacks by the immune system cause injuries to the cells and tissues in the abovementioned organs. In the US, 480,000 people are afflicted with lupus erythematosus.

What Are the Symptoms of Lupus Erythematosus?
- Muscle pain (sometimes even breathing can lead to chest pain)
- Anemia, fatigue, and malaise
- Lack of appetite
- Sensitivity to sun exposure
- Scaly rashes on the skin
- Joint stiffness

- Bloody urine
- Skin rashes on the cheekbones
- Dry mouth and ulceration in the oral cavity
- Hair loss
- Edema in the hands and feet

What Are the Causes of Lupus Erythematosus?

The cause of lupus erythematosus is not clear at present. Both genes and environment are thought to play roles in the cause of the disease. Since 90% of lupus erythematosus patients are women, hormonal involvement cannot be ignored. Lupus erythematosus is also likely linked to environmental factors that stimulate the expression of predisposed disease-causing genes.

What Are the Risk Factors for Lupus Erythematosus?

- *Gender.* About 90% of lupus erythematosus patients are women of childbearing age. However, postmenopausal women have only a 2.5 times increased risk of the disease compared to men.
- *Ultraviolet B.* People whose skin turns red and swollen instead of darkening after sun exposure have a higher risk of lupus erythematosus.
- *Family and genetics.* Having a parent or sibling who has suffered from lupus erythematosus increases your risk. Gene mutations in human lymphocyte antigens, or HLAs, increase the incidence of lupus erythematosus. HLAs are responsible for differentiating self from nonself. Gene mutations of HLAs dismantle this defense mechanism, leading to immune cells erroneously attacking their own cells and tissues, causing lupus erythematosus.
- *Thrombotic thrombocytopenia purpura.* Thrombotic thrombocytopenia purpura is a rare genetic disease in children. Thrombotic thrombocytopenia purpura is common in children who suffer from lupus erythematosus.

- *Medications.* More than 40 drugs—including hydrochlorothiazide- and angiotensin-converting enzyme inhibitors and the like—are known to increase the risk of lupus erythematosus.
- *Viral infection.* Viral infections—such as Epstein-Barr virus, cytomegalovirus, and parvovirus B-19—heighten the risk of lupus erythematosus.
- *Chemicals.* Crystalline silica and chlorinated pesticides are two known chemicals that may induce lupus erythematosus.

What Is the Association between Vitamin D and Lupus Erythematosus?

- Lupus erythematosus patients have lower blood levels of vitamin D compared to healthy individuals. Studies have shown that low blood levels of vitamin D significantly elevated the risk of lupus erythematosus. Lupus erythematosus patients with sufficient blood levels of vitamin D have fewer flares and better control over the disease's symptoms.
- Lupus erythematosus patients tend to avoid outdoor activities because of sensitivity to sun exposure. However, avoidance of sun exposure can exacerbate vitamin D deficiency as well as the symptoms of the disease.
- Vitamin D inhibits the immune system's ability to produce autoimmune antibodies, enhances innate immunity, and prevents adaptive immunity. Adaptive immunity disorder is the major cause of lupus erythematosus.

Meta-analysis

- *Vitamin D.* A meta-analysis of 11 research articles explored the relationship between vitamin D and lupus erythematosus. Analysis confirmed that low blood levels of vitamin D exacerbated the symptoms of lupus erythematosus, while high blood levels of vitamin D alleviated the symptoms of the disease.

Recommendation
- *Prevention.* For people at risk of lupus erythematosus, take daily 800 IU vitamin D3 (11).
- *Treatment.* For lupus erythematosus patients, take daily 2,000 IU vitamin D3 (11).

84

AGE-RELATED MACULAR DEGENERATION

The macula is an oval-shaped pigmented area near the center of the retina, a highly light-sensitive region located at the back of the eye. Its role is to present the images of an object to the retina before transmitting them to the brain via the optic nerve. The macula is responsible for sharp central vision for daily activities like reading, driving, and differentiating faces and details, whereas other parts of the retina are responsible for peripheral vision. Aging accelerates macular degeneration, causing blurred vision and, in severe cases, blindness. Age-related macular degeneration is the leading cause of blindness in elderly people. The incidence rate is higher in the US and Europe compared to other regions of the world. In the US, 10 million people are afflicted with age-related macular degeneration.

Age-related macular degeneration can be divided into two types:

- *"Dry" macular degeneration.* About 85–90% of age-related macular degeneration belongs to this type.
- *"Wet" macular degeneration.* About 10–15% of age-related macular degeneration belongs to this type.

What Are the Symptoms of Age-Related Macular Degeneration?

Symptoms of "dry" macular degeneration
- Need bright light to see objects close up
- Words or sentences become blurred while reading
- Colors do not look as bright as before
- Images are blurred near the center of one's vision

Symptoms of "wet" age-related macular degeneration
- Straight lines become curved or bent
- Closeup objects seem small in size and look as if they are distant
- A blind spot appears in images near the center of vision

What Are the Risk Factors for Age-Related Macular Degeneration?
- *Age.* Aging accelerates pathological changes to the macula. As we age, our bodies produce fewer antioxidants to defend against the surge of harmful free radicals that damage organs and tissues, including the macula. Free radical–induced oxidative damage is the culprit in age-related macular degeneration.
- *Smoking.* Cigarette smoke contains toxic chemicals that enter the bloodstream and travel to the eyes. These harmful chemicals injure blood vessels near the macula. Tar, a toxic chemical from the smoke, enters the retina and causes pathological changes, including to the macula.
- *Ultraviolet B.* Ultraviolet B radiation from the sun's rays induces a surge of free radical production in the eyes. If unabated, these harmful free radicals can damage the eyes. Although the

cornea and lens provide certain shielding protection, ultraviolet radiation can reach the retina and macula at the back of the eye. Excessive sun exposure increases the risk of age-related macular degeneration.

- *Cardiovascular disease.* Hypertension and atherosclerosis are common in patients with cardiovascular diseases. Hypertension and atherosclerosis damage the blood vessels of the eyes and heighten the risk of age-related macular degeneration.
- *Race.* People with light-colored eyes and fair skin have a higher risk of age-related macular degeneration compared to people with darker eyes and darker skin.
- *Obesity.* Obesity is associated with chronic inflammation, hypercholesterolemia, and cardiovascular disease, all of which are risk factors for age-related macular degeneration.
- *Lack of exercise.* Regular exercise reduces abdominal fat; prevents hypertension, inflammation, and endothelial dysfunction; and boosts "good" cholesterol levels in the blood, thus reducing the risk of age-related macular degeneration. Lack of physical activity increases the risk of age-related macular degeneration in elderly people.
- *Hypertension.* Hypertension induces the formation of new blood vessels in the choroid layer of the eye, leading to epithelial atrophy in the eyes and increasing the risk of age-related macular degeneration.
- *Pathological myopia.* Pathological or degenerative myopia is different from ordinary myopia. The former is when an individual is severely nearsighted and has a noticeably elongated eyeball. About 2% of people have pathological myopia in the US. The incidence rates in China, Japan, the Middle East, and Israel are higher than in the US. An elongated eyeball causes a fissure near the bottom of the retina. Frequent bleeding in the fissure region leads to scar formation and growth of new blood vessels. Structural changes to the macula in pathological myopia resemble those in age-related macular degeneration.

What Is the Association between Vitamins B9 and B12 and Age-Related Macular Degeneration?

- Vitamin B9 and vitamin B12 can lower the blood level of homocysteine. High blood levels of homocysteine are a known risk factor for age-related macular degeneration.
- Homocysteine is a strong oxidant that can induce atherosclerosis and other cardiovascular diseases, increasing the risk of age-related macular degeneration. Supplementation with vitamins B9 and B12 lowers the blood level of homocysteine and reduces the risk of age-related macular degeneration.

Meta-analysis

- *Vitamin B9 and vitamin B12.* A meta-analysis of 11 research articles studied the association between vitamins B9 and B12 and age-related macular degeneration in 1,072 patients with age-related macular degeneration and 1,202 healthy individuals. Analysis confirmed that patients with age-related macular degeneration had higher blood levels of homocysteine and lower blood levels of vitamin B9 and vitamin B12 compared to healthy controls.

Recommendation

- *Prevention.* For people aged 55 and older at risk of age-related macular degeneration, take daily 400 mcg vitamin B9 (8) and 100 mcg vitamin B12 (9).
- *Treatment.* For age-related macular degeneration patients, take daily 800 mcg vitamin B9 (8) and 400 mcg vitamin B12 (9).

85

MALE INFERTILITY

Infertility is defined as the inability to conceive after sexual intercourse with the same partner within one year. Infertility affects about 12% of couples, and male infertility is the cause of 50% of those cases. Almost 4 million people aged 15–45 suffer from male infertility in the US. The cause of male infertility may include low sperm count, poor sperm quality, or the occlusion of sperm ducts. Globally, 47 million couples have infertility problems.

What Are the Symptoms of Male Infertility?
- Low sperm count in ejaculate
- Diluted appearance of semen
- Impotence
- Premature ejaculation
- Lack of libido
- Pain in testicles
- Loss of sense of smell

- Enlarged breasts
- Hairless face and body

What Are the Risk Factors for Male Infertility?

- *Smoking.* Cigarette smoke contains harmful chemicals that enter the bloodstream and travel to the male reproductive organs, where these toxic chemicals can directly injure sperm and reduce sperm quality. Smoking is a major risk factor for male infertility.
- *Alcohol.* The male reproductive system consists of the hypothalamus, the pituitary gland, and the testicles. Alcohol from alcoholic beverages interferes with normal functioning of these organs and induces impotence and infertility. In the testicles, alcohol lowers testosterone production from Leydig cells. Heavy consumption of alcohol reduces the blood level of testosterone. Alcohol also blocks the maturation of sperm and decreases sperm quality. In the hypothalamus and pituitary gland, alcohol inhibits the production of hormones related to male reproduction and brings on impotence and male infertility.
- *Obesity.* Obesity increases the risk of male infertility. Obesity reduces semen quality, alters protein contents in the sperm, and leads to erectile dysfunction. In addition, obesity can change the ratio of hormones in the male reproductive system and raise the temperature in the scrotum, both of which are risk factors for male infertility.

What Is the Association between Zinc and Male Infertility?

- Zinc ions have antioxidant functions. They prevent free radical–induced damage to the sperm and maintain sperm quality.
- Sufficient zinc ions in semen enhance membrane fluidity and the mobility of sperm. Zinc ions help maintain proper functioning of the prostate gland.

Meta-analysis

- *Zinc.* A meta-analysis of 20 research articles investigated the association between zinc and male infertility in 2,600 male infertility patients and 867 healthy individuals. The analysis confirmed that male infertility patients had lower zinc levels in their semen compared to healthy controls. Supplementation with zinc was found to increase ejaculation volume, vitality of sperm, the percentage of normal sperm, and the quality of sperm in the semen significantly.

Recommendation

- *Prevention.* For men at risk of infertility, take daily 10 mg zinc (20).
- *Treatment.* For male infertility patients, take daily 20 mg zinc (20).

86

MELANOMA

Melanoma is a type of skin cancer that develops from the transformation of pigment-containing cells, called melanocytes, to cancerous cells in the skin. The skin consists of three layers—namely, the epidermis, dermis, and subcutaneous layers. The epidermis layer consists of several types of cells, including melanocytes. Melanocytes produce melanin, a dark pigment that makes the color of the skin darken upon sun exposure. Melanoma is caused by the abnormal growth and proliferation of melanocytes. Certain kinds of melanoma continue to produce melanin, causing the tumors to appear black, but others cannot produce melanin, so the tumors appear pink or white. Melanoma affects various areas of the body, such as the face and neck. Melanoma is often found on the chest and back in men and on the legs in women. In the US, it is estimated that 760,000 people will be afflicted with melanoma this year.

What Are the Symptoms of Melanoma?

Moles on the skin are common and harmless. They are either brown or black in color and round or oval in shape. However, if some moles are different sizes, shapes, and colors compared to the others, it is imperative that you seek medical examination to rule out the possibility of melanoma.

- The edge of mole is blurred and irregular in shape and rough and dented in texture.
- The mole changes in size, shape, and color.
- The mole contains multiple colors, including brown, black, pink, and white.
- The color of mole bleeds onto neighboring skin.
- The mole is red and swollen and affects the peripheral region of the skin, turning it red and swollen as well.
- The mole is ulcerative and slow to heal.

What Are the Risk Factors for Melanoma?

- *Ultraviolet exposure.* Ultraviolet exposure from the sun's rays and tanning beds increases the risk of melanoma. Ultraviolet radiation induces a surge of free radical production in the skin, which damages DNA and causes gene mutations in the chromosomes of melanocytes, leading to melanoma. People with fair skin have a higher risk of melanoma compared to people with darker skin.
- *Moles.* Individuals who have more than 50 moles on their bodies have an increased risk of melanoma. The majority of moles are harmless and do not affect daily life activities, but a small number of moles may be susceptible to transforming into cancerous cells. For example, atypical moles—which are larger and abnormally shaped—are of particular concern, because they can develop into melanoma.
- *Family and genetics.* About 90% of melanoma is attributed to environmental factors, and only 10% is linked to genetics. Having a parent or sibling who has suffered from melanoma

increases your risk of the disease twofold. CDKN2A gene polymorphic variants are associated with melanoma. The CDKN2A gene encodes a protein that is responsible for controlling cell division. Mutations of the CDKN2A gene lead to uncontrollable cell division and increase the risk of melanoma.

What Is the Association between Vitamin A and Melanoma?

- Vitamin A repairs damage to the skin caused by ultraviolet radiation and reduces the risk of melanoma. Retinoid, a derivative of vitamin A, is an antioxidant that protects the skin and prevents the formation of melanoma.
- Melanoma patients have low blood levels of vitamin A compared to healthy individuals. Sufficient dietary intake of vitamin A can prevent melanoma.

What Is the Association between Vitamin D and Melanoma?

- Blood levels of vitamin D are lower in melanoma patients compared to healthy individuals. Maintaining higher blood levels of vitamin D decreases the risk of melanoma. Sun exposure makes the skin produce vitamin D, but excessive sun exposure can lead to melanoma.
- Vitamin D inhibits the proliferation and migration of melanoma cells. A low blood level of vitamin D exacerbates the production of inflammatory cytokines and the proliferation and migration of melanoma cells.

Meta-analysis

- *Vitamin A.* A meta-analysis of 10 research papers explored the relationship between vitamin A and melanoma in 233,295 participants, including 3,328 melanoma patients. The analysis confirmed that sufficient dietary intake of vitamin A curtailed the risk of melanoma.
- *Vitamin D.* Twenty research papers investigated the association between vitamin D and melanoma in 1,420 melanoma

patients. A lower blood level of vitamin D was found to be associated with a higher risk of melanoma.

Recommendation
- *Prevention.* For people at risk of melanoma, take daily 2,000 IU vitamin A (1) and 800 IU vitamin D3 (11).
- *Treatment.* For melanoma patients, take daily 5,000 IU vitamin A (1) and 2,000 IU vitamin D3 (11).

87

METABOLIC SYNDROME

Metabolic syndrome is not a disease but a collection of conditions related to physiological disorders, characterized by obesity, high blood pressure, high blood glucose, high cholesterol, and high triglycerides. People with three or more of these conditions are said to have metabolic syndrome, resulting in an increased risk of heart attack, stroke, and type 2 diabetes. Metabolic syndrome is also known as "insulin resistance syndrome." In the US, 52 million people are afflicted with metabolic syndrome, which is equivalent to 24% of all adults in the country.

Who Is at Risk of Metabolic Syndrome?
- *Obesity.* Obesity is associated with type 2 diabetes, hypertension, and hypercholesterolemia, all of which are risk factors for metabolic syndrome.

- *Little physical exercise.* Lack of regular exercise is linked to obesity, hypertension, and hypercholesterolemia, increasing the risk of metabolic syndrome.
- *High blood glucose levels and cardiovascular disease.* Hypertension and hypercholesterolemia are common in patients with high blood glucose levels and cardiovascular disease, both of which heighten the risk of metabolic syndrome.
- *Fatty liver disease.* Fatty liver disease is common in patients with insulin resistance. Insulin resistance leads to diabetes, hypercholesterolemia, and chronic kidney disease, raising the risk of metabolic syndrome.
- *Chronic kidney disease.* Chronic kidney disease is associated with hypertension, insulin resistance, and hypercholesterolemia, all of which elevate the risk of metabolic syndrome.

What Is the Association between Magnesium and Metabolic Syndrome?

- Magnesium deficiency is associated with metabolic disorder, a warning sign of metabolic syndrome.
- Magnesium concentrations in the blood are lower in patients with metabolic syndrome compared to healthy individuals. A low blood level of magnesium stimulates cortisol production, leading to metabolic disorders in the liver.

Meta-analysis

- *Magnesium.* A meta-analysis of 10 research articles studied the association between magnesium intake and metabolic syndrome in 30,092 participants aged 18–72. The analysis revealed that increasing daily dietary intake of magnesium by 150 mg reduced the risk of metabolic syndrome by 12%.
- *Magnesium.* Six observational study reports evaluated the relationship between magnesium intake and metabolic syndrome in 24,473 participants, including 6,311 metabolic syndrome patients. Increasing daily dietary intake of magnesium by 100 mg was found to decrease the risk of metabolic syndrome by 17%.

Recommendation
- *Prevention.* For people at risk of metabolic syndrome, take daily 100 mg magnesium (17).
- *Treatment.* For metabolic syndrome patients, take daily 200 mg magnesium (17).

88

MIGRAINE

A migraine is a recurrent, severe headache that often begins on one side of the head and then spreads to the other side of the head. The pain eventually engulfs the whole head. Migraine attacks are associated with nausea, vomiting, and an aversion to light, noise, or smells. In the US, 3 million people suffer from migraines, and the root cause is still unknown.

Migraines can be divided into two types:

- *Flashing aura migraines.* Flashing aura migraines are also known as "ocular migraines." About 30 minutes prior to a migraine attack, sufferers see a small blind spot with flashing lights or bent lines surrounding the blind spot.
- *Non–flashing aura migraines.* No small blind spot with flashing lights is seen before the migraine attack. Instead, sufferers might crave sweets and feel thirsty, lethargic, and depressed.

What Are the Symptoms of a Migraine Attack?
- Mood swings, confusion, and anxiety
- Stiffness in the neck
- Constipation or diarrhea
- Thirst and frequent urination

Symptoms of a flashing aura migraine attack include
- Seeing a small blind spot with flashing lights and zigzag lines near it
- Loss of vision
- Needle-like, piercing pains in the hands and feet
- Weakness and numbness in the face
- Inability to speak

Symptoms of non–flashing aura migraine attack might include
- Waves of pulsing pain in the head
- A headache that begins from one side of head and spreads to the other side and eventually to the whole head (sometimes the headache affects only one side of the head)
- Nausea and vomiting
- Dizziness
- Inability to stand still
- Fatigue and malaise
- Sensitivity to bright lights or noises

What Are the Risk Factors for Migraines?
- *Gender and age.* Migraines affect predominantly women. In the teenage years, the incidence rate of migraines is similar between girls and boys. At ages 25–45, migraines affect women three times more often compared to men. Female hormonal fluctuations during the perimenopausal period is a major risk factor for migraines.
- *Family and genetics.* About 70–80% of migraine patients have family members who also suffer from migraines. Genes are

linked to migraines. Gene polymorphic variants may cause neurological and vascular pathological changes in the brain of migraine sufferers.

- *Diet.* Foods that trigger migraine attacks include canned meat, hot dogs, ham, aged cheese, wine, artificial sweeteners, nuts, onions, papaya, monosodium glutamate, and chocolate.
- *Depression and anxiety.* Depression and anxiety are common in migraine sufferers; among them, 25% have depression, while 50% have anxiety. Depression and anxiety exacerbate migraines. Likewise, migraines aggravate depression and anxiety.
- *Stress.* Daily stress can trigger a migraine attack. Stress causes the brain to produce corticotropin-releasing hormones, which in turn stimulate the release of epinephrine and glucocorticoid in the bloodstream. These hormones reduce blood glucose levels, raise blood pressure, and increase the risk of migraines.

What Is the Association between Magnesium and Migraines?
- Magnesium ions prevent the optic nerve from transmitting erroneous messages to the brain that lead to a migraine attack.
- The constriction of blood vessels associated with a migraine attack can be prevented by magnesium ions that relax the constricted blood vessels in the brain. In addition, magnesium ions inhibit the production of glutamate, which is known to aggravate pain during a migraine attack.

Meta-analysis
- *Magnesium.* A meta-analysis of 10 clinical research reports studied the association between magnesium supplements and migraines in 789 participants. Analysis confirmed that supplementation with magnesium curtailed the incidence rate of migraines and alleviated pain during migraine attacks.

Recommendation

- *Prevention.* For people at risk of migraine, take daily 200 mg magnesium (17).
- *Treatment.* For migraine patients, take daily 400 mg magnesium (17).

89

MULTIPLE SCLEROSIS

Multiple sclerosis—characterized by the immune cells attacking myelin, mistaking it as foreign—is an autoimmune disorder. Myelin, a fatty white substance surrounding the outermost layer of nerve fibers, forms an electrically insulating layer necessary for proper signal transmission in the nervous system. The function of myelin resembles that of the insulating plastic layer wrapped around electric wires. Destruction of myelin in the nerve fiber disrupts signal transmission from the brain to other parts of the body and causes the deterioration of the nerve fiber as well as the permanent loss of its function. In severe cases, multiple sclerosis patients have problems with simple daily tasks, such as walking, eating, reading, and urinating. Multiple sclerosis is not contagious or fatal. The cause of the disease is still largely unknown. Both genetics and viral infections are linked to the disease. In the US, about 400,000 people are afflicted with multiple sclerosis.

What Are the Symptoms of Multiple Sclerosis?

The symptoms of multiple sclerosis vary individually depending on which areas in the nervous system are destroyed by the disease.

- In the early stages, blurred vision, double vision, distortion of the colors red and green, and even blindness in one eye
- Degenerated muscles in the extremities and thus the inability to stand or walk; in severe cases, paralysis
- Attention deficit and memory decline
- Trembling and slurred speech

What Are the Risk Factors for Multiple Sclerosis?

- *Age.* Multiple sclerosis often occurs at age 20–40. Almost 85% of multiple sclerosis patients have the relapsing-remitting form, in which the symptoms of the disease are mild and in a cycle of recurrence and remission. The condition may persist for 10–15 years. After that, 95% of the patients develop secondary progressive multiple sclerosis, which worsens the symptoms of the disease.
- *Family and genetics.* Having a parent or sibling who has suffered from multiple sclerosis increases your risk of the disease. Gene polymorphic variants are associated with multiple sclerosis, among which HLA-RB1 variants are the most well documented. HLA genes encode a group of proteins known as the human leukocyte antigen complex, which are responsible for differentiating self from nonself. Mutations of HLA-RB1 genes cause the immune cells to attack the myelin shield of the nerve fiber, mistaking it as foreign, leading to multiple sclerosis.
- *Infection.* The majority of multiple sclerosis patients were infected previously by the Epstein-Barr virus. Infection by the Epstein-Barr virus alone does not lead to any serious illness. However, mutations of HLA-RB1 genes together with the infection increase the risk of multiple sclerosis.

- *Vitamin D.* People who live at higher latitudes have an increased risk of multiple sclerosis. The higher the latitude, the lower the strength of ultraviolet B from the sun's rays, and the weaker the ability of the skin to produce vitamin D. Multiple sclerosis patients often have lower blood levels of vitamin D compared to healthy individuals. Vitamin D regulates immune functions and prevents autoimmune disorders. Vitamin D deficiency increases the risk of multiple sclerosis.
- *Smoking.* The role of the blood-brain barrier is to prevent harmful substances from getting into the brain. Toxic chemicals from cigarette smoke can injure the structural integrity of the blood-brain barrier, allowing leukocytes to enter the nerve cells and cause damage to the myelin shield, increasing the risk of multiple sclerosis. Smoking cigarettes can exacerbate the risk of multiple sclerosis, particularly in individuals with HLA-RB1 gene variants.

What Is the Association between Vitamin B12 and Multiple Sclerosis?

- Vitamin B12 can lower the blood level of homocysteine. A high blood level of homocysteine damages DNA and causes the premature death of nerve cells.
- Multiple sclerosis patients have low blood levels of vitamin B12 compared to healthy individuals.

What Is the Association between Vitamin D and Multiple Sclerosis?

- Lack of sun exposure may be linked to the cause of multiple sclerosis. People who live in higher-latitude regions where ultraviolet B from the sun's rays is weak produce less vitamin D from the skin. On the other hand, children with sufficient sun exposure have a lower risk of multiple sclerosis in adulthood. Moderate exposure to ultraviolet B from the sun's rays may prevent multiple sclerosis.

- Maintaining a high blood level of vitamin D alleviates the symptoms of multiple sclerosis.

Meta-analysis
- *Vitamin B12.* A meta-analysis of six research articles explored the relationship between blood levels of vitamin B12 and homocysteine and multiple sclerosis in 639 multiple sclerosis patients and 430 healthy individuals. The analysis confirmed that multiple sclerosis patients had a low blood level of vitamin B12 and a high blood level of homocysteine compared to healthy controls. In addition, vitamin B12 deficiency was found to increase the risk of multiple sclerosis.
- *Vitamin D.* Eleven research papers investigated the association between vitamin D and multiple sclerosis in 1,007 multiple sclerosis patients and 829 healthy individuals. The meta-analysis revealed that multiple sclerosis patients had a lower blood level of vitamin D compared to healthy controls.

Recommendation
- *Prevention.* For people at risk of multiple sclerosis, take daily 100 mcg vitamin B12 (9) and 800 IU vitamin D3 (11).
- *Treatment.* For multiple sclerosis patients, take daily 400 mcg vitamin B12 (9) and 2,000 IU vitamin D3 (11).

90

NEURAL TUBE DEFECTS

Neural tube defects are a collection of malformations of the brain and spinal cord during gestation. Under normal conditions, the neural tube of an infant is formed at 28 days after conception. A neural tube defect, characterized by the exposure of the brain and spinal cord, is a malformation of the neural tube. The majority of infants with neural tube defects die either in the womb or right after birth. The few that survive after birth often have multiple organ failure problems and live short lives. In the US, 1 in 1,000 new babies develops a neural tube defect. Globally, 300,000 infants are afflicted with neural tube defects every year.

What Are the Risk Factors for Neural Tube Defects?
- *Family and genetics.* Neural tube defects are linked to genetics. Genes have been identified to be associated with the cause of

neural tube defects, among which MTHFR gene mutations are well documented. The MTHFR gene encodes an enzyme that is responsible for converting homocysteine to methionine. Mutations in the gene disrupt this biochemical pathway and result in the accumulation of homocysteine in the fetal brain. Homocysteine is a neurotoxin. High concentrations of homocysteine in the brain increase the risk of neural tube defects.

- *Folic acid (vitamin B9).* Folic acid deficiency increases the risk of neural tube defects. Supplementation with folic acid for women before conception and during gestation reduces the risk of neural tube defects by 70%. Folic acid is involved in one-carbon metabolism, which supports the synthesis and repair of DNA in the neurons. Folic acid deficiency causes errors in the synthesis and repair of DNA, leading to gene mutations, increasing the risk of neural tube defects. One-carbon metabolic pathways convert homocysteine to methionine and decrease homocysteine contents in the brain.

- *Obesity.* Obese pregnant women have a twofold increased risk of giving birth to infants with neural tube defects compared to nonobese pregnant women.

- *Diabetes.* Pregnant women who have diabetes and have high blood glucose levels have an increased risk of giving birth to babies with neural tube defects. Glucose at high concentrations is a teratogen that disturbs the development of the fetus, increasing the risk of neural tube defects in the infants of pregnant women with diabetes.

- *Anticonvulsant drugs.* Pregnant women who take anticonvulsant drugs—such as phenytoin, carbamazepine, valproic acid, and aminopterin—have a greater risk of giving birth to infants with neural tube defects.

What Is the Association between Folic Acid
(Vitamin B9) and Neural Tube Defects?

- Folic acid is involved in the one-carbon metabolism that supports the conversion of homocysteine to methionine and prevents the accumulation of homocysteine in the fetal brain. The buildup of homocysteine, a known neurotoxin, in the brain increases the risk of neural tube defects.

- Sufficient dietary intake of folic acid during gestation prevents neural tube defects. Women who gave birth to infants with neural tube defects were found to have folic acid deficiency during gestation. But the neural tube is formed at 28 days after conception, and the majority of women could not even have known that they were pregnant during that first month of pregnancy. Even if they had known that they were pregnant near the end of the first month of pregnancy, it could have already been too late to supplement with folic acid. As such, it is recommended that women consider taking folic acid supplements before conception.

- Many countries have mandated food manufacturers to fortify certain food items—such as cereals, bread, and flour—with folic acid to prevent neural tube defects.

Meta-analysis

- *Folic acid (vitamin B9).* A meta-analysis of 123 research papers evaluated the relationship between folic acid fortification and neural tube defects. The analysis confirmed that the fortification of folic acid in foods such as bread and flour reduced the incidence rate of neural tube defects.

- *Folic acid (vitamin B9).* Five research papers explored the association between supplementation with folic acid in women of various races before gestation and the incidence rate of neural tube defects in infants in England. The meta-analysis has shown that European women gave birth to fewer infants with neural tube defects compared to Asian or Hispanic women. In these studies, European women were found to be more likely to follow the instructions to take daily folic acid supplements compared to Asian or Hispanic women.

Recommendation

- *Prevention.* For women at risk of having babies with neural tube defects, take daily 400 mcg vitamin B9 (8).
- *Prevention.* For pregnant women, before getting pregnant and during pregnancy, take daily 800 mcg vitamin B9 (8).

91

OBESITY

Obesity is a chronic disease in which the body stores an excessive amount of fat that causes a multitude of deleterious health effects. Obesity has the highest incidence rate, highest mortality rate, and highest medical expenditure of all diseases and illnesses known to humankind. In the US, 78 million people are obese, which is equivalent to almost one-third of the adult population. Obesity can lead to heart attack, stroke, hypertension, type 2 diabetes, and cancer, as well as a shortened life-span.

What Are the Causes of Obesity?
- *Energy imbalance.* The body converts food into energy. Energy balance means energy from food intake is equal to the energy needed for the body. Obesity occurs when energy from food intake is more than the energy needed for the body. Contrary to that, weight loss occurs when energy from food intake is

less than the energy needed for the body. Energy balance is required for body weight to be stable.

- *Little physical exercise.* Lack of physical exercise is common in modern lifestyles, as people watch television for hours, spend time on their computers, and drive instead of walk whenever possible. Lack of physical exercise induces energy imbalance and obesity.

- *Sweets.* Various food items and beverages contain high levels of sugar. Sucrose is the most commonly found sugar in foods and beverages. Sucrose is made of glucose and fructose. Glucose is converted to energy in all organs and tissues, including the brain, heart, liver, muscles, and others. Fructose is metabolized only in the liver, where it is converted into fat, part of which is accumulated in the liver, potentially causing fatty liver disease, and part of which is transported via the bloodstream and stored in fat tissues, such as in the abdomen and hips, causing obesity.

- *Family and genetics.* Obesity is caused by the interplay between genes and lifestyle, including eating disorders. Individuals who inherit obesity-related genes may have an increased risk of obesity, but it does not mean that they will inevitably suffer from the disease. Obesity is caused by both genetics and environmental factors. For example, habitual consumption of fried foods can trigger the expression of predisposed obesity-related genes and increase the risk of obesity.

What Are the Complications Associated with Obesity?

- *Type 2 diabetes.* Obesity increases the incidence of insulin resistance and type 2 diabetes. Fat tissues in obese people release a large amount of fatty acids, glycerol, inflammatory cytokines, and other chemicals into the bloodstream, which can lead to insulin resistance. Chronic insulin resistance injures insulin-producing beta cells in the pancreas. Insulin resistance and the death of beta cells are both associated with type 2 diabetes.

- *Myocardial infarction.* Obese people tend to suffer from hypertension and hypercholesterolemia, heightening the risk of blood clot formation and myocardial infarction.
- *Hypertension.* Obesity increases vasoconstrictor contents like renin, angiotensin, and aldosterone in the bloodstream, causing hypertension.
- *Cancer.* Obesity increases the incidence rate and mortality of colorectal cancer, pancreatic cancer, breast cancer, lymphatic cancer, and prostate cancer. It triggers the body to produce cancer risk factors, such as leptin, adiponectin, interleukin-6, and tumor necrosis factor-alpha. The abovementioned obesity-related cancers tend to develop near white adipose tissues in the digestive tract, pancreas, breast, lymphatic gland, and prostate gland. White adipose tissues cause cancerous cells to grow, proliferate, and migrate into neighboring cells.
- *Stroke.* Excessive abdominal fat increases the risk of ischemic stroke. Body mass index is often used in predicting the risk of stroke. However, recent studies have shown that abdominal fat is more accurate in predicting the risk of stroke compared to body mass index, particularly in young people. Obesity also raises cerebral blood pressure, reduces blood flow, and diminishes cerebral perfusion, all of which are risk factors for stroke.
- *Fatty liver disease.* Obesity is associated with fatty liver disease. In obese people, excessive fat is stored in the liver, leading to fatty liver disease.

What Is the Association between Vitamin D and Obesity?
- Vitamin D deficiency is common in obese individuals. Lipid-soluble vitamin D tends to be stored in fat tissues. Fat tissues may store a large amount of vitamin D, while the rest of the body is void of vitamin D. Weight loss can release vitamin D from fat tissues in obese people.
- Vitamin D deficiency triggers the parathyroid gland to produce parathyroid hormone, which causes the body to store fat

406 | The Vitamin Cure

in fat tissues. Vitamin D deficiency also stimulates appetite and leads to binge eating and obesity.

What Is the Association between Chromium and Obesity?

- Chromium has antioxidant functions. It reduces chronic inflammation in obesity. Chromium also raises insulin sensitivity and increases energy expenditure.
- Obese people have low blood levels of chromium compared to individuals at normal weights. Supplementation with chromium reduces body weight and prevents obesity.

Meta-analysis

- *Vitamin D.* A meta-analysis of 15 research articles studied the association between vitamin D and obesity in 3,867 obese people and 9,342 normal-weight individuals. Analysis confirmed that the majority of obese people were vitamin D deficient. Moreover, people who were vitamin D deficient were more likely to be obese compared to normal-weight individuals.
- *Chromium.* Eleven randomized controlled trials explored the relationship between chromium supplements and obesity. The meta-analysis confirmed that chromium supplementation significantly reduced body weight in obese people. The side effects of chromium supplementation were watery stools and headaches.

Recommendation

- *Prevention.* For people at risk of obesity, take daily 800 IU vitamin D3 (11) and 50 mg chromium (25).
- *Treatment.* For obese people, take daily 2,000 IU vitamin D3 (11) and 200 mg chromium (25).

92

ORAL CLEFT

Oral cleft is characterized by the lip or roof of the mouth not forming properly in the fetus. In an oral-cleft fetus, the deformation of the lip or roof of the mouth occurs during this critical period. Oral cleft, a birth defect, is linked to both genetics and environment. In Asia, 1 in 500 new babies has an oral cleft birth defect, while in the US, 1 in 2,500 new babies has an oral cleft birth defect.

What Are the Risk Factors for Oral Cleft?
- *Age.* Fathers who are aged 40 and older at conception increase the risk of oral cleft in their new babies by 58%. Likewise, mothers who are aged 40 and older at conception heighten the risk of oral cleft in their new babies by 56%.
- *Family and genetics.* Oral cleft is associated with genetics. Having a family member, even a third-degree blood relative, who has suffered from oral cleft increases your risk of giving birth to a baby with oral cleft.

- *Smoking.* A meta-analysis of 24 research articles confirmed that pregnant women who smoke cigarettes had a greater risk of giving birth to babies with oral cleft.
- *Diabetes.* Diabetic pregnant women have an increased risk of giving birth to babies with oral cleft. High blood glucose is a known teratogenic agent that induces pathological changes in the growth and development of the fetus in the womb, heightening the risk of oral cleft.
- *Anticonvulsant drugs.* Anticonvulsant drugs for treating epilepsy are often prescribed to treat neuropathic pain, migraines, and mental illness in pregnant women. Anticonvulsant drugs increase the risk of pregnant women giving birth to babies with oral cleft.

What Is the Association between Vitamin B9 and Oral Cleft?
- Intake of sufficient amounts of vitamin B9 may prevent pregnant women from giving birth to babies with oral cleft.
- Supplementation with vitamin B9 after conception curtails the risk of pregnant women giving birth to babies with oral cleft.
- Supplementation with vitamin B9 greatly reduces the risk of oral cleft in the babies of women who previously gave birth to babies with oral cleft.

Meta-analysis
- *Vitamin B9.* A meta-analysis of five research articles examined the relationship between vitamin B9 and oral cleft. The analysis revealed that vitamin B9 supplements, taken after conception and throughout pregnancy, significantly reduced the incidence of upper-lip cleft by 49% and roof-of-the-mouth cleft by 45% in newborn babies.

Recommendation
- *Prevention.* For pregnant women whose babies may be at risk of oral cleft, take daily 400 mcg vitamin B9 (8); the first and second months of pregnancy are particularly critical times.

93

ORTHOSTATIC HYPOTENSION

If you feel dizzy or faint when you stand up after sitting or lying down, you may have orthostatic hypotension. Mild orthostatic hypotension needs no treatment. However, if fainting occurs frequently, you will need to seek medical attention. Orthostatic hypotension can be diagnosed by measuring changes in blood pressure when moving from a seated or lying-down position to a standing position. You may have orthostatic hypotension if, within three minutes after standing, your systolic pressure drops by 20 mmHg or your diastolic pressure drops by 10 mmHg. About 5–30% of American elderly people suffer from orthostatic hypotension. An estimated 80,000 severe orthostatic hypotension patients require in-hospital care in the US each year.

What Are the Symptoms of Orthostatic Hypotension?
- Dizziness when standing after sitting or lying down
- Legs that are bent and weak
- Nausea and vomiting
- Fainting
- Blurred vision
- Fatigue
- Headaches

What Are the Risk Factors for Orthostatic Hypotension?
- *Age.* The older your age, the greater the risk of orthostatic hypotension. Orthostatic hypotension is common among people aged 65 and older. The heart and neck contain special cells that sense and regulate blood pressure. Aging deteriorates the function of those specific cells in the heart and neck and increases the risk of orthostatic hypotension.
- *Medications.* Many medications increase the risk of orthostatic hypotension, such as diuretics, beta blockers, calcium channel blockers, angiotensin-converting enzyme inhibitors, antidepressant drugs, anti–Parkinson's disease drugs, and drugs for treating erectile dysfunction.
- *Heart disease.* Patients with heart disease—such as myocardial infarction, heart failure, heart valve dysfunction, or irregular heartbeat—are unable to adapt to sudden changes in the position of the body.
- *Parkinson's disease.* The inability to regulate blood pressure is common in patients with Parkinson's disease. Parkinson's disease patients have high blood pressure when they lie down on their backs, and they suffer from orthostatic hypotension when they stand up. About 40% of Parkinson's disease patients have orthostatic hypotension.
- *Dehydration.* Fever, severe diarrhea, and extreme exercise may cause orthostatic hypotension. Insufficient intake of water on a hot day leads to dehydration, resulting in dizziness, fatigue, weakness, and orthostatic hypotension.

What Are the Complications Associated with Orthostatic Hypotension?

- *Falling down.* Falls and injuries can be caused by severe dizziness and unconsciousness.
- *Stroke.* Drastic changes in blood pressure lead to insufficient cerebral blood perfusion and stroke.
- *Cardiovascular disease.* Orthostatic hypotension increases the risk of cardiovascular disease.

What Is the Association between Vitamin D and Orthostatic Hypotension?

- Vitamin D and its receptor support the regulation of blood pressure in the cardiovascular system.
- Individuals with vitamin D deficiency have an elevated risk of orthostatic hypotension. Supplementation with vitamin D alleviates the symptoms of orthostatic hypotension.

Meta-analysis

- *Vitamin D.* A meta-analysis of five research papers explored the relationship between vitamin D and orthostatic hypotension in 3,646 participants, including 1,270 people with vitamin D deficiency and 2,376 healthy individuals. The analysis confirmed that orthostatic hypotension patients had lower blood levels of vitamin D compared to healthy controls.

Recommendation

- *Prevention.* For people at risk of orthostatic hypotension, take daily 800 IU vitamin D3 (11).
- *Treatment.* For orthostatic hypotension patients, take daily 2,000 IU vitamin D3 (11).

94

OSTEOPOROSIS

Osteoporosis is a chronic bone disease characterized by low bone density and fragile bones. Osteoporosis occurs when bone loss is excessive and the amount of newly synthesized bone is not able to replace it in the body. The back, forearm, and hip bones are most susceptible to fracture in patients with osteoporosis. The bones of osteoporosis patients are highly porous and look like beehives under a microscope. In the US, 44 million people aged 50 and older or about 55% of the adult population aged 50 and older are afflicted with osteoporosis. Osteoporosis is one of the major public health problems in the US.

What Are the Symptoms of Osteoporosis?
- A hunched back
- Reduction in height
- Back pain
- Neck and lower back pain
- Bone fractures

What Are the Risk Factors for Osteoporosis?

- *Age.* The bone is living tissue, where bone formation and bone destruction are taking place to actively maintain the homeostasis of the bone structure. Osteoblasts increase bone density, while osteoclasts lower bone density. In youth, osteoblasts are more active than osteoclasts, and bones become elongated and hardened. In old age, osteoclasts are more active than osteoblasts, and bones gradually lose density and become weak. Aging accelerates bone loss and increases the major risk of osteoporosis.

- *Gender.* Women have a fourfold increased risk of osteoporosis compared to men. Women with smaller frames have a greater risk of osteoporosis because any amount of bone loss can have a detrimental impact on the body. Likewise, men with smaller frames have a higher risk of osteoporosis. Low blood estrogen levels heighten the risk of osteoporosis in postmenopausal women.

- *Alcohol.* Consumption of alcohol in moderation may not be harmful to bone health. However, heavy consumption of alcohol during youth and adulthood can damage bones and lead to osteoporosis at older ages. Injuries to the bones during youth and adulthood are permanent and cannot be repaired, even abstinence from alcohol in later stages of life. Alcohol can inflict irreversible damage to the bones.

- *Lack of exercise.* Lack of regular exercise augments the risk of osteoporosis. Exercise strengthens the muscles, which can enhance the support and protection of the bones. Bone fractures from falls occur more often in elderly people who are not physically active.

- *Medications.* Glucocorticoids are a group of chemically related steroid drugs that include cortisone, hydrocortisone, prednisone, and dexamethasone. These drugs are commonly prescribed for treating asthma, allergies, and autoimmune diseases like rheumatoid arthritis, lupus erythematosus, and inflammatory bowel disease. Glucocorticoids are lifesaving drugs for more than 30 million asthma patients in the US. However, long-term use of glucocorticoids damages the bones and leads to osteoporosis. Other medications that may exacerbate osteoporosis include cyclosporine, thyroid hormone, heparin, methotrexate, and phenobarbital.

- *Family and genetics.* Osteoporosis is related to genetics. Having a parent or grandparent who has suffered from osteoporosis increases your risk of the disease. Gene polymorphic variants of vitamin D receptors and estrogen receptors heighten the risk of osteoporosis.
- *Vitamin D.* Vitamin D deficiency elevates the risk of osteoporosis. Vitamin D deficiency can lead to osteomalacia, characterized by weak and fragile bones. Vitamin D increases calcium absorption and mitigates bone loss.
- *Diseases.* Some chronic diseases like anorexia, chronic liver disease, chronic kidney disease, hypercalcemia, hyperparathyroidism, hyperthyroidism, and hemochromatosis heighten the risk of osteoporosis.

How Is Osteoporosis Diagnosed?
- Osteoporosis is often diagnosed by using a DXA (double-energy X-ray absorptiometry) scanner, which measures bone density in the hip, spine, forearm, and leg bones. By analyzing scanned data, health-care professionals can diagnose osteoporosis. Each DXA scan takes about 5–15 minutes and is rather safe because of low X-ray radiation exposure.

What Is the Association between Vitamin D and Osteoporosis?
- Vitamin D enhances bone density and strength and prevents osteoporosis.
- Calcium is the most important essential element in the bones. About 99% of calcium is stored in teeth and bones in the body. Calcium increases the strength and hardness of bones. Bones that contain sufficient amounts of calcium are less likely to break or fracture. Vitamin D is required for the absorption

of calcium in the intestines and for the deposition of calcium into bones. Without vitamin D, the body cannot absorb calcium from foods or deposit calcium into bones.

- Osteoporosis patients have lower blood levels of vitamin D compared to healthy individuals.

What Is the Association between Zinc and Osteoporosis?

- Zinc enhances the mineralization of calcium phosphates in the bone, increasing bone density and strength. Zinc is an essential trace element that supports calcium metabolism.
- Zinc deficiency induces bone loss and lowers bone density. Insufficient dietary intake of zinc is a serious global public health issue.

What Is the Association between Copper or Iron and Osteoporosis?

- Copper is an essential trace element that supports normal growth and development of the bones in the body.
- Iron is an essential trace element that supports the synthesis of collagen, a protein that makes up 99% of all proteins involved in supporting and maintaining the integrity and structure of the bones.

Meta-analysis

- *Vitamin D.* A meta-analysis of eight clinical research reports examined the association between vitamin D and osteoporosis in 30,970 participants. The analysis has shown that supplementation with vitamin D and calcium curtailed the risk of bone fractures, particularly in the hip bone.
- *Zinc/copper/iron.* Eight research articles investigated the relationship between zinc/copper/iron content and osteoporosis in 2,188 people. The result revealed that osteoporosis patients had lower blood levels of zinc/copper/iron compared to healthy controls.

Recommendation
- *Prevention.* For people at risk of osteoporosis, take daily 800 IU vitamin D3 (11), 500 mg calcium (14), 1 mg copper (22), 10 mg zinc (20), and 8 mg iron (19).
- *Treatment.* For osteoporosis patients, take daily 2,000 IU vitamin D3 (11), 1,000 mg calcium (14), 2 mg copper (22), 20 mg zinc (20), and 16 mg iron (19).

95

PANCREATIC CANCER

Pancreatic cancer occurs when malignant cells emerge in the tissues of the pancreas. Pancreatic cells can be divided into two major types, exocrine cells and endocrine cells. Exocrine cells are responsible for the production of pancreatic enzymes to support the digestion of foods in the small intestines, and endocrine cells are responsible for the production of insulin and glucagon, both of which are involved in controlling blood glucose levels. About 95% of all pancreatic cancers originate from the tumorigenesis of exocrine cells. In the US, an estimated 50,000 people will suffer from pancreatic cancer this year. The five-year survival rate of pancreatic cancer is only 3–7%.

What Are the Symptoms of Pancreatic Cancer?
- Jaundice (an early sign)
- Brown urine due to high bilirubin content
- Light-colored, oily stools

- Abdominal pain and back pain due to an enlarged tumor exerting pressure on neighboring organs and nerves
- Diabetes
- Venous thrombosis
- Itching all over the body
- Weight loss and lack of appetite
- Nausea and vomiting

What Are the Risk Factors for Pancreatic Cancer?

- *Smoking.* Smokers have a twofold increase in the risk of pancreatic cancer compared to nonsmokers. About 20% of pancreatic cancer is linked to cigarette smoking. Carcinogens in the smoke enter the bloodstream, travel to pancreatic tissues, and alter genes in the chromosomes. NNK (nicotine-derived nitrosamine ketone) is a known carcinogen that can cause point mutation in the DNA of pancreatic cells and elevate the risk of pancreatic cancer.
- *Obesity.* Obesity increases the risk of pancreatic cancer. It stimulates the production of growth factors such as insulin and insulin-like growth factors as well as the production of tumor growth factors such as leptin and adiponectin. Obesity is a chronic inflammatory condition, which facilitates the growth and proliferation of cancerous cells.
- *Type 2 diabetes.* Type 2 diabetes is the third-highest risk factor for pancreatic cancer. The first and the second are cigarette smoking and obesity. Type 2 diabetes is associated with insulin resistance, high blood insulin, and chronic inflammation, all of which can stimulate the growth and proliferation of cancerous pancreatic cells.
- *Age.* The older you are, the higher the risk of pancreatic cancer. Almost all pancreatic cancer patients are 45 years old or older, and 70% of all pancreatic cancer patients are 65 years old or older.

What Is the Association between Vitamin C and Pancreatic Cancer?

- Vitamin C can neutralize free radicals, prevent oxidative damage to DNA, and mitigate inflammation. Chronic inflammation is a risk factor for pancreatic cancer.
- Sufficient dietary intake of vitamin C curtails the risk of pancreatic cancer. Supplementation with vitamin C was found to prevent pancreatic cancer.
- High-dose IV vitamin C therapy may be an effective treatment for certain types of cancers. High concentrations of vitamin C generate hydrogen peroxide, which kills cancerous cells. (See chapter 47, "Breast Cancer," for details.)

What Is the Association between Vitamin E and Pancreatic Cancer?

- Lipid-soluble vitamin E quenches free radicals in the cell membrane, prevents free radical–induced oxidative damage to the cell membrane and genetic material of DNA, and reduces the risk of tumorigenesis. Vitamin E has anti-inflammatory and anticancer functions. It mitigates inflammation and inhibits the growth and proliferation of cancerous pancreatic cells.
- Pancreatic cancer patients have low blood levels of vitamin E compared to healthy individuals. Supplementation with vitamin E reduces the risk of pancreatic cancer.

What Is the Association between Folic Acid (Vitamin B9) and Pancreatic Cancer?

- Folic acid is an essential vitamin that supports one-carbon metabolism, a biochemical pathway that is crucial for the synthesis and repair of DNA. Folic acid deficiency precipitates errors in the synthesis of DNA and increases the risk of gene mutation and tumorigenesis.

- Pancreatic cancer patients have low blood levels of folic acid compared to healthy individuals. Sufficient blood levels of folic acid reduce the risk of pancreatic cancer.

Meta-analysis
- *Vitamin C.* A meta-analysis of 17 research articles studied the relationship between vitamin C and pancreatic cancer in 4,827 pancreatic cancer patients. Sufficient dietary intake of vitamin C was found to curtail the risk of pancreatic cancer.
- *Vitamin E.* Ten research papers examined the association between vitamin E and pancreatic cancer in 254,393 participants, including 2,976 pancreatic cancer patients. The meta-analysis revealed that sufficient dietary intake of vitamin E decreased the risk of pancreatic cancer by 19%.
- *Vitamin B9.* A meta-analysis of 10 research papers investigated the relationship between vitamin B9 and pancreatic cancer. The analysis revealed that sufficient dietary intake of vitamin B9 reduced the risk of pancreatic cancer. Increasing daily intake of vitamin B9 by 100 mcg was shown to curtail the risk of pancreatic cancer.

Recommendation
- *Prevention.* For people at risk of pancreatic cancer, take daily 200 mg vitamin C (10), 30 IU vitamin E (12), and 400 mcg vitamin B9 (8).
- *Treatment.* For pancreatic cancer patients, take daily 500 mg vitamin C (10), 100 IU vitamin E (12), and 800 mcg vitamin B9 (8).

96

PARKINSON'S DISEASE

Parkinson's disease is a chronic neurodegenerative disease. It progressively hampers daily activities, such as speaking and reading, and motor functions of arms and legs, such as standing and walking. Parkinson's disease can be divided into primary and secondary Parkinson's disease. The root cause of primary Parkinson's disease is still unclear, although it is likely linked to genetics. Secondary Parkinson's disease is caused by environmental exposure to toxic substances, such as pesticides and herbicides. In the US, 1 million people are afflicted with Parkinson's disease. Globally, 55 million people suffer from Parkinson's disease.

What Are the Symptoms of Parkinson's Disease?
- *Trembling.* It often starts with the hands or fingers. The patient involuntarily rubs his thumb against his index finger back

and forth. Trembling hands are a characteristic of Parkinson's disease.

- *Motor function decline.* As time goes on, patients experience decreased mobility. They tend to take shorter steps and, in severe cases, walk with one leg dragging the other immobile leg along.
- *Muscle stiffness.* Muscles in any part of the body can become stiff, affecting the range of motion.
- *Posture change.* Posture change causes a bent spine, making it harder to stand or walk.
- *Disappearance of automatic functions.* Automatic functions, such as blinking and smiling, gradually diminish.
- *Altered speech.* Speech becomes weaker, faster paced, and harder to comprehend.
- *Altered writing style.* It becomes difficult for patients to write even simple words, and written words become smaller.

What Are the Risk Factors for Parkinson's Disease?
- *Age.* Aging accelerates the degeneration of neurons and the impairment of repair functions, and it is the major risk factor for Parkinson's disease. Aging diminishes dopamine production and increases Lewy body disease and pathological changes in the nervous and vascular systems in the brain, all of which elevate the risk of Parkinson's disease.
- *Gender.* The incidence rate of Parkinson's disease in men is about 1.5 to 2 times higher compared to that in women. Estrogen hormones also seem to provide protective effects on women patients' brains. Women with Parkinson's disease are more likely to have trembling hands, but other degenerative conditions in women are milder compared to those in men. All in all, women with Parkinson's disease are less likely to be as affected compared to men with Parkinson's disease.
- *Family and genetics.* Having a parent or sibling who has suffered from Parkinson's disease increases your risk. About 15% of Parkinson's disease is linked to gene polymorphic variants,

such as LRRK2, PARK2, PARK7, and PINK1 gene variants. These genes encode proteins that support dopamine production and mitochondrial functions. Gene mutations affecting mitochondrial dysfunction can cause the loss of energy production and the surge of free radical production, leading to free radical–induced oxidative damage to neurons and Parkinson's disease.

- *Toxic chemicals.* Frequent contact with toxic chemicals, such as pesticides and herbicides, increases the risk of Parkinson's disease. Farmers have a greater risk of Parkinson's disease compared to city dwellers.

What Is the Association between Sun Exposure and Parkinson's Disease?

- Studies from Denmark have shown that people who worked outdoors in the sun were less likely to suffer from Parkinson's disease compared to people who predominantly worked indoors. Exposure to ultraviolet B from the sun's rays causes the skin to produce vitamin D. Vitamin D sufficiency reduces the risk of Parkinson's disease.
- The higher the latitude of one's home, the greater the risk of Parkinson's disease, because ultraviolet B is weaker at higher latitudes.

What Is the Association between Vitamin D and Parkinson's Disease?

- A lower blood level of vitamin D is common in patients with Parkinson's disease compared to healthy individuals. People with higher blood levels of vitamin D have a reduced risk of Parkinson's disease.
- Vitamin D reduces the risk of Parkinson's disease by activating the brain to produce BDNF (brain-derived neurotropic factor), nitric oxide synthase, and monoamine. In addition, vitamin D also supports the immune system and enhances the antioxidant capacity of the brain.

What Is the Association between Vitamin E and Parkinson's Disease?

- Vitamin E protects the cell membranes of neurons and prevents free radical–induced oxidative damage to the nervous system. Oxidative damage to phospholipids in the cell membranes of neurons causes the death of those neurons, increasing the risk of Parkinson's disease. Parkinson's disease patients have lower blood levels of vitamin E compared to healthy individuals.

What Is the Association between Vitamin B6 and Parkinson's Disease?

- Vitamin B6 lowers the blood level of homocysteine, a known neurotoxin. Overaccumulation of homocysteine in the brain can damage neurons and increase the risk of Parkinson's disease. Higher blood levels of homocysteine exacerbated the degenerative conditions of the disease.

Meta-analysis

- *Vitamin D.* A meta-analysis of seven research papers studied the relationship between vitamin D and Parkinson's disease in 1,008 Parkinson's disease patients and 4,536 healthy individuals. The analysis has shown that Parkinson's disease patients had lower blood levels of vitamin D compared to healthy controls. In addition, individuals with vitamin D deficiency (< 20 ng/ml) were found to have a twofold increased risk of Parkinson's disease compared to people with vitamin D sufficiency.
- *Vitamin B6.* Ten research papers examined the association between vitamin B6 and Parkinson's disease. The meta-analysis has shown that Parkinson's disease patients had a lower blood level of vitamin B6 compared to healthy individuals.
- *Vitamin E.* A meta-analysis of eight research articles explored the relationship between vitamin E and Parkinson's disease.

The meta-analysis confirmed that sufficient dietary intake of vitamin E reduced the risk of Parkinson's disease.

Recommendation

- *Prevention.* For people at risk of Parkinson's disease, take daily 800 IU vitamin D3 (11), 2 mg vitamin B6 (6), and 30 IU vitamin E (12).
- *Treatment.* For Parkinson's disease patients, take daily 2,000 IU vitamin D3 (11), 10 mg vitamin B6 (6), and 100 IU vitamin E (12).

97

PREECLAMPSIA

Preeclampsia, formerly called toxemia, is characterized by high blood pressure and high protein content in the urine and is a disease developed during pregnancy. The symptoms of preeclampsia usually occur around 20 weeks after conception. The majority of pregnant women with preeclampsia are able to give birth to healthy babies. However, the symptoms of some pregnant women with preeclampsia may be exacerbated to the extent that it threatens their own lives and the lives of their infants. In the US, 140,000 pregnant women suffer from preeclampsia during pregnancy.

What Are the Symptoms of Preeclampsia?
Initially, preeclampsia may be symptomless. High blood pressure is the most obvious symptom of preeclampsia. Other symptoms include

- Proteinuria, characterized by an excessive amount of proteins in the urine

- Edema in the hands, feet, and face
- Blurred vision, which gets worse with time
- Abdominal pain, particularly under the right side of the rib cage
- Nausea and vomiting

What Are the Risk Factors for Preeclampsia?

- *Diabetes.* About 20% of women with diabetes suffer from preeclampsia during pregnancy. High blood glucose leads to pathological changes in the cytotrophoblast layer situated in the connection region between mother and infant in the placenta and results in an abnormal placenta, placenta ischemia, and preeclampsia.
- *Obesity.* Obese women have a threefold increased risk of preeclampsia during pregnancy compared to nonobese women. Obesity stimulates the body to produce asymmetric dimethylarginine, an inhibitor of nitric oxide synthase. Nitric oxide is the strongest vasodilator in the body. Inhibition of nitric oxide synthase by asymmetric dimethylarginine diminishes nitric oxide production, leading to high blood pressure and preeclampsia.
- *Family and genetics.* Preeclampsia is related to gene polymorphic variants, such as CORIN, EPHX1, and STOX1 gene variants. Having a grandmother, mother, or sister who has suffered from preeclampsia increases your risk of preeclampsia during pregnancy. First-time pregnant women also have a higher risk of preeclampsia.
- *Autoimmune disease.* Preeclampsia may be related to autoimmune disorder, a condition that is common in women with preeclampsia. In addition, patients with autoimmune diseases, such as lupus erythematosus and rheumatoid arthritis, have a twofold greater risk of preeclampsia.

What Is the Association between Vitamin D and Preeclampsia?

- Vitamin D lowers blood pressure, boosts immune functions, and prevents the immune system from erroneously attacking the placenta and infant.
- Incidences of preeclampsia occur more often in the winter months than in the summer months because blood levels of vitamin D are higher in the summer compared to those in the winter. Vitamin D deficiency is linked to an elevated risk of preeclampsia in pregnant women.
- Supplementation with vitamin D at a dose of 600–800 IU daily was found to reduce the risk of preeclampsia in pregnant women.

What Is the Association between Calcium and Preeclampsia?

- Insufficient dietary intake of calcium may cause high blood pressure. Pregnant women with preeclampsia often have a low blood level of calcium. Supplementation with calcium at a dose of 1 g daily was found to lower blood pressure and prevent preeclampsia in pregnant women.
- Supplementation with calcium may alleviate the symptoms of preeclampsia by reducing blood pressure and preventing endothelial dysfunction, insufficient perfusion, and inflammation of the placenta in pregnant women.

What Is the Association between Selenium and Preeclampsia?

- Pregnant women with preeclampsia have low blood levels of selenium. Supplementation with selenium reduces the risk of preeclampsia during pregnancy.
- The symptoms of preeclampsia include high blood pressure, proteinuria, oxidative damage to the placenta, and inadequate body weight of the infant. Supplementation with selenium was found to reduce blood pressure and proteinuria and prevent oxidative damage to the placenta.

Meta-analysis

- *Vitamin D.* Seven research papers evaluated the relationship between vitamin D supplements and preeclampsia. The meta-analysis confirmed that supplementation with vitamin D reduced the risk of preeclampsia in pregnant women.
- *Calcium.* A meta-analysis of four randomized controlled trials investigated the association between calcium supplements and preeclampsia. The analysis has shown that supplementation with calcium lowered blood pressure in pregnant women, but it was not effective in preventing other symptoms of preeclampsia, such as premature birth and inadequate body weight of the infant.
- *Selenium.* Three randomized controlled trials examined the relationship between selenium and preeclampsia in 439 pregnant women. The meta-analysis has shown that supplementation with selenium reduced the risk of preeclampsia by 72% in pregnant women.

Recommendation

- *Prevention.* For pregnant women at risk of preeclampsia, take daily 800 IU vitamin D3 (11), 500 mg calcium (14), and 50 mcg selenium (26).
- *Treatment.* For pregnant women with preeclampsia, take daily 2,000 IU vitamin D3 (11), 1,000 mg calcium (14), and 100 mcg selenium (26).

98

PREMATURE MORTALITY

Premature mortality, or premature death, occurs when a deceased person's age is below the life expectancy of the country. For example, the life expectancy is 78.7 years in the US; therefore, if someone dies at age 50, he dies prematurely by 28.7 years. The research on contributing factors that lead to premature mortality, particularly in young people, is crucial for implementing effective public health policies. The five major causes of premature mortality are heart attack, cancer, chronic respiratory disease, stroke, and accidental injuries. In the US, 900,000 people die prematurely each year. About 40% of all premature mortality is preventable.

What Is the Association between Vitamin D and Premature Mortality?

- The relationship between vitamin D and the incidence and mortality of chronic diseases is a hot research topic. One billion people are known to be vitamin D deficient globally. Vitamin D deficiency contributes to many chronic diseases, including cardiovascular disease, diabetes, chronic obstructive pulmonary disease, Alzheimer's disease, lung cancer, breast cancer, and autoimmune diseases, such as rheumatoid arthritis and lupus erythematosus. Vitamin D has a multitude of functions; including regulating calcium and phosphorus homeostatis, strengthening the immune system, and stimulating secretion of insulin.

- Studies confirmed that people with lower blood levels of vitamin D had shorter life-spans and increased all-cause mortality by 15% compared to people with higher blood levels of vitamin D. Except accidental injuries, the other four contributing factors of premature death—heart attack, cancer, chronic respiratory disease, and stroke—are all related to vitamin D deficiency.

Meta-analysis

- *Vitamin D.* A meta-analysis of 12 research papers studied the relationship between vitamin D and premature mortality in 32,142 participants, including 6,921 people who died during the study period. The analysis confirmed that individuals with a lower blood level of vitamin D were more likely to die prematurely compared to individuals with a higher blood level of vitamin D. Supplementation with vitamin D to maintain the blood level of vitamin D at 20–34 ng/ml was found to significantly prevent premature death.

Recommendation

- *Prevention.* For people at risk of premature mortality, take daily 800 IU vitamin D3 (11).
- *Treatment.* For chronic disease patients, take daily 2,000 IU vitamin D3 (11).

99

PROSTATE CANCER

Prostate cancer occurs when prostate cells transform into cancerous cells in the prostate gland. The prostate gland is located beneath the urinary bladder and in front of the rectum. In youth, the prostate gland is about the size of a walnut. The older one gets, the larger the prostate gland becomes. The prostate gland secretes fluids that constitute a part of semen. Prostate cancer is caused by the tumorigenesis of fluid-producing glandular cells in the prostate gland. In the US each year, 250,000 men suffer from prostate cancer, the most common cancer in men. It is estimated that 1 out of every 39 men will die from prostate cancer in the US.

What Are the Symptoms of Prostate Cancer?
- Frequent urination, particularly at night
- Difficulty urinating (the urine does not come out or is difficult to stop once flowing)
- Urine comes out choppy and slow

- Pain when urinating
- Erectile dysfunction; pain when ejaculating
- Blood in the urine or semen
- Pain in the back and hips

What Are the Risk Factors for Prostate Cancer?

- *Age.* The size of the prostate gland increases with age. Aging elevates the risk of prostate cancer due to increasing gene mutation, decreasing immune functions, and declining prostate functions.
- *Family and genetics.* Genetics is linked to prostate cancer. About 5–10% of prostate cancer is hereditary. If your father has suffered from prostate cancer, it increases your risk of the disease by 2.4 times. Having a sibling who has suffered from prostate cancer increases your risk of the disease 3 times, and having two or more first-degree blood relatives who have the disease increases your risk 4.4 times.
- *Diet.* High consumption of polysaturated fats, such as fried foods, raises the risk of prostate cancer. Diets that lack antioxidant vitamins—including vitamin C, vitamin E, and omega-3 fatty acids—also exacerbate the risk of prostate cancer.
- *Chemicals.* Exposure to pesticides and herbicides elevates the risk of prostate cancer. Exposure to toxic chemicals and heavy metals, such as cadmium in the workplace, increases the risk of prostate cancer.
- *Smoking.* Toxic chemicals from cigarette smoke can elevate the testosterone level in the blood. Testosterone is needed for normal growth of the prostate, but an excessive amount of testosterone can induce abnormal growth and proliferation of cancerous prostate cells.
- *Prostate tumor.* People with prostate tumors have a greater risk of prostate cancer. Almost 50% of men have benign prostate tumors, which are mostly symptomless.

What Is the Association between Vitamin C and Prostate Cancer?

- Water-soluble vitamin C can inhibit the activation of carcinogens, such as nitrosamines, and the growth and proliferation of cancerous prostate cells. Sufficient dietary intake of vitamin C reduces the risk of prostate cancer.
- High-dose IV vitamin C therapy may be an effective therapy for treating cancer patients. High concentrations of vitamin C generate hydrogen peroxide, which in turn can kill cancerous cells in the body. (See chapter 47, "Breast Cancer," for details.)

What Is the Association between Vitamin E and Prostate Cancer?

- Sufficient dietary intake of vitamin E decreases the risk of prostate cancer. Prostate cancer patients often have a lower blood level of vitamin E compared to healthy individuals.
- Vitamin E has antioxidant functions. It quenches free radicals and prevents oxidative damage to the cell membrane and DNA in prostate cells, thus reducing the risk of prostate cancer.

What Is the Association between Selenium and Prostate Cancer?

- Selenium-dependent enzymes inactivate carcinogens and prevent carcinogenesis. Selenium-dependent enzymes can also degrade hydrogen peroxide and prevent it from causing oxidative damage to DNA and gene mutation, reducing the risk of prostate cancer.

Meta-analysis

- *Vitamin C.* A meta-analysis of 18 research papers studied the association between vitamin C and prostate cancer in 103,658 participants. The analysis confirmed that sufficient dietary intake of vitamin C reduced the risk of prostate cancer. Increasing daily intake of vitamin C by 150 mg was shown to significantly curtail the risk of prostate cancer.
- *Vitamin E.* Nine research articles investigated the relationship between vitamin E and prostate cancer in 4,004 prostate

cancer patients and 6,890 healthy individuals. The meta-analysis confirmed that sufficient dietary intake of vitamin E lowered the risk of prostate cancer.

- *Selenium.* A meta-analysis of 12 research papers evaluated the relationship between selenium and prostate cancer in 14,254 participants, including 5,007 prostate cancer patients. Higher blood levels of selenium were found to reduce the risk of prostate cancer.

Recommendation

- *Prevention.* For people at risk of prostate cancer, take daily 200 mg vitamin C (10), 30 IU vitamin E (12), and 50 mcg selenium (26).
- *Treatment.* For prostate cancer patients, take daily 500 mg vitamin C (10), 100 IU vitamin E (12), and 100 mcg selenium (26).

100

RENAL CELL CANCER

Renal cell cancer is a form of kidney cancer in which cancerous cells emerge in the tissues of the kidneys. The kidneys are two bean-shaped, fist-size organs located on either side of the back of the abdomen, just beneath the ribcage. The main function of the kidneys is to filter excessive water, salt, and wastes out of the blood and into the urine. Other functions of the kidneys include regulating blood pressure and assisting the bone marrow in producing new red blood cells. Renal cell cancer is the most common kidney cancer in adults, while Wilms tumor is the most common kidney tumor in children. In the US, 60,000 people will suffer from renal cell cancer this year.

What Are the Symptoms of Renal Cell Cancer?
At early stages, renal cell cancer is symptomless. Symptoms appear only at a later stage. Renal cell cancer is often diagnosed using ultrasounds, CT scans, or MRIs.

- Waist and abdominal pain, particularly pain in between the upper abdomen and the back, lasting for several months
- Anemia
- Blood in the urine (pink, red, or brown)
- Weight loss
- Fatigue
- Persistent fever (not related to the common cold)

What Are the Risk Factors for Renal Cell Cancer?

- *Smoking.* Smokers have a twofold increased risk of renal cell cancer compared to nonsmokers. About 30% of renal cell cancer cases in men and 25% in women are linked to cigarette smoking. Carcinogens from cigarette smoke enter the bloodstream, travel to the kidneys, and cause injuries to renal cells, increasing the risk of renal cell cancer.
- *Gender and age.* The incidence rate of renal cell cancer in men is two to three times greater than in women. The disease often occurs from age 50 to 70.
- *Obesity.* Obese people have an elevated risk of renal cell cancer compared to individuals at normal weights. The greater your BMI, the higher the risk of renal cell cancer. The risk is the highest among individuals with BMIs over 30. Obesity is linked to chronic inflammation, high blood pressure, and diabetes. It stimulates insulin and insulin-like growth factor production. Obesity also augments glomerular hyperfiltration rates, causing damage to renal cells and heightening the risk of renal cell cancer.
- *Hypertension.* Hypertensive patients have a higher risk of renal cell cancer compared to normotensive individuals. Systolic blood pressure of patients with renal cell cancer is about 140 mmHg, which is 20 mmHg higher than that in healthy individuals. Hypertension induces a chronic hypoxic condition, which stimulates the kidneys to produce hypoxia-induced factors that support the growth and proliferation of renal cell cancer.

- *Medications.* Painkillers like aspirin, phenacetin, and ibuprofen can increase the risk of renal cell cancer.
- *Cadmium.* Exposure to cadmium in workplaces like battery, paint, and welding factories increases the risk of renal cell cancer.

What Is the Association between Vitamin B6 and Renal Cell Cancer?

- A low blood level of vitamin B6 is associated with a higher risk of renal cell cancer. Low blood levels of vitamin B6 exacerbate the symptoms of renal cell cancer.
- Vitamin B6 supports one-carbon metabolism, a biochemical pathway that is crucial in the synthesis and repair of DNA in chromosomes. Vitamin B6 deficiency causes one-carbon metabolism disorder, which leads to errors in the synthesis of DNA and increases the risk of renal cell cancer.

What Is the Association between Vitamin C and Renal Cell Cancer?

- A lower blood level of vitamin C is common in patients with renal cell cancer. Sufficient dietary intake of vitamin C can reduce the risk of renal cell cancer.
- High-dose IV vitamin C therapy generates hydrogen peroxide, which can kill cancerous cells in the body. (See chapter 47, "Breast Cancer," for details.)

What Is the Association between Vitamin D and Renal Cell Cancer?

- Vitamin D enhances the immune system's ability to defend against the growth and proliferation of cancerous cells. A high blood level of vitamin D was found to decrease the risk of renal cell cancer by 21%.
- Anticancer functions of vitamin D include inhibiting the formation of new blood vessels and preventing the migration of cancerous cells to neighboring cells.

What Is the Association between Vitamin E and Renal Cell Cancer?

- Lipid-soluble vitamin E quenches free radicals and prevents oxidative damage to the cell membrane and DNA in the nucleus and mitochondria. Oxidative damage to these cellular organelles in renal cells heightens the risk of renal cell cancer.
- Renal cell cancer patients have lower blood levels of vitamin E compared to healthy individuals. Sufficient dietary intake of vitamin E reduced the risk of renal cell cancer by 42%.

Meta-analysis

- *Vitamin B6.* A meta-analysis of five research papers explored the relationship between vitamin B complex and renal cell cancer in 133,995 participants, including 244 renal cell carcinoma patients. The analysis confirmed that sufficient dietary intake of vitamin E curtailed the risk of renal cell cancer by 17%.
- *Vitamin C.* Ten research articles investigated the association between vitamin C and renal cell cancer in 4,439 renal cell cancer patients and 10,580 healthy individuals. The meta-analysis revealed that sufficient dietary intake of vitamin C reduced the risk of renal cell cancer.
- *Vitamin D.* A meta-analysis of nine research papers evaluated the relationship between vitamin D and renal cell cancer in 130,609 participants, including 1,815 renal cell cancer patients. The analysis confirmed that individuals with sufficient blood levels of vitamin D were less likely to suffer from renal cell cancer compared to individuals with insufficient blood levels of vitamin D.
- *Vitamin E.* Thirteen research articles evaluated the relationship between vitamin E and renal cell cancer in 6,944 renal cell cancer patients and 465,275 healthy individuals. The meta-analysis confirmed that sufficient dietary intake of vitamin E lowered the risk of renal cell cancer.

Recommendation

- *Prevention.* For people at risk of renal cell cancer, take daily 2 mg vitamin B6 (6), 200 mg vitamin C (10), 800 IU vitamin D3 (11), and 30 IU vitamin E (12).
- *Treatment.* For renal cell cancer patients, take daily 10 mg vitamin B6 (6), 500 mg vitamin C (10), 2,000 IU vitamin D3 (11), and 100 IU vitamin E (12).

101

RESPIRATORY INFECTIONS

Respiratory infections generally include viral infections of the sinuses, throat, bronchi, trachea, and lungs. The major viral pathogens that commonly infect the respiratory tract are rhinovirus, influenza virus, adenovirus, and coronavirus. Respiratory infections are among the most common illnesses that cause people to seek medical attention. Travel-acquired infections account for about 20% of all respiratory infections. In the US, an estimated 62 million people are afflicted with the common cold, and 50 million people suffer from influenza viral infections each year. Among them, 40 million people are afflicted with respiratory infections.

Respiratory infections can be divided into two types:

- Upper respiratory infections, which include infections of the nose, sinuses, and throat, leading to tonsillitis, sinusitis, and laryngitis
- Lower respiratory infections, which include infections of the bronchi and lungs, leading to bronchitis and pneumonia

Infants are particularly susceptible to upper respiratory infections due to immature immune defense systems. Viral infections are contagious, and pathogens can easily spread through the cough or sneeze of an infected individual. Accidentally inhaling mucous fluids containing viruses from an infected individual can lead to respiratory infection.

What Are the Symptoms of Respiratory Infections?
- *Early stage.* Nasal congestion, runny nose, cough, sore throat, and fatigue
- *Later stage.* Difficulty breathing, dizziness, and confusion

What Are the Risk Factors for Respiratory Infections?
- *Poor sanitation.* Respiratory bacteria or viruses spread via person-to-person infections. People who do not regularly wash their hands are prone to catch influenza virus–related illnesses. Touching the nose, mouth, or eyes with dirty hands increases the risk of respiratory infections.
- *Malaise.* Lethargy caused by heart conditions, kidney disease, immune dysfunction, allergies, asthma, and pregnancy, for example, increases the risk of respiratory infections.
- *Smoking.* Cigarette smoking elevates the risk of respiratory infections. Harmful chemicals from the smoke inhibit the anti-infection functions of epithelial cells, macrophages, and dendritic cells in the respiratory tract. These smoke-related chemicals can also exacerbate the lethality and drug resistance of pathogens in the respiratory tract.
- *Age.* The older you get, the greater the risk of respiratory infections. Aging decreases air flow, weakens the muscles, and diminishes immune defense in the respiratory tract.

- *Air pollution.* Both outdoor and indoor air pollution raise the risk of respiratory infections. The sources of indoor air pollution include fuels used for cooking and heating, dust, and humidity-related molds. The sources of outdoor air pollution include exhaust from automobiles and dust haze, such as PM2.5 particulate matter.

What Is the Association between Vitamin D and Respiratory Infections?

- Vitamin D enhances the production of cathelicidin in the defense against pathogens. Cathelicidin exerts antibacterial properties by destroying the cell membrane of bacteria. Cathelicidin can also recruit immune cells to heal wounds caused by infections.
- Insufficient blood levels of vitamin D increase the risk of respiratory infections, particularly in elderly people and children. People with sufficient blood levels of vitamin D generally recover faster from respiratory infections compared to people with insufficient blood levels of vitamin D.

Meta-analysis

- *Vitamin D.* A meta-analysis of five randomized controlled trials studied the association between vitamin D and respiratory infections. The analysis confirmed that supplementation with vitamin D3 at a dose of 400–2,000 IU daily prevented respiratory infections.

Recommendation

- *Prevention.* For people at risk of respiratory infections, take daily 800 IU vitamin D3 (11).
- *Treatment.* For respiratory infection patients (including children), take daily 2,000 IU vitamin D3 (11).

102

RHEUMATOID ARTHRITIS

Rheumatoid arthritis is an autoimmune disease characterized by chronic inflammation of the joints, leading to deformity and immobility. Rheumatoid arthritis is caused by the immune system attacking the joints and other organs in the body, mistaking them as foreign, leading to painful and swollen joints, especially in the fingers, wrists, ankles, and feet. Chronic inflammatory arthritis can also damage the skin, eyes, lungs, heart, blood vessels, and the like. In the US, 1.5 million people are afflicted with rheumatoid arthritis.

What Are the Symptoms of Rheumatoid Arthritis?
- Joints become stiff, inflamed, and painful. Symptoms persist for a few weeks and suddenly stiffness and pain may go away. When symptoms recur after that, the disease begins worsening.

- Inflamed, stiff, and swollen joints often start in the fingers, wrists, and feet and gradually spread to the shoulders, arms, ankles, and knees.
- Common symptoms also include fatigue, malaise, depression, and light fever.

What Are the Risk Factors for Rheumatoid Arthritis?

- *Family and genetics.* Genes are linked to rheumatoid arthritis. People who carry PADI4 and PTPN22 gene polymorphic variants are prone to suffer from rheumatoid arthritis. The PADI4 gene encodes peptidyl arginine deiminase, an enzyme that supports the conversion of arginine to citrulline, and the PTPN22 gene encodes tyrosine phosphatase, an enzyme that supports signaling pathways associated with immune response.
- *Smoking.* Smoking cigarettes aggravates autoimmune diseases. Harmful chemicals from cigarette smoke can trigger the expression of genes related to rheumatoid arthritis. Besides rheumatoid arthritis, smoking increases the incidence of lupus erythematosus, multiple sclerosis, and Crohn's disease. Pregnant women who smoke have a higher risk of giving birth to babies that have an increased risk of rheumatoid arthritis during adulthood.
- *Breastfeeding.* Breastfed babies have a lowered risk of rheumatoid arthritis during adulthood.
- *Menstruation.* Premenopausal women with irregular menstruation and postmenopausal women have a higher risk of rheumatoid arthritis compared to healthy premenopausal women.
- *Gender and age.* The incidence rate of rheumatoid arthritis in women is three times higher than in men. Regardless of gender, rheumatoid arthritis often occurs at age 60 and older.

What Is the Association between Vitamin D and Rheumatoid Arthritis?

- Low blood levels of vitamin D exacerbate the symptoms of rheumatoid arthritis. Supplementation with vitamin D was found to alleviate muscle and bone pain in patients with rheumatoid arthritis.

- Vitamin D regulates both innate immunity and adaptive immunity and inhibits the autoimmune system. Vitamin D deficiency raises the risk of rheumatoid arthritis.

What Is the Association between Selenium and Rheumatoid Arthritis?

- Rheumatoid arthritis patients have lower blood levels of selenium compared to healthy individuals. Selenium-dependent enzymes display antioxidant functions by boosting immune functions and accelerating repair of injured tissues and organs in patients with rheumatoid arthritis.
- Selenium is an essential trace element that supports the synthesis of glutathione peroxidase, an enzyme that degrades hydrogen peroxide in cells. Excessive accumulation of hydrogen peroxide in the joints aggravates the symptoms of rheumatoid arthritis.

What Is the Association between Zinc and Rheumatoid Arthritis?

- Lower blood levels of zinc are common in patients with rheumatoid arthritis. Zinc supports growth, development, and repair in the body. Individuals with sufficient blood levels of zinc are less likely to suffer from rheumatoid arthritis.
- Zinc supports the anti-inflammatory and immune functions of leukocytes. Zinc deficiency affects the anti-inflammatory and immune functions of leukocytes and exacerbates the degeneration of joints in patients with rheumatoid arthritis.

What Is the Association between Omega-3 Fatty Acids and Rheumatoid Arthritis?

- Rheumatoid arthritis patients have lower blood levels of omega-3 fatty acids compared to healthy individuals. Supplementation with omega-3 fatty acid mitigates muscle and bone pain in patients with rheumatoid arthritis.

- High contents of omega-3 fatty acids in the synovial cells of the joints reduce the production of inflammatory cytokines and mitigate painful and swollen joints in rheumatoid arthritis patients.

Meta-analysis

- *Vitamin D.* A meta-analysis of 24 research papers conducted with 3,489 rheumatoid arthritis patients studied the relationship between vitamin D and rheumatoid arthritis. The analysis revealed that blood levels of vitamin D in rheumatoid arthritis patients were 5 ng/ml lower compared to those in healthy individuals.

- *Selenium.* Fourteen research articles investigated selenium contents in the blood along with rheumatoid arthritis in 716 participants. The meta-analysis confirmed that blood levels of selenium were lower in rheumatoid arthritis patients compared to those in healthy controls.

- *Zinc.* A meta-analysis of 26 research papers explored the relationship between blood zinc contents and rheumatoid arthritis in 1,444 rheumatoid arthritis patients and 1,241 healthy individuals. The analysis confirmed that rheumatoid arthritis patients had lower blood contents of zinc compared to healthy controls.

- *Omega-3 fatty acids.* Ten randomized controlled trials evaluated the relationship between omega-3 fatty acids and rheumatoid arthritis in 183 rheumatoid arthritis patients and 187 healthy individuals. Glucocorticoids are commonly prescribed medications for the treatment of rheumatoid arthritis. In this meta-analysis, supplementation with omega-3 fatty acids was found to reduce the amount of glucocorticoid medication needed to control painful and swollen joints in patients with rheumatoid arthritis. The dose of omega-3 fatty acids was 2.7 g daily for 3 months.

Recommendation

- *Prevention.* For people at risk of rheumatoid arthritis, take daily 800 IU vitamin D3 (11), 50 mcg selenium (26), 10 mg zinc (20), and 1 g omega-3 fatty acids (27).
- *Treatment.* For rheumatoid arthritis patients, take daily 2,000 IU vitamin D3 (11), 100 mcg selenium (26), 20 mg zinc (20), and 2 g omega-3 fatty acids (27).

103

RICKETS

Rickets is a bone disease characterized by bowed legs in children due to an extreme and prolonged vitamin D deficiency. Infants are most susceptible to developing rickets at 3–18 months. Abnormal bone development results in softened bones and deformity, particularly in the legs. Rickets is one of the most common childhood diseases in developing countries.

What Are the Causes of Rickets?
Rickets is caused by vitamin D deficiency. Vitamin D supports calcium absorption by the intestines. Vitamin D deficiency affects calcium intake, leading to retardation of the growth and development of the bones, as well as bone deformities, in infants.

Recommendation
Here are recommendations from the American Academy of Pediatrics:

- *Prevention.* For breastfed infants at risk of rickets, take daily 400 IU vitamin D3 (11).
- *Prevention.* For infants or children who consume less than one liter of formulated infant milk powders or whole milk at risk of rickets, take daily 400 IU vitamin D3 (11).
- *Prevention.* For adolescents who don't drink milk or have insufficient dietary intake of vitamin D and are at risk of rickets, take daily 400 IU vitamin D3 (11).

104

SCHIZOPHRENIA

Schizophrenia is a chronic mental disorder characterized by hallucinations, delusions, chaotic thinking and speech, and behavior that seems out of touch with reality. Eccentricities, disheveled clothing, poor sanitation, and lack of willpower and judgment are common in patients with schizophrenia. The onset of schizophrenia often occurs at age 16–30. In the US, 200,000 people are afflicted with schizophrenia. Almost 50% of schizophrenia patients don't admit they are ill and refuse to accept any prescribed medications from physicians.

What Are the Symptoms of Schizophrenia?
- Hallucinations, delusions, disorganized thinking, and deranged behavior
- Lack of facial expressions; joylessness
- Poor executive function, attention deficit, and lack of motivation

What Are the Risk Factors for Schizophrenia?

- *Family and genetics.* Schizophrenia is linked to genetics. Having a parent who has suffered from schizophrenia increases your risk of the disease by 47%. At least 100 gene polymorphic variants are associated with schizophrenia, but how these genes interact with environmental factors and lead to schizophrenia is still largely unknown.
- *Environmental factors.* Environmental factors such as stress, malnutrition, diabetes, viral infections, and smoking during pregnancy heighten the risk of children developing schizophrenia during adulthood.

What Is the Association between Omega-3 Fatty Acids and Schizophrenia?

- Omega-3 fatty acids support normal growth and development of the fetal nervous system in the womb. Omega-3 fatty acids have antioxidant functions and prevent oxidative damage to the neurons in the fetal brain.
- Schizophrenia patients have low blood levels of omega-3 fatty acids compared to healthy individuals. Insufficient blood levels of omega-3 fatty acids cause inflammation in neurons, increasing the risk of schizophrenia.

Meta-analysis

- *Omega-3 fatty acids.* A meta-analysis of 10 randomized controlled trials evaluated the relationship between omega-3 fatty acids and schizophrenia. The analysis revealed that supplementation with omega-3 fatty acids alleviated the symptoms in patients with early stages of schizophrenia. However, omega-3 fatty acids were shown to be not as effective in patients with late stages of schizophrenia.

Recommendation

- *Prevention.* For people at risk of schizophrenia, take daily 1 g omega-3 fatty acids (27).
- *Treatment.* For schizophrenia patients, take daily 2 g omega-3 fatty acids (27).

105

SEPSIS

Sepsis is a collection of complications caused by systemic bacterial infections. If untreated, it can lead to multiple organ failure and, in severe cases, death. Chronic illness or major surgeries can weaken immune defenses and allow bacteria to grow and proliferate in the bloodstream, resulting in systemic bacterial infections. Systematic bacterial infections trigger a strong immune response from the body. This can include the release of inflammatory cytokines like tumor necrosis factor-alpha and interleukin-2 and vasodilators, such as nitric oxide, in the bloodstream, which manifest as systemic hypotension, causing multiple organ failure and even death. Besides bacterial infections, infections by viruses and fungi can also lead to sepsis and septic shock. In the US, 900,000 people suffer from sepsis and septic shock each year.

What Are the Symptoms of Sepsis?
- Body temperature either too high (above 38.3°C) or too low (below 36°C)

- Heartbeat faster than 90 beats per minute
- Respiratory rate of more than 20 breaths per minute
- Leukocyte count either too high or too low
- Oliguria (reduced urine output)
- Thrombocytopenia (low platelet count)

What Are the Risk Factors for Sepsis?
- *Infection.* Bacterial infections in the lungs, abdominal cavity, digestive tract, reproductive system, and urinary system increase the risk of sepsis.
- *Illness.* Chronic illnesses—such as cancer, chronic obstructive pulmonary disease, diabetes, liver disease, and Parkinson's disease—increase the chances for bacteria to invade the bloodstream and cause sepsis.
- *Surgery.* Traumas or major surgeries that require intravenous infusions or artificial ventilators increase the risk of sepsis and septic shock.

What Is the Association between Vitamin D and Sepsis?
- Sepsis patients have low blood levels of vitamin D compared to healthy individuals. Low blood levels of vitamin D increase the mortality rate of patients with sepsis. Individuals with insufficient blood levels of vitamin D are susceptible to systemic bacterial infection.
- Vitamin D supports the production of defensins and LL-37 antibacterial peptides, both of which can kill bacteria and reduce the risk of sepsis.

What Is the Association between Selenium and Sepsis?
- Selenium-dependent enzymes have anti-inflammatory and antibacterial functions. Supplementation with selenium improves the survival rate of patients with sepsis.
- Selenium-dependent enzymes can degrade hydrogen peroxide and prevent free radical–induced oxidative damage to organs and tissues in patients with sepsis.

Meta-analysis
- *Vitamin D.* A meta-analysis of 10 research papers studied the relationship between vitamin D and sepsis in 33,810 hospitalized patients. The analysis confirmed that patients with vitamin D deficiency had an increased risk of sepsis during hospitalization.
- *Selenium.* Nine randomized controlled trials investigated the association between selenium supplements and the mortality rate of sepsis in 792 sepsis patients. The meta-analysis has shown that selenium supplementation reduced the mortality rate of sepsis patients compared to the placebo group.

Recommendation
- *Prevention.* For people who need to stay in the hospital for major surgeries or severe illnesses who are at risk of nosocomial infection and sepsis, take 10,000 IU vitamin D3 (11) for three days before hospitalization, and after that, take daily 2,000 IU vitamin D3 (11) during the entire hospital stay.
- *Prevention.* For chronic disease patients at risk of sepsis, take daily 800 IU vitamin D3 (11) and 50 mcg selenium (26).
- *Treatment.* For sepsis patients, take daily 400 mcg selenium (26) during the entire hospital stay.

106

SLEEP APNEA

Sleep apnea is a serious sleep disorder characterized by repetitive interruptions or pauses in breathing during sleep. The duration of the pause in breathing can be just a few seconds or a few minutes, and it may occur more than 30 times per hour. Sleep apnea causes poor sleep quality, sleepiness during the day, and poor work efficiency. In the US, 25 million people suffer from sleep apnea.

What Are the Causes of Sleep Apnea?
In the daytime, the larynx supports the trachea for smooth air passage to the lungs. In sleep, the larynx relaxes and the trachea becomes narrower. In healthy individuals, the narrowing of the trachea during sleep normally does not affect air passage to the lungs. In individuals with sleep apnea, the severe narrowing of the trachea during sleep can lead to obstruction and difficulty breathing. These factors contribute to sleep apnea:

- The muscles of the trachea and tongue are more flaccid in people with sleep apnea.
- Fat buildup in the respiratory tract causes the narrowing of the trachea in obese individuals.

What Are the Symptoms of Sleep Apnea?
- Loud snoring during sleep (however, not all those who snore have sleep apnea)
- Sleepiness during the daytime
- Headaches in the morning
- Dry mouth and tongue when waking up in the morning
- Irritability and mood swings

What Are the Risk Factors for Sleep Apnea?
- *Obesity.* The collapse of the upper respiratory tract during sleep leads to difficulty breathing in patients with sleep apnea. Structural changes as well as signal-transmission disorders between nerves and muscles in the upper respiratory tract contribute to the collapse of the upper respiratory tract during sleep. Obesity induces structural changes in the upper respiratory tract, making it easier for the trachea to collapse during sleep. Fat tissues in obese people also release adipokine, a protein that affects the signal transmission between nerves and muscles in the upper respiratory tract. Obesity increases the risk of sleep apnea.
- *Neck size.* The larger a person's neck size, the greater the risk of sleep apnea. Men with a neck size greater than 17 inches and women with a neck size greater than 16 inches have an increased risk of sleep apnea. Individuals born with narrow tracheas also have a higher risk of sleep apnea.
- *Hypertension.* Hypertension increases the risk of sleep apnea. Likewise, sleep apnea leads to hypertension. Patients with sleep apnea have higher systolic and diastolic pressure during sleep, and their blood pressure remains high during the daytime. Hypertension and sleep apnea are a vicious cycle.

Hypertension cannot be properly controlled if one's sleep apnea problem is not resolved.

- *Smoking.* Cigarette smoking elevates the risk of sleep apnea. Nicotine from cigarette smoke enters the bloodstream and travels to the brain, where nicotine causes the brain to relax the muscles in the respiratory tract and allows air passage to the lungs. During the day, nicotine enhances the breathing capacity of a smoker, but blood levels of nicotine precipitously drop during sleep. The lack of nicotine leads to the contraction of the muscles in the respiratory tract, causing smokers to have difficulty breathing during sleep. The rebound effect of nicotine withdrawal can lead to sleep apnea in smokers.

- *Diabetes.* About 50% of patients with diabetes, particularly men, are afflicted with sleep apnea. Insulin resistance and hypertension, both of which are common among patients with diabetes, add to the risk of sleep apnea.

- *Family and genetics.* About 40% of sleep apnea can exacerbate genetics. Craniofacial structure, distribution of fat in the body, and neural control of the muscles in the upper respiratory tract are gene-related contributing factors to the risk of sleep apnea.

What Is the Association between Vitamin D and Sleep Apnea?

- People with sleep apnea have a lower blood level of vitamin D compared to healthy individuals. Low blood levels of vitamin D aggravate the symptoms of sleep apnea.

- Vitamin D reduces the risk of sleep apnea by blocking the production of tumor necrosis factor-alpha, an inflammatory cytokine that is related to sleep apnea.

Meta-analysis

- *Vitamin D.* A meta-analysis of 11 clinical research reports examined the relationship between vitamin D and sleep apnea in 506 participants. The analysis confirmed that people with sleep apnea had lower blood levels of vitamin D compared to healthy controls.

Recommendation

- *Prevention.* For people at risk of sleep apnea, take daily 800 IU vitamin D3 (11).
- *Treatment.* For sleep apnea patients, take daily 2,000 IU vitamin D3 (11).

107

STOMACH CANCER

Stomach cancer, or gastric cancer, is caused by the emergence of malignant cells in the tissues of the stomach. The stomach wall consists of five different layers, and each layer contains a specific cell type. The innermost layer is the mucosa layer, which produces stomach acid. Stomach cancer often occurs when mucosa cells transform into malignant cells. Stomach cancer grows slowly, often without apparent symptoms in the early stages. Hence people suffering from stomach cancer may not know it until the cancer has already progressed to the late stages. In the US, about 26,000 people suffer from stomach cancer each year.

What Are the Symptoms of Stomach Cancer?
- Lack of appetite and weight loss
- Abdominal pain, particularly in areas above the navel
- Feeling of fullness after eating only a small amount of food
- Nausea, vomiting, and indigestion
- Low hemoglobin count

The above symptoms resemble those of the common stomachache. Seek medical attention to rule out any possibility of stomach cancer if symptoms persist for months.

What Are the Risk Factors for Stomach Cancer?

- *Age.* Stomach cancer often occurs at age 65 and older; in fact, about 60% of stomach cancer patients are age 65 and older. The older you get, the greater the risk of stomach cancer.

- *Helicobacter pylori infection.* Infection by *Helicobacter pylori* increases the risk of stomach cancer. About 95% of all stomach cancer patients are infected by *Helicobacter pylori*, which can cause inflammation in the mucosa layer and damage the DNA of mucosa cells. This may trigger the transformation of mucosa cells to malignant cells.

- *Smoking.* Cigarette smokers have a twofold increased risk of stomach cancer compared to nonsmokers. The smoke from cigarettes contains at least 60 known carcinogens, including nicotine. In the stomach, nicotine is converted to nitrosamines, which are known to induce stomach cancer.

- *Pernicious anemia.* Patients with pernicious anemia have a higher risk of stomach cancer. The nitrite level in the stomach of pernicious anemia patients is 50 times higher than that in healthy individuals. The high amount of nitrite induces the formation of nitrosamines, carcinogens that cause stomach cancer.

- *Blood type A.* People with blood type A have an elevated risk of stomach cancer, although the reason is not known at present. The risk is particularly higher in Asians, Hispanics, and Africans compared to Europeans.

- *Diet.* Habitual consumption of ham, hot dogs, and salted fish, as well as food items containing preservatives, such as nitrates and nitrites, increases the risk of stomach cancer.

What Is the Association between Vitamin A and Stomach Cancer?

- Vitamin A enhances cell division and inhibits cell proliferation and migration, reducing the risk of stomach cancer. Stomach cancer patients have lower blood levels of vitamin A compared to healthy individuals. Sufficient dietary intake of vitamin A was found to decrease the risk of stomach cancer by 40%.

- Vitamin A prevents oxidative damage to the cell membrane and protects the integrity of the mucosa cells. Vitamin A exhibits anti-inflammatory effects by inhibiting the production of inflammatory cytokines. The latter fosters chronic inflammation and heightens the risk of cancer formation.

What Is the Association between Vitamin C and Stomach Cancer?

- Vitamin C prevents the production of cancer-causing nitrosamines in the stomach. Supplementation with vitamin C reduced the risk of stomach cancer by 30–70%.

- *Helicobacter pylori* infections increase the risk of stomach cancer. Vitamin C inhibits *Helicobacter pylori* infections in the stomach. A low blood level of vitamin C is common among people infected with *Helicobacter pylori* compared to healthy individuals.

- High-dose IV vitamin C therapy may be an effective treatment for certain types of cancers. High concentrations of vitamin C generate hydrogen peroxide, which kills cancerous cells in the body. (See chapter 47, "Breast Cancer," for details.)

What Is the Association between Vitamin E and Stomach Cancer?

- Vitamin E forces cancerous cells to commit apoptosis (cell death) and inhibits the growth and proliferation of cancerous cells. Autophagy is a normal cellular process in which a cell dies and recycles its cellular components. Cancerous cells frequently use autophagy to elude immune defenses and allow neighboring cancerous cells to survive by absorbing the recycled cellular components of the dead cancerous cell. Vitamin E inhibits the autophagy of cancerous cells and decreases the risk of cancer.

- Stomach cancer patients have a lower blood level of vitamin E compared to healthy individuals. Sufficient dietary intake of vitamin E can reduce the risk of stomach cancer.

What Is the Association between Selenium and Stomach Cancer?

- Selenium-dependent enzymes exert anticancer functions by inactivating carcinogens, regulating cell division and inhibiting the migration of cancerous cells and the formation of new blood vessels in cancerous lesions.
- A low blood level of selenium is common in patients with stomach cancer compared to healthy individuals. Supplementation with selenium could curtail the risk of stomach cancer.

Meta-analysis

- *Antioxidant vitamins.* A meta-analysis of 47 research papers conducted with 1,221,392 participants studied the relationship between antioxidant vitamins and stomach cancer. The analysis confirmed that sufficient dietary intake of antioxidant vitamins decreased the risk of stomach cancer. Based on the dose-response analysis, the result revealed that antioxidant vitamins and their respective daily doses reduced the risk of stomach cancer as follows:
  - Vitamin A at a daily dose of 1.5 mg or 5,000 IU reduced the risk by 29%.
  - Vitamin C at a daily dose of 100 mg reduced the risk by 26%.
  - Vitamin E at a daily dose of 10 mg or 15 IU reduced the risk by 24%.

  The result from this meta-analysis confirmed that supplementation with relatively low doses of antioxidant vitamins could be a safe and effective approach to preventing stomach cancer.

- *Selenium.* Eight research articles investigated the association between blood selenium levels and stomach cancer in 17,834 participants. The meta-analysis has shown that individuals with high blood levels of selenium had a decreased risk of stomach cancer of 38%, and stomach cancer patients with low blood levels of selenium had an increased incidence rate of death from the cancer.

Recommendation

- *Prevention.* For people at risk of stomach cancer, take daily 2,000 IU vitamin A (1), 200 mg vitamin C (10), 30 IU vitamin E (12), and 50 mcg selenium (26).
- *Treatment.* For stomach cancer patients, take daily 5,000 IU vitamin A (1), 500 mg vitamin C (10), 100 IU vitamin E (12), and 100 mcg selenium (26).

108

STROKE

Stroke occurs when blood flow to the brain is blocked or a blood vessel is ruptured in the brain, leading to ischemia and the death of neurons in the affected regions of the brain. The severity of the stroke depends on the region of the brain where the stroke occurs and the degree of ischemic damage incurred. Minor strokes lead to temporary numbness in the hands or feet. Major strokes can lead to complete paralysis of one side of the body. Partial or even full recovery from strokes is now possible, given long-term rehabilitation. In the US, 800,000 people suffer from strokes each year, which is equal to one stroke every 40 seconds.

Stroke can be divided into two major types:

- *Ischemic stroke.* Blood flow to the brain is occluded by a blood clot, resulting in the depletion of the supply of blood and oxygen in a specific region of the brain. About 85% of strokes are ischemic strokes.

- *Cerebral hemorrhagic stroke.* The rupture of a blood vessel in the brain triggers cerebral hemorrhage and increases the cranial pressure of the brain, causing brain edema. Cerebral hemorrhagic stroke is linked to uncontrollable hypertension. About 15% of strokes are cerebral hemorrhagic strokes, but 40% of deaths from stroke are due to cerebral hemorrhagic strokes.

What Are the Symptoms of Stroke and How Should Bystanders React to Such Urgent Situations?

If someone near you experiences the following symptoms, you should recognize them and react to the situation as instructed:

- *Face drooping.* Ask the person to smile and see whether he has facial symmetry.
- *Numbness in the hand.* Ask the person to raise both hands and see whether he can do so.
- *Slurred speech.* Ask the person to repeat a simple sentence and see whether he can say it clearly.

If someone around you suddenly cannot perform any of the above items, call 9-1-1 right away.

What Are the Risk Factors for Stroke?

- *Age.* Stroke can affect any age group. After age 55, there is a twofold increase in your risk of stroke every 10 years. Almost 75% of strokes occur at age 65 and older.
- *Smoking.* Smokers have a two to four times higher risk of stroke compared to nonsmokers. The more cigarettes one smokes, the higher the risk of stroke. The relationship between the number of cigarettes smoked and the increased incidence rate of stroke is as follows:
  - 1–10 cigarettes daily increases it by 2.2 times
  - 11–20 cigarettes daily increases it by 2.5 times
  - 21–35 cigarettes daily increases it by 4.3 times
  - more than 40 cigarettes daily increases it by 9.1 times

Cigarette smoking can lead to blood clot formation and atherosclerosis, both of which are the major risk factors for stroke.

- *Hypertension.* Hypertension increases the risk of stroke. Hypertension damages the blood-brain barrier, leading to regional edema in the brain. Hypertension also injures the arterial wall in the brain and leads to the formation of brain aneurysms, heightening the risk of cerebral hemorrhagic stroke.

- *Heart failure.* Patients with heart failure have a two to three times higher risk of stroke. Heart failure is associated with blood coagulation and clot formation, increasing the risk of ischemic stroke.

- *Diabetes.* Patients with diabetes have a twofold increased risk of stroke compared to healthy individuals. Insulin resistance, blood clot formation, and atherosclerosis are contributing factors of stroke, and they are common among patients with type 2 diabetes.

- *Stroke.* Stroke patients who do not improve their diets and/or lifestyles have a greater risk of suffering from a second stroke.

What Is the Association between Milk Consumption and Stroke?

- A meta-analysis of 10 research articles evaluated the relationship between the calcium content of milk and the incidence of stroke in 371,495 participants, including 10,408 stroke patients for 14 years. The analysis has shown that people who consumed milk regularly reduced the incidence rate of stroke by 24%.

What Is the Association between Vitamin B Complex and Stroke?

- Vitamin B6, folic acid (vitamin B9), and vitamin B12 support the conversion of homocysteine to methionine and lower the blood level of homocysteine. Homocysteine is a known neurotoxin that damages the blood vessels and causes blood clot formation in the brain. A high blood level of homocysteine is a risk factor for stroke.

- Stroke patients have lower blood levels of B vitamins compared to healthy individuals. Supplementation with vitamin B6 and vitamin B9 reduced the incidence rate of both ischemic stroke and cerebral hemorrhagic stroke.

What Is the Association between Vitamin C and Stroke?

- Ischemic stroke causes cerebral damage by inducing cerebral ischemia—manifested by neuronal excitotoxicity and acute inflammation, leading to the death of neurons—and by ischemic reperfusion injury. Ischemic reperfusion injury occurs when oxygenated blood flows back into previously infarct regions, causing a surge of reactive oxygen radical production and subsequent oxidative damage to the infarct regions of the brain. Vitamin C quenches reactive oxygen species and reduces the risk of ischemic reperfusion injury as well as the rupture of the blood-brain barrier.
- Sufficient dietary intake of vitamin C decreases the risk of stroke. Supplementation with vitamin C reduced the incidence rate of stroke.

What Is the Association between Potassium/ Magnesium and Stroke?

- Hypertension is a major risk factor for stroke. Potassium and magnesium ions can lower systolic pressure as well as diastolic pressure.
- Stroke patients have lower blood levels of potassium and magnesium compared to healthy individuals. Sufficient dietary intake of potassium lowered the risk of stroke by 9%, and sufficient dietary intake of magnesium lowered the risk of stroke by 13%.

What Is the Association between Omega-3 Fatty Acids and Stroke?

- Omega-3 fatty acids boost the brain to produce brain-derived neurotropic factor (BDNF), a protein that nourishes the neurons and maintains neuronal functions, including memory, learning, and cognition. Omega-3 fatty acids also increase the membrane fluidity of the neurons to allow proper transport of nutrients and transmission of neural signals. Omega-3 fatty acids also reduce the production of inflammatory cytokines in the brain.

- Omega-3 fatty acid deficiency increases the risk of stroke. Supplementation with omega-3 fatty acids reduced the risk of stroke.

Meta-analysis

- *Vitamin B complex.* A meta-analysis of 17 randomized controlled trials evaluated the relationship between vitamin B complex and stroke in 86,393 participants. The analysis confirmed that vitamin B complex was effective in preventing ischemic stroke and cerebral hemorrhagic stroke. In order from highest to lowest, these were the most effective B vitamins in the prevention of stroke: a combination of vitamin B9 and vitamin B6; Vitamin B9 alone; a combination of vitamin B9, vitamin B6, and vitamin B12; vitamin B3 alone; and vitamin B6 alone.

  The analysis confirmed that vitamin B9 combined with vitamin B6 was the most effective vitamin B complex in preventing ischemic stroke and cerebral hemorrhagic stroke.

- *Vitamin B complex.* Eleven randomized controlled trials studied the relationship between vitamin B complex and stroke in 4,643 high-risk cardiovascular disease patients, including stroke survivors but excluding patients who took antiplatelet medications. The meta-analysis revealed that stroke patients with sufficient dietary intake of vitamin B6, vitamin B9, and vitamin B12 curtailed their risk of suffering from a second stroke.

- *Vitamin C.* A meta-analysis of 12 research papers conducted with 217,454 participants investigated the association between vitamin C and stroke. Daily vitamin C daily ranged from 45 to 376 mg for 6 to 30 years. The analysis confirmed that vitamin C supplementation significantly reduced the risk of stroke.

- *Potassium/magnesium.* Two major research papers studied the relationship between potassium/magnesium and stroke in 180,864 women. The study durations, including a subsequent observation period, ranged from 22 to 30 years. During the study period, 3,780 stroke incidences occurred among participants. The analysis confirmed that increasing daily intake of potassium by 1,000 mg reduced the risk of stroke by 9%, while increasing daily intake of magnesium by 100 mg reduced the risk of stroke by 13%.
- *Omega-3 fatty acids.* A meta-analysis of eight research articles evaluated the relationship between omega-3 fatty acids and stroke in 242,076 participants, including 5,238 stroke patients. The result revealed that supplementation with omega-3 fatty acids reduced the risk of stroke. The effect was particularly robust in women.

Recommendation
- *Prevention.* For people at risk of stroke, take daily 2 mg vitamin B6 (6), 400 mcg vitamin B9 (8), 200 mg vitamin C (10), 500 mg potassium (15), 50 mg magnesium (17), and 1 g omega-3 fatty acids (27).
- *Treatment.* For stroke patients, take daily 10 mg vitamin B6 (6), 800 mcg vitamin B9 (8), 500 mg vitamin C (10), 1,000 mg potassium (15), 100 mg magnesium (17), and 2 g omega-3 fatty acids (27).

109

TUBERCULOSIS

Tuberculosis is an infectious disease caused by infections of *Mycobacterium tuberculosis*, a bacterium also known as mycobacterium. This pathogen most often attacks the lungs, but it also targets the brain, central nervous system, circulatory system, urinary system, skeletal system, and joints, as well as the skin. If untreated, tuberculosis can lead to death. Every year, 1 million people die from tuberculosis globally. It is estimated that one-third of the world's population is afflicted with tuberculosis, and the majority of them become latent carriers of *Mycobacterium tuberculosis*. Latent tuberculosis or inactive tuberculosis may become active tuberculosis in immunodeficient individuals. In the US, about 9,400 people suffer from tuberculosis each year.

Tuberculosis can be divided into two types:

- *Latent tuberculosis.* Patients with latent tuberculosis do not show any symptoms of the disease.

- *Active tuberculosis.* Patients become ill from the infection. Active tuberculosis is contagious.

What Are the Symptoms of Active Tuberculosis?
- Persistent cough lasting longer than three weeks
- Blood in phlegm
- Chest pain from breathing or coughing
- Weight loss
- Fatigue
- Chills and fever
- Poor appetite

Who Is at Risk for Tuberculosis?
- Intravenous illicit drug users
- Health-care professionals
- Workers in homeless facilities, prisons, or nursing homes

Individuals who work with or live in close proximity to active tuberculosis patients have an increased chance of encountering the airborne infection through phlegm containing the pathogen.

What Conditions May Cause Inactive Tuberculosis to Become Active Tuberculosis?
- *HIV.* HIV infections can trigger inactive tuberculosis to become active tuberculosis. Patients with HIV have a 20 times higher risk of converting inactive tuberculosis to active tuberculosis. HIV patients are also susceptible to *Mycobacterium tuberculosis* infections, as are tuberculosis patients to HIV infections. Coinfection is common among patients with tuberculosis and HIV.
- *Diabetes.* Patients with diabetes tend to have a weakened immune defense system and are more prone to infections like tuberculosis. Diabetes causes latent tuberculosis to become active tuberculosis. About 5–30% of tuberculosis patients are afflicted with type 2 diabetes.

- *Leukemia.* Leukemia patients are often immunodeficient and at risk of converting their inactive tuberculosis to active tuberculosis.
- *Medications.* Glucocorticoid drugs for treating rheumatoid arthritis and lupus erythematosus can inhibit the immune system and exacerbate the risk of tuberculosis.

What Is the Association between Vitamin D and Tuberculosis?

- Vitamin D enhances immune defense and reduces the risk of infections. People with low blood levels of vitamin D are more susceptible to tuberculosis infection and more likely to convert their inactive tuberculosis to active tuberculosis. Supplementation with vitamin D alleviates the symptoms of tuberculosis.
- Before the era of antibiotics, sun exposure was used clinically to treat tuberculosis. Physicians in the distant past suspected some substance in the sun's rays could cure tuberculosis. We, of course, know that that substance is ultraviolet B, which can induce the skin to produce vitamin D. Indeed, at present, vitamin D produced from the skin upon sun exposure is still an effective and indispensable approach for treating tuberculosis.
- Tuberculosis patients who took antibiotics together with vitamin D sped up their recovery from the disease.

Meta-analysis

- *Vitamin D.* A meta-analysis of 15 research articles studied the relationship between vitamin D and tuberculosis in 1,440 tuberculosis patients and 2,558 healthy individuals. The analysis revealed that people with blood levels of vitamin D below 10 ng/ml had the highest risk of tuberculosis. The incidence rate was also higher in people with blood levels of vitamin D between 10 to 20 ng/ml. The analysis confirmed that people with blood levels of vitamin D at 21–30 ng/ml had a lowered risk of tuberculosis.

Recommendation

- *Prevention.* For people at risk of tuberculosis, take daily 800 IU vitamin D3 (11).
- *Treatment.* For tuberculosis patients, take daily 2,000 IU vitamin D3 (11).

110

VENOUS THROMBOSIS

Venous thrombosis is a condition characterized by blood clot (thrombus) formation inside a vein. The most common type is deep vein thrombosis, in which a blood clot is formed in a deep vein of the leg. When a thrombus from a deep vein of the leg travels through the heart and enters the lungs, it can cause pulmonary thrombosis. Pulmonary thrombosis is a serious and life-threatening condition, and it is the third most common cardiovascular disease. The first and second are heart attack and stroke. In the US, each year 1 million people are afflicted with venous thrombosis, including deep vein thrombosis and pulmonary thrombosis. Almost two-thirds of venous thrombosis patients require hospitalization, and each year, 300,000 people die from venous thrombosis.

What Are the Symptoms of Venous Thrombosis?

- *Deep vein thrombosis.* The leg becomes painful and swollen (it often affects only one leg).
- *Pulmonary thrombosis.* The patient experiences sudden shortness of breath, chest pain, dizziness, racing heartbeat, and blood in phlegm.

What Are the Risk Factors for Venous Thrombosis?

- *Age.* Aging is a risk factor for venous thrombosis. Aging causes veins to become fragile. Aging also increases blood coagulation, damages venous valves, and reduces innate anticoagulation, as well as causes a decline in physical activity.
- *Family and genetics.* Genes are linked to venous thrombosis. G20210A gene variants are functional mutations of the gene encoding for prothrombin, a protein that supports normal blood coagulation. Mutations in prothrombin genes can result in abnormal blood coagulation and lead to venous thrombosis.
- *Obesity.* Among all metabolic disorders caused by obesity, chronic inflammation and fibrinolysis are two factors that are closely related to venous thrombosis. The consequence of chronic inflammation is the activation of blood coagulation in the venous blood vessel. Chronic inflammation also stimulates platelet activity, lessens the activity of anticoagulation factors, and promotes blood clot formation. Fibrinolysis is a normal enzymatic process that degrades fibrin and prevents blood clot formation. Obesity weakens fibrinolysis and precipitates blood clot formation.
- *Oral contraceptives.* The main ingredients of oral contraceptives are estrogen and progestin. Estrogen elevates blood levels of coagulation factors V, VIII, and X. About 25% of women of childbearing age use oral contraceptives. Although certain health benefits are associated with oral contraceptives, such as alleviating pain during menstruation and reducing the risk of ovarian cancer and endometrial cancer, long-term use of oral contraceptives increases the risk of venous thrombosis.

- *Smoking.* Toxic chemicals in cigarette smoke can aggravate blood coagulation and elevate the risk of venous thrombosis. Women who smoke cigarettes and use oral contraceptives have a greater risk of venous thrombosis. Studies have shown that women smokers who used oral contraceptives were at an 8.8 times greater risk of venous thrombosis compared to women smokers who did not use oral contraceptives.
- *Cancer.* In patients with cancer, the blood vessels produce tissue factors that promote blood coagulation and blood clot formation. In addition, coagulation-inducing fat particles are released into the bloodstream and can block blood flow, increasing the risk of venous thrombosis.
- *Sitting or lying down.* Lack of muscle contraction is common in patients with paralysis lying in bed or travelers sitting on an airplane during a long-haul flight, both of which augment the risk of venous thrombosis. In an airplane, one should stand up and walk around every four hours or so during a long journey to avoid venous thrombosis.

What Is the Association between Vitamin B6 and Venous Thrombosis?

- Vitamin B6 inhibits platelet coagulation and reduces the risk of venous thrombosis. Vitamin B6 deficiency increases the risk of venous thrombosis.
- Vitamin B6 is a safe and effective natural anticoagulant, and vitamin B6 supplements are used clinically to replace vitamin K–related synthetic anticoagulants.

What Is the Association between Vitamin B9 and Venous Thrombosis?

- Vitamin B9 deficiency reduces vitamin K–related coagulation factors and exacerbates blood clot formation.
- Vitamin B9 deficiency increases free radical production and oxidative stress–induced damage to the blood vessels and

leads to the enlargement of the muscle layer in blood vessels, increasing the risk of venous thrombosis.

What Is the Association between Vitamin B12 and Venous Thrombosis?

- Vitamin B12 lowers the blood level of thrombin–antithrombin complexes, reducing the risk of blood clot formation and venous thrombosis.
- Vitamin B complexes consisting of vitamin B6, vitamin B9, and vitamin B12 are safer and more effective than steroid anti-inflammatory drugs in preventing venous thrombosis.
- Deficiencies in vitamin B6, vitamin B9, and vitamin B12 heighten the risk of venous thrombosis. High blood levels of homocysteine are common in people with deficiencies in vitamin B6, vitamin B9, and vitamin B12. Homocysteine can damage the structural integrity of the blood vessels and lead to venous thrombosis.

Meta-analysis

- *Vitamin B complex.* A meta-analysis of 19 research articles studied the relationship between vitamin B complex and venous thrombosis. The analysis revealed that people with low blood levels of vitamin B6, vitamin B9, and vitamin B12 had a greater risk of venous thrombosis compared to healthy individuals.

Recommendation

- *Prevention.* For people at risk of venous thrombosis, take daily 2 mg vitamin B6 (6), 400 mcg vitamin B9 (8), and 100 mcg vitamin B12 (9).
- *Treatment.* For venous thrombosis patients, take daily 10 mg vitamin B6 (6), 800 mcg vitamin B9 (8), and 400 mcg vitamin B12 (9).

111

VITILIGO

Vitiligo is a skin disease in which areas of the skin lose pigmentation, causing whitish patches. Vitiligo can affect any area of the skin—including the hair, oral cavity, and eyes—but it most commonly affects areas of the skin that are exposed to the sun, such as the face, neck, and hands. The color of our hair, skin, and eyes is determined by the amount of melanin—the pigment—produced from melanocytes in the scalp, skin, or eyes. Africans' skin produces more melanin, so the color of their skin is dark brown. Caucasians' skin produces less melanin, so the color of their skin is fair. The melanin content in the skin of Asians and Hispanics is between Africans and Caucasians. Vitiligo is caused by the death of melanocytes, causing the skin of the affected area to not produce any melanin. It can affect people of any race and any skin color. People with darker skin colors have a lower risk of vitiligo compared to people with fair skin. In the US, 2 million people are afflicted with vitiligo.

What Are the Symptoms of Vitiligo?
- Loss of pigmentation in areas or patches of the skin
- Changes to the color of the retina in the eyes
- White patches in the hair

What Are the Risk Factors for Vitiligo?
- *Autoimmune disease.* Vitiligo is an autoimmune disorder in which the immune system erroneously attacks melanin-producing melanocytes in the skin, mistaking them as foreign. Vitiligo patients often are afflicted with other autoimmune diseases, such as Hashimoto's disease, rheumatoid arthritis, type 1 diabetes, psoriasis, pernicious anemia, and lupus erythematosus.
- *Family and genetics.* Vitiligo is a hereditary disease. A multitude of genes are linked to vitiligo, although the exact mechanism is still not clear at present.

What Is the Association between Vitamin D and Vitiligo?
- Vitamin D enhances melanocytes' ability to produce melanin. Vitamin D deficiency diminishes immune functions and melanin production. Vitiligo patients often are vitamin D deficient. Supplementation with vitamin D curtails the risk of vitiligo.
- Autoimmune disorders activate the skin to produce inflammatory cytokines that can lead to vitiligo. Vitamin D decreases the symptoms of autoimmune disorders and may prevent vitiligo.

What Is the Association between Copper/Zinc and Vitiligo?
- Zinc-dependent enzymes promote melanin production in the skin. Zinc together with topical steroid drugs is used clinically to treat vitiligo.
- Copper and zinc are the two essential trace elements that support the synthesis of superoxide dismutase, an enzyme that

can degrade reactive oxygen species generated by sun exposure and prevent oxidative damage to melanocytes in the skin.

Meta-analysis

- *Vitamin D.* A meta-analysis of 17 research articles studied the relationship between vitamin D and vitiligo. The analysis has shown that blood levels of vitamin D in vitiligo patients were 7.45 ng/ml lower compared to those in healthy controls.
- *Copper/zinc.* Sixteen research papers investigated the association between copper/zinc contents and vitiligo in 891 vitiligo patients and 1,682 healthy individuals. The meta-analysis confirmed that vitiligo patients had lower blood contents of copper/zinc compared to healthy controls.

Recommendation

- *Prevention.* For people at risk of vitiligo, take daily 800 IU vitamin D3 (11), 1 mg copper (22), and 10 mg zinc (20).
- *Treatment.* For vitiligo patients, take daily 2,000 IU vitamin D3 (11), 2 mg copper (22), and 20 mg zinc (20).

PART FIVE

Summary of Recommended Daily
Doses of Vitamins and Essential
Elements for Prevention and Treatment
of 75 Diseases and Conditions

Alzheimer's Disease (page 181)

- *Prevention.* For people at risk of dementia and Alzheimer's disease, take daily 2,000 IU vitamin A (1), 200 mg vitamin C (10), 800 IU vitamin D3 (11), 30 IU vitamin E (12), and 10 mg zinc (20).
- *Treatment.* For dementia and Alzheimer's patients, take daily 5,000 IU vitamin A (1), 500 mg vitamin C (10), 2,000 IU vitamin D3 (11), 100 IU vitamin E (12), and 20 mg zinc (20).

Asthma (page 188)

- *Prevention.* For children at risk of asthma, take daily 1,000 IU vitamin A (1), 80 mg vitamin C (10), and 400 IU vitamin D3 (11).
- *Prevention.* For adults at risk of asthma, take daily 2,000 IU vitamin A (1), 200 mg vitamin C (10), and 800 IU vitamin D3 (11).
- *Treatment.* For children with asthma, take daily 4,000 IU vitamin A (1), 300 mg vitamin C (10), and 1,000 IU vitamin D3 (11).
- *Treatment.* For adults with asthma, take daily 5,000 IU vitamin A (1), 500 mg vitamin C (10), and 2,000 IU vitamin D3 (11).

Atherosclerosis (page 192)

- *Prevention.* For people at risk of atherosclerosis, take daily 400 mcg vitamin B9 (8).
- *Treatment.* For atherosclerosis patients, take daily 800 mcg vitamin B9 (8).

Atrial Fibrillation (page 196)

- *Prevention.* For people at risk of atrial fibrillation, take daily 200 mg vitamin C (10) and 1 g omega-3 fatty acids (27).
- *Treatment.* For atrial fibrillation patients, take daily 500 mg vitamin C (10) and 2 g omega-3 fatty acids (27).

Attention-Deficit/Hyperactivity Disorder (page 200)

- *Prevention.* For children at risk of attention-deficit/hyperactivity disorder, take daily 1 g omega-3 fatty acids (27).
- *Treatment.* For children with attention-deficit/hyperactivity disorder, take daily 2 g omega-3 fatty acids (27).

Autism Spectrum Disorder (page 204)

- *Prevention.* For pregnant women and breastfeeding women whose children may be at risk of autism, take daily 1,000 IU vitamin D3 (11).
- *Prevention.* For newborn babies at risk of autism, take daily 400 IU vitamin D3 (11).
- *Treatment.* For children with autism, take daily 2,000 IU vitamin D3 (11).

Autoimmune Thyroid Disease (page 208)

- *Prevention.* For people at risk of autoimmune thyroid disease, take daily 800 IU vitamin D3 (11) and 50 mcg selenium (26).
- *Treatment.* For autoimmune thyroid disease patients, take daily 2,000 IU vitamin D3 (11) and 100 mcg selenium (26).

Bladder Cancer (page 212)

- *Prevention.* For people at risk of bladder cancer, take daily 2,000 IU vitamin A (1), 200 mg vitamin C (10), 800 IU vitamin D3 (11), 30 IU vitamin E (12), 400 mcg vitamin B9 (8), 50 mcg selenium (26), and 10 mg zinc (20).
- *Treatment.* For bladder cancer patients, take daily 5,000 IU vitamin A (1), 500 mg vitamin C (10), 2,000 IU vitamin D3

(11), 100 IU vitamin E (12), 800 mcg vitamin B9 (8), 100 mcg selenium (26), and 20 mg zinc (20).

Blood Cancers (page 217)

- *Prevention.* For people at risk of blood cancer, take daily 800 IU vitamin D3 (11).
- *Treatment.* For blood cancer patients, take daily 2,000 IU vitamin D3 (11).

Bone Fracture (page 221)

- *Prevention.* For people at risk of bone fracture, take daily 500 mg calcium (14) and 800 IU vitamin D3 (11).
- *Treatment.* For bone fracture patients, take daily 1,000 mg calcium (14) and 2,000 IU vitamin D3 (11).

Breast Cancer (page 224)

- *Prevention.* For women at risk of breast cancer, take daily 2 mg vitamin B6 (6), 200 mg vitamin C (10), 800 IU vitamin D3 (11), 30 IU vitamin E (12), 400 mcg vitamin B9 (8), 50 mcg selenium (26), and 1 g omega-3 fatty acids (27).
- *Treatment.* For women with breast cancer, take daily 10 mg vitamin B6 (6), 500 mg vitamin C (10), 2,000 IU vitamin D3 (11), 100 IU vitamin E (12), 800 mcg vitamin B9 (8), 100 mcg selenium (26), and 2 g omega-3 fatty acids (27).

Cardiovascular Disease (page 232)

- *Prevention.* For people at risk of cardiovascular disease, take daily 200 mg vitamin C (10), 800 IU vitamin D2 (11), 30 IU vitamin E (12), 100 mg magnesium (17), and 1 g omega-3 fatty acids (27).
- *Treatment.* For cardiovascular disease patients, take daily 500 mg vitamin C (10), 2,000 IU vitamin D3 (11), 100 IU vitamin E (12), 200 mg magnesium (17), and 2 g omega-3 fatty acids (27).

Cataracts (page 239)

- *Prevention.* For people at risk of cataracts, take daily 2,000 IU vitamin A (1), 200 mg vitamin C (10), and 30 IU vitamin E (12).
- *Treatment.* For cataract patients, take daily 5,000 IU vitamin A (1), 500 mg vitamin C (10), and 100 IU vitamin E (12).

Cervical Cancer (page 244)

- *Prevention.* For women at risk of cervical cancer, take daily 2,000 IU vitamin A (1), 100 mcg vitamin B12 (9), and 200 mg vitamin C (10).
- *Treatment.* For cervical cancer patients, take daily 5,000 IU vitamin A (1), 400 mcg vitamin B12 (9), and 500 mg vitamin C (10).

Cervical Intraepithelial Neoplasia (page 248)

- *Prevention.* For women at risk of cervical intraepithelial neoplasia, take daily 200 mg vitamin C (10).
- *Treatment.* For cervical intraepithelial neoplasia patients, take daily 500 mg vitamin C (10).

Chronic Kidney Disease (page 251)

- *Prevention.* For people at risk of chronic kidney disease, take daily 800 IU vitamin D3 (11) and 400 mcg vitamin B9 (8).
- *Treatment.* For chronic kidney disease patients, take daily 2,000 IU vitamin D3 (11) and 800 mcg vitamin B9 (8).

Chronic Obstructive Pulmonary Disease (page 255)

- *Prevention.* For people at risk of chronic obstructive pulmonary disease, take daily 800 IU vitamin D3 (11).
- *Treatment.* For chronic obstructive pulmonary disease patients, take daily 2,000 IU vitamin D3 (11).

Chronic Pancreatitis (page 260)

- *Prevention.* For people at risk of chronic pancreatitis, take daily 50 mcg selenium (26), 2,000 IU vitamin A (1), 200 mg vitamin C (10), and 30 IU vitamin E (12).
- *Treatment.* For chronic pancreatitis patients, take daily 100 mcg selenium (26), 5,000 IU vitamin A (1), 500 mg vitamin C (10), and 100 IU vitamin E (12).

Cognitive Impairment (page 263)

- *Prevention.* For people at risk of cognitive impairment, take daily 800 IU vitamin D3 (11) and 1 g omega-3 fatty acids (27).
- *Treatment.* For cognitively impaired patients, take daily 2,000 IU vitamin D3 (11) and 2 g omega-3 fatty acids (27).

Colorectal Cancer (page 267)

- *Prevention.* For people at risk of colorectal cancer, take daily 2 mg vitamin B2 (3), 2 mg vitamin B6 (6), 100 mcg vitamin B12 (9), 800 IU vitamin D3 (11), 400 mcg vitamin B9 (8), 500 mg calcium (14), 100 mg magnesium (17), 50 mcg selenium (26), and 10 mg zinc (20).
- *Treatment.* For colorectal cancer patients, take daily 10 mg vitamin B2 (3), 10 mg vitamin B6 (6), 400 mcg vitamin B12 (9), 2,000 IU vitamin D3 (11), 800 mcg vitamin B9 (8), 1,000 mg calcium (14), 200 mg magnesium (17), 100 mcg selenium (26), and 20 mg zinc (20).

Coronary Artery Disease (page 275)

- *Prevention.* For people at risk of coronary artery disease, take daily 400 mcg vitamin B9 (8) and 1 g omega-3 fatty acids (27).
- *Treatment.* For coronary disease patients, take daily 5 mg vitamin B9 (8) and 2 g omega-3 fatty acid (27) for one month, and after that, take daily 800 mcg vitamin B9 (8) and 2 g omega-3 fatty acids (27).

Depression (page 279)

- *Prevention.* For people at risk of depression, take daily 100 mcg vitamin B12 (9), 800 IU vitamin D3 (11), 400 mcg vitamin B9 (8), and 1 g omega-3 fatty acids (27).
- *Treatment.* For depression patients, take daily 400 mcg vitamin B12 (9), 2,000 IU vitamin D3 (11), 800 mcg vitamin B9 (8), and 2 g omega-3 fatty acids (27).

Type 1 Diabetes (page 285)

- *Prevention.* For new babies at risk of type 1 diabetes, take daily 400 IU vitamin D3 (11).
- *Prevention.* For adults at risk of type 1 diabetes, take daily 800 IU vitamin D3 (11).
- *Treatment.* For type 1 diabetes patients, take daily 2,000 IU vitamin D3 (11).

Type 2 Diabetes (page 289)

- *Prevention.* For people at risk of type 2 diabetes, take daily 800 IU vitamin D3 (11), 100 mg magnesium (17), 10 mg zinc (20), 50 mg chromium (25), and 1 g omega-3 fatty acids (27).
- *Treatment.* For type 2 diabetes patients, take daily 2,000 IU vitamin D3 (11), 200 mg magnesium (17), 20 mg zinc (20), 200 mg chromium (25), and 2 g omega-3 fatty acids (27).

Dry Eyes (page 295)

- *Prevention.* For people at risk of dry eyes, take daily 1 g omega-3 fatty acids (27).
- *Treatment.* For dry eye patients, take daily 2 g omega-3 fatty acids (27).

Eczema (page 298)

- *Prevention.* For people at risk of eczema, take daily 800 IU vitamin D3 (11).
- *Treatment.* For eczema patients in remission, take daily 1,000 IU vitamin D3 (11).

- *Treatment.* For eczema patients, take daily 2,000 IU vitamin D3 (11).

Endometrial Cancer (page 301)
- *Prevention.* For women at risk of endometrial cancer, take daily 2,000 IU vitamin A (1), 200 mg vitamin C (10), and 30 IU vitamin E (12).
- *Treatment.* For female endometrial cancer patients, take daily 5,000 IU vitamin A (1), 500 mg vitamin C (10), and 100 IU vitamin E (12).

Esophageal Cancer (page 305)
- *Prevention.* For people at risk of esophageal cancer, take daily 200 mg vitamin C (10) and 400 mcg vitamin B9 (8).
- *Treatment.* For esophageal cancer patients, take daily 500 mg vitamin C (10), and 800 mcg vitamin B9 (8).

Exercise-Induced Bronchoconstriction (page 308)
- *Prevention.* For people at risk of exercise-induced bronchoconstriction, take 500 mg vitamin C (10) before exercise.

Fatty Liver Disease (page 310)
- *Prevention.* For people at risk of fatty liver disease, take daily 800 IU vitamin D3 (11), 30 IU vitamin E (12), and 1 g omega-3 fatty acids (27).
- *Treatment.* For fatty liver disease patients, take daily 2,000 IU vitamin D3 (11), 100 IU vitamin E (12), and 2 g omega-3 fatty acids (27).

Fibromyalgia (page 315)
- *Prevention.* For people at risk of fibromyalgia, take daily 800 IU vitamin D3 (11).
- *Treatment.* For fibromyalgia patients, take daily 2,000 IU vitamin D3 (11).

Gestational Diabetes (page 318)

- *Prevention.* For women at risk of gestational diabetes, take daily 2,000 IU vitamin D3 (11) and 100 mcg selenium (26).

Glaucoma (page 321)

- *Prevention.* For people at risk of glaucoma, take daily 400 mcg vitamin B9 (8).
- *Treatment.* For glaucoma patients, take daily 800 mcg vitamin B9 (8).

Glioma (page 324)

- *Prevention.* For people at risk of glioma, take daily 2,000 IU vitamin A (1) and 200 mg vitamin C (10).
- *Treatment.* For glioma patients, take daily 5,000 IU vitamin A (1) and 500 mg vitamin C (10).

Gout (page 327)

- *Prevention.* For people at risk of gout, take daily 200 mg vitamin C (10).
- *Treatment.* For gout patients, take daily 500 mg vitamin C (10).

Graves' Disease (page 330)

- *Prevention.* For people at risk of Graves' disease, take daily 800 IU vitamin D3 (11).
- *Treatment.* For Graves' disease patients, take daily 2,000 IU vitamin D3 (11).

Heart Disease (page 333)

- *Prevention.* For people at risk of heart attack, take daily 30 IU vitamin E (12) and 100 mg magnesium (17).
- *Treatment.* For heart attack patients, take daily 100 IU vitamin E (12) and 200 mg magnesium (17).

Heart Failure (page 337)

- *Prevention.* For people at risk of heart failure, take daily 5 mg vitamin B1 (2) and 1 g omega-3 fatty acids (27).
- *Treatment.* For heart failure patients, take daily 100 mg vitamin B1 (2) and 2 g omega-3 fatty acids (27).

Hemodialysis (page 341)

- *Treatment.* For hemodialysis patients, take daily 500 mg vitamin C (10), 2,000 IU vitamin D3 (11), and 2 g omega-3 fatty acids (27).

Hepatitis C (page 345)

- *Prevention.* For people at risk of hepatitis C, take daily 800 IU vitamin D3 (11).
- *Treatment.* For hepatitis C patients, take daily 2,000 IU vitamin D3 (11).

Hypercholesterolemia (page 348)

- *Prevention.* For people at risk of hypercholesterolemia, take daily 200 mg vitamin C (10).
- *Treatment.* For hypercholesterolemia patients, take daily 500 mg vitamin C (10).

Hypertension (page 352)

- *Prevention.* For people at risk of hypertension, take daily 200 mg vitamin C (10), 800 IU vitamin D3 (11), 400 mcg vitamin B9 (8), 500 mg potassium (15), 100 mg magnesium (17), and 1 g omega-3 fatty acids (27).
- *Treatment.* For hypertension patients, take daily 500 mg vitamin C (10), 2,000 IU vitamin D3 (11), 800 mcg vitamin B9 (8), 1,000 mg potassium (15), 200 mg magnesium (17), and 2 g omega-3 fatty acids (27).

Inflammatory Bowel Disease (page 359)
- *Prevention.* For people at risk of inflammatory bowel disease, take daily 800 IU vitamin D3 (11).
- *Treatment.* For inflammatory bowel disease patients, including those with ulcerative colitis and Crohn's disease, take 5,000 IU vitamin D3 (11) for 6 months, and after that, take daily 2,000 IU vitamin D3 (11).

Kashin-Beck Disease (page 363)
- *Prevention.* For children in Kashin-Beck disease regions, take daily 50 mcg selenium (26).
- *Treatment.* For Kashin-Beck disease patients, take daily 100 mcg selenium (26).

Liver Cancer (page 365)
- *Prevention.* For people at risk of liver cancer, take daily 1 g omega-3 fatty acids (27).
- *Treatment.* For cirrhosis patients, take daily 2 g omega-3 fatty acids (27).
- *Treatment.* For liver cancer patients, take daily 2 g omega-3 fatty acids (27).

Lung Cancer (page 368)
- *Prevention.* For people at risk of lung cancer, take daily 2,000 IU vitamin A (1), 200 mg vitamin C (10), 800 IU vitamin D3 (11), 30 IU vitamin E (12), and 400 mcg vitamin B9 (8).
- *Prevention.* For smokers at risk of lung cancer, take daily 2,000 IU vitamin A (1), 300 mg vitamin C (10), 1,000 IU vitamin D3 (11), 30 IU vitamin E (12), and 800 mcg vitamin B9 (8).
- *Treatment.* For lung cancer patients, take daily 5,000 IU vitamin A (1), 500 mg vitamin C (10), 2,000 IU vitamin D3 (11), 100 IU vitamin E (12), and 800 mcg vitamin B9 (8).

95

Lupus Erythematosus (page 373)
- *Prevention.* For people at risk of lupus erythematosus, take daily 800 IU vitamin D3 (11).
- *Treatment.* For lupus erythematosus patients, take daily 2,000 IU vitamin D3 (11).

Age-Related Macular Degeneration (page 377)
- *Prevention.* For people aged 55 and older at risk of age-related macular degeneration, take daily 400 mcg vitamin B9 (8) and 100 mcg vitamin B12 (9).
- *Treatment.* For age-related macular degeneration patients, take daily 800 mcg vitamin B9 (8) and 400 mcg vitamin B12 (9).

Male Infertility (page 381)
- *Prevention.* For men at risk of infertility, take daily 10 mg zinc (20).
- *Treatment.* For male infertility patients, take daily 20 mg zinc (20).

Melanoma (page 384)
- *Prevention.* For people at risk of melanoma, take daily 2,000 IU vitamin A (1) and 800 IU vitamin D3 (11).
- *Treatment.* For melanoma patients, take daily 5,000 IU vitamin A (1) and 2,000 IU vitamin D3 (11).

Metabolic Syndrome (page 388)
- *Prevention.* For people at risk of metabolic syndrome, take daily 100 mg magnesium (17).
- *Treatment.* For metabolic syndrome patients, take daily 200 mg magnesium (17).

Migraine (page 391)
- *Prevention.* For people at risk of migraine, take daily 200 mg magnesium (17).

- *Treatment.* For migraine patients, take daily 400 mg magnesium (17).

Multiple Sclerosis (page 395)
- *Prevention.* For people at risk of multiple sclerosis, take daily 100 mcg vitamin B12 (9) and 800 IU vitamin D3 (11).
- *Treatment.* For multiple sclerosis patients, take daily 400 mcg vitamin B12 (9) and 2,000 IU vitamin D3 (11).

Neural Tube Defects (page 399)
- *Prevention.* For women at risk of having babies with neural tube defects, take daily 400 mcg vitamin B9 (8).
- *Prevention.* For pregnant women, before getting pregnant and during pregnancy, take daily 800 mcg vitamin B9 (8).

Obesity (page 403)
- *Prevention.* For people at risk of obesity, take daily 800 IU vitamin D3 (11) and 50 mg chromium (25).
- *Treatment.* For obese people, take daily 2,000 IU vitamin D3 (11) and 200 mg chromium (25).

Oral Cleft (page 407)
- *Prevention.* For pregnant women whose babies may be at risk of oral cleft, take daily 400 mcg vitamin B9 (8); the first and second months of pregnancy are particularly critical times.

Orthostatic Hypotension (page 409)
- *Prevention.* For people at risk of orthostatic hypotension, take daily 800 IU vitamin D3 (11).
- *Treatment.* For orthostatic hypotension patients, take daily 2,000 IU vitamin D3 (11).

Osteoporosis (page 412)

- *Prevention.* For people at risk of osteoporosis, take daily 800 IU vitamin D3 (11), 500 mg calcium (14), 1 mg copper (22), 10 mg zinc (20), and 8 mg iron (19).
- *Treatment.* For osteoporosis patients, take daily 2,000 IU vitamin D3 (11), 1,000 mg calcium (14), 2 mg copper (22), 20 mg zinc (20), and 16 mg iron (19).

Pancreatic Cancer (page 417)

- *Prevention.* For people at risk of pancreatic cancer, take daily 200 mg vitamin C (10), 30 IU vitamin E (12), and 400 mcg vitamin B9 (8).
- *Treatment.* For pancreatic cancer patients, take daily 500 mg vitamin C (10), 100 IU vitamin E (12), and 800 mcg vitamin B9 (8).

Parkinson's Disease (page 421)

- *Prevention.* For people at risk of Parkinson's disease, take daily 800 IU vitamin D3 (11), 2 mg vitamin B6 (6), and 30 IU vitamin E (12).
- *Treatment.* For Parkinson's disease patients, take daily 2,000 IU vitamin D3 (11), 10 mg vitamin B6 (6), and 100 IU vitamin E (12).

Preeclampsia (page 426)

- *Prevention.* For pregnant women at risk of preeclampsia, take daily 800 IU vitamin D3 (11), 500 mg calcium (14), and 50 mcg selenium (26).
- *Treatment.* For pregnant women with preeclampsia, take daily 2,000 IU vitamin D3 (11), 1,000 mg calcium (14), and 100 mcg selenium (26).

Premature Mortality (page 430)

- *Prevention.* For people at risk of premature mortality, take daily 800 IU vitamin D3 (11).

- *Treatment.* For chronic disease patients, take daily 2,000 IU vitamin D3 (11).

Prostate Cancer (page 432)
- *Prevention.* For people at risk of prostate cancer, take daily 200 mg vitamin C (10), 30 IU vitamin E (12), and 50 mcg selenium (26).
- *Treatment.* For prostate cancer patients, take daily 500 mg vitamin C (10), 100 IU vitamin E (12), and 100 mcg selenium (26).

Renal Cell Cancer (page 436)
- *Prevention.* For people at risk of renal cell cancer, take daily 2 mg vitamin B6 (6), 200 mg vitamin C (10), 800 IU vitamin D3 (11), and 30 IU vitamin E (12).
- *Treatment.* For renal cell cancer patients, take daily 10 mg vitamin B6 (6), 500 mg vitamin C (10), 2,000 IU vitamin D3 (11), and 100 IU vitamin E (12).

Respiratory Infections (page 441)
- *Prevention.* For people at risk of respiratory infections, take daily 800 IU vitamin D3 (11).
- *Treatment.* For respiratory infection patients (including children), take daily 2,000 IU vitamin D3 (11).

Rheumatoid Arthritis (page 444)
- *Prevention.* For people at risk of rheumatoid arthritis, take daily 800 IU vitamin D3 (11), 50 mcg selenium (26), 10 mg zinc (20), and 1 g omega-3 fatty acids (27).
- *Treatment.* For rheumatoid arthritis patients, take daily 2,000 IU vitamin D3 (11), 100 mcg selenium (26), 20 mg zinc (20), and 2 g omega-3 fatty acids (27).

Rickets (page 449)
- *Prevention.* For breastfed infants at risk of rickets, take daily 400 IU vitamin D3 (11).

- *Prevention.* For infants or children who consume less than one liter of formulated infant milk powders or whole milk at risk of rickets, take daily 400 IU vitamin D3 (11).
- *Prevention.* For adolescents who don't drink milk or have insufficient dietary intake of vitamin D and are at risk of rickets, take daily 400 IU vitamin D3 (11).

Schizophrenia (page 451)
- *Prevention.* For people at risk of schizophrenia, take daily 1 g omega-3 fatty acids (27).
- *Treatment.* For schizophrenia patients, take daily 2 g omega-3 fatty acids (27).

Sepsis (page 454)
- *Prevention.* For people who need to stay in the hospital for major surgeries or severe illnesses who are at risk of nosocomial infection and sepsis, take 10,000 IU vitamin D3 (11) for three days before hospitalization, and after that, take daily 2,000 IU vitamin D3 (11) during the entire hospital stay.
- *Prevention.* For chronic disease patients at risk of sepsis, take daily 800 IU vitamin D3 (11) and 50 mcg selenium (26).
- *Treatment.* For sepsis patients, take daily 400 mcg selenium (26) during the entire hospital stay.

Sleep Apnea (page 457)
- *Prevention.* For people at risk of sleep apnea, take daily 800 IU vitamin D3 (11).
- *Treatment.* For sleep apnea patients, take daily 2,000 IU vitamin D3 (11).

Stomach Cancer (page 461)
- *Prevention.* For people at risk of stomach cancer, take daily 2,000 IU vitamin A (1), 200 mg vitamin C (10), 30 IU vitamin E (12), and 50 mcg selenium (26).

- *Treatment.* For stomach cancer patients, take daily 5,000 IU vitamin A (1), 500 mg vitamin C (10), 100 IU vitamin E (12), and 100 mcg selenium (26).

Stroke (page 466)
- *Prevention.* For people at risk of stroke, take daily 2 mg vitamin B6 (6), 400 mcg vitamin B9 (8), 200 mg vitamin C (10), 500 mg potassium (15), 50 mg magnesium (17), and 1 g omega-3 fatty acids (27).
- *Treatment.* For stroke patients, take daily 10 mg vitamin B6 (6), 800 mcg vitamin B9 (8), 500 mg vitamin C (10), 1,000 mg potassium (15), 100 mg magnesium (17), and 2 g omega-3 fatty acids (27).

Tuberculosis (page 472)
- *Prevention.* For people at risk of tuberculosis, take daily 800 IU vitamin D3 (11).
- *Treatment.* For tuberculosis patients, take daily 2,000 IU vitamin D3 (11).

Venous Thrombosis (page 476)
- *Prevention.* For people at risk of venous thrombosis, take daily 2 mg vitamin B6 (6), 400 mcg vitamin B9 (8), and 100 mcg vitamin B12 (9).
- *Treatment.* For venous thrombosis patients, take daily 10 mg vitamin B6 (6), 800 mcg vitamin B9 (8), and 400 mcg vitamin B12 (9).

Vitiligo (page 480)
- *Prevention.* For people at risk of vitiligo, take daily 800 IU vitamin D3 (11), 1 mg copper (22), and 10 mg zinc (20).
- *Treatment.* For vitiligo patients, take daily 2,000 IU vitamin D3 (11), 2 mg copper (22), and 20 mg zinc (20).

AUTHOR'S PUBLICATIONS

Lai C-S and Piette LH, Hydroxyl radical production involved in lipid peroxidation of rat liver microsomes. Biochemical and Biophysical Research Communication 1977; 78:51–59.

Lai C-S and Piette LH, Spin trapping studies of hydroxyl radical production involved in lipid peroxidation. Archives of Biochemistry and Biophysics 1978; 190:27.

Lai C-S and Piette LH, Further evidence for OH radical production in Fenton's reagent. Tetrahedron Letters 1979; 9:775–78.

Lai C-S, Grover TA and Piette LH, Hydroxyl radical production in a purified NADPH Cytochrome C (P-450) reductase systems. Archives of Biochemistry and Biophysics 1979; 193:373.

REFERENCES

References are in alphabetical order by disease.

Alzheimer's Disease

Shen L, Ji HF, Association between homocysteine, folic acid, vitamin B12 and Alzheimer's disease: Insight from meta-analyses. J Alzheimer's Dis 2015; 46(3): 777–90

Shen L, Ji HF, Vitamin D deficiency is associated with increased risk of Alzheimer's disease and dementia: Evidence from meta-analysis. Nutr Journal 2015; 14:76

Ventriglia M, Brewer GJ, Simonelli I, Mariani S, Siotto M, Bucossi S, Squitti R, Zinc in Alzheimer's disease: A meta-analysis of serum, plasma and cerebrospinal fluid studies. J Alzheimer's Dis 2015; 46(1): 75–87

Zhao Y, Sun Y, Ji HF, Shen L, Vitamin D levels in Alzheimer's and Parkinson's disease: A meta-analysis. Nutrition 2013; 29(6): 828–32

Anemia

Liu T, Zhong S, Liu L, Liu S, Li X, Zhou T, Zhang J, Vitamin D deficiency and the risk of anemia: A meta-analysis of observational studies. Renal Fail 2015; 37(6): 929–34

Anorexia

Veronese N, Solmi M, Rizza W, Manzato E, Sergi G, Santonastaso P, Caregaro L, Favaro A, Correll CU, Vitamin D status in anorexia nervosa: A meta-analysis. Int J Eat Disord 2015; 48(7): 803–13

Asthma

Allen S, Britton JR, Leonardi-Bee JA, Association between antioxidant vitamins and asthma outcome measures: Systematic review and meta-analysis. Thorax 2009; 64(7): 610–19

Man L, Zhang, Z, Zhang M, Zhang Y, Li J, Zheng N, Cao Y, Chi M, Chao Y, Huang Q, Song C, Xu B, Association between vitamin D deficiency and insufficiency and the risk of childhood asthma: Evidence from a meta-analysis. Int J Clin Exp Med 2015; 8(4): 5699–706

Riverin BD, Maguire JL, Li P, Vitamin D supplementation for childhood asthma: A systematic review and meta-analysis. PLoS One 2015; 10(8): e0136841

Atherosclerosis

Qin X, Xu M, Zhang Y, Li J, Xu X, Wang X, Xu X, Huo Y, Effect of folic acid supplementation on the progression of carotid intima-media thickness: A meta-analysis of randomized controlled trials. Atherosclerosis 2012; 222(2): 307–13

Atrial Fibrillation

He Z, Yang L, Tian J, Yang K, Wu J, Yao Y, Efficacy and safety of omega-3 fatty acids for the prevention of atrial fibrillation: A meta-analysis. Can J Cardiol 2013; 29(2): 196–203

Hemila H, Suonsyrja T, Vitamin C for preventing atrial fibrillation in high risk patients: A systematic review and meta-analysis. BMC Cardiovasc Disord 2017; 17(1): 49

Hu X, Yuan L, Wang H, Li C, Cai J, Hu Y, Ma C, Efficacy and safety of vitamin C for atrial fibrillation after cardiac surgery: A meta-analysis with trial sequential analysis of randomized controlled trials. Int J Surg 2017; 37:58–64

Violi F, Pastori D, Pignatelli P, Loffredo L, Antioxidants for prevention of atrial fibrillation: A potentially useful future therapeutic approach? A review of the literature and meta-analysis. Europace 2014; 16(8): 1107–16

Attention-Deficit/Hyperactivity Disorder

Bloch MH, Qawasmi A, Omega-3 fatty acid supplementation for the treatment of children with attention-deficit/hyperactivity disorder symptomatology: Systematic review and meta-analysis. J Am Acad Child Adolesc Psychiatry 2011; 50(10): 991–1000

Hawkey E, Nigg JT, Omega-3 fatty acid and ADHD: Blood level analysis and meta-analytic extension of supplementation trials. Clin Psychol Rev 2014; 34(6): 496–505

Autism Spectrum Disorder

Wang T, Shan L, Du L, Feng J, Xu Z, Staal WG, Jia F, Serum concentration of 25-hydroxyvitamin D in autism spectrum disorder: A systematic review and meta-analysis. Eur Child Adolesc Psychiatry 2015; doi: 10.1007/s00787-015-0786-1

Autoimmune Thyroid Disease

Fan Y, Xu S, Zhang H, Cao W, Wang K, Chen G, Di H, Cao M, Liu C, Selenium supplementation for autoimmune thyroiditis: A systematic review and meta-analysis. Int J Endocrinol 2014: 904573

Wang J, Lv S, Chen G, Gao C, He J, Zhong H, Xu Y, Meta-analysis of the association between vitamin D and autoimmune thyroid disease. Nutrients 2015; 7(4): 2485–98

Bladder Cancer

Amaral AF, Cantor KP, Silverman DT, Malats N, Selenium and bladder cancer risk: A meta-analysis. Cancer Epidemiol Biomarker Prev 2010; 19(9): 2407–15

He H, Shui B, Folate intake and risk of bladder cancer: A meta-analysis of epidemiological studies. Int J Food Sci Nutr 2014; 65(3): 286–92

Mao S, Huang S, Zinc and copper levels in bladder cancer: A systematic review and meta-analysis. Biol Trace Elem Res 2013; 153(1–3): 5–10

Tang JE, Wang RJ, Zhong H, Yu B, Chen Y, Vitamin A and risk of bladder cancer: A meta-analysis of epidemiological studies. World J Surg Oncol 2014; 12:130

Wang YY, Wang XL, Yu ZJ, Vitamin C and E intake and risk of bladder cancer: A meta-analysis of observational studies. Int J Clin Exp Med 2014; 7(11): 4154–64

Zhang H, Zhang H, Wen X, Zhang Y, Wei X, Liu T, Vitamin D deficiency and increased risk of bladder carcinoma: A meta-analysis. Cell Physiol Biochem 2015; 37(5): 1686–92

Zhao Y, Chen C, Pan W, Gao M, He W, Mao R, Lin T, Huang J, Comparative efficacy of vitamin D status in reducing the risk of bladder cancer: A systematic review and network meta-analysis. Nutrition 2016; 32(5): 515–23

Blood Cancers

Wang W, Li G, He X, Gao J, Wang R, Wang Y, Zhao W, Serum 25-hydroxyvitamin D levels and prognosis in hematological malignancies: A systematic review and meta-analysis. Cell Physiol Biochem 2015; 35(5): 1999–2005

Bone Fracture

Weaver CM, Alexander DD, Boushey CJ, Dawson-Hughes B, Lappe JM, LeBoff MS, Liu S, Looker AC, Wallace TC, Wang DD, Calcium plus vitamin D supplementation and risk of fractures: An updated meta-analysis from the National Osteoporosis Foundation. Osteoporos Int 2016; 27(1): 367–76

Breast Cancer

Babaknejad N, Sayehmiri F, Sayehmiri K, Rahimifar P, Bahrami S, Delpesheh A, Hemati F, Alizadeh S, The relationship between selenium levels and breast cancer: A systematic review and meta-analysis. Biol Trace Elem Res 2014; 159(1–3): 1–7

Chen P, Li C, Li X, Li J, Chu R, Wang H, Higher dietary folate intake reduces the breast cancer risk: A systematic review and meta-analysis. Br J Cancer 2014; 110(9): 2327–38

Harris HR, Orsini N, Wolk A, Vitamin C and survival among women with breast cancer: A meta-analysis. Eur J Cancer 2014; 50(7): 1223–31

Hu F, Wu Z, Li G, Teng C, Liu Y, Wang F, Zhao Y, Pang D, The plasma level of retinol, vitamins A, C and alpha-tocopherol could reduce breast cancer risk? A meta-analysis and meta-regression. J Cancer Res Clin Oncol 2015; 141(4): 601–14

Wu W, Kang S, Zhang D, Association of vitamin B6, vitamin B12 and methionine with risk of breast cancer: A dose-response meta-analysis. Br J Cancer 2013; 109(7): 1926–44

Zheng JS, Hu XJ, Zhao YM, Yang J, Li D, Intake of fish and marine n-3 polyunsaturated fatty acids and risk of breast cancer: Meta-analysis of data from 21 independent prospective cohort studies. BMJ 2013; 346: f3706

Cardiovascular Disease

Ashor AW, Lara J, Mathers JC, Siervo M, Effect of vitamin C on endothelial function in health and disease: A systematic review and meta-analysis of randomized controlled trials. Atherosclerosis 2014; 235(1): 9–20

Ashor AW, Siervo M, Lara J, Oggioni C, Afshar S, Mathers JC, Effect of vitamin C and vitamin E supplementation on endothelial function: A systematic review and meta-analysis of randomized controlled trials. Br J Nutr 2015; 113(8): 1182–94

Casula M, Soranna D, Catapano AL, Corrao G, Long-term effect of high dose omega-3 fatty acid supplementation for secondary prevention of cardiovascular outcomes: A meta-analysis of randomized, placebo controlled trials. Atheroscer Suppl 2013; 14(2): 243–51

Chen N, Wan Z, Chen N, Wan Z, Han SF, Li BY, Zhang ZL, Qin LQ, Effect of vitamin D supplementation on the level of circulating high-sensitivity C-reactive protein: A meta-analysis of randomized controlled trials. Nutrients 2014; 6(6): 2209–16

Qin X, Huo Y, Langman CB, Hou F, Chen Y, Matossian D, Xu X, Wang X, Folic acid therapy and cardiovascular disease in ESRD or advanced chronic kidney disease: A meta-analysis. Clin J Am Soc Nephrol 2011; 6(3): 482–88

Qu X, Jin F, Hao Y, Li H, Tang T, Wang H, Yan W, Dai K, Magnesium and the risk of cardiovascular events: A meta-analysis of prospective cohort studies. PLoS One 2013; 8(3): e57720

Saboori S, Shab-Bidar S, Speakman JR, Yousefi Rad E, Djafarian K, Effect of vitamin E supplementation on serum C-reactive protein level: A meta-analysis of randomized controlled trials. Eur J Clin Nutr 2015; 69(8): 867–73

Wang L, Song Y, Manson JE, Pilz S, Marz W, Michaelsson K, Lundqvist A, Jassal SK, Barrett-Connor E, Zhang C, Eaton CB, May HT,

Anderson JL, Sesso HD, Circulating levels of 25-hydroxy-vitamin D and risk of cardiovascular disease: A meta-analysis of prospective studies. Circ Cardiovasc Qual Outcomes 2012; 5(6): 819–29

Cataracts

Wang A, Han J, Jiang Y, Zhang D, Association of vitamin A and beta-carotene with risk for age-related cataract: A meta-analysis. Nutrition 2014; 30(10): 1113–21

Wei L, Liang G, Cai C, Lv J, Association of vitamin C with the risk of age-related cataract: A meta-analysis. Acta Ophthalomol 2016; 94(3): e170–76

Zhang Y, Jiang W, Xie Z, Wu W, Zhang D, Vitamin E and risk of age-related cataract: A meta-analysis. Public Health Nutr 2015; 18(15): 2804–14

Zhao LQ, Li LM, Zhu H, The effect of multivitamin/mineral supplements on age-related cataracts: A systematic review and meta-analysis. Nutrients 2014; 6(3): 931–49

Cervical Cancer

Cao D, Shen K, Li Z, Xu Y, Wu D, Association between vitamin C intake and the risk of cervical neoplasia: A meta-analysis. Nutr Cancer 2016; 68(1): 48–57

Myung SK, Ju W, Kim SC, Kim H, Korean meta-analysis (KORMA) study group, Vitamin or antioxidant intake (or serum level) and risk of cervical neoplasm: A meta-analysis. BJOG 2011; 118(11): 1285–91

Zhang X, Dai B, Zhang B, Wang Z, Vitamin A and risk of cervical cancer: A meta-analysis. Gynecol Oncol 2012; 124(2): 366–73

Chronic Kidney Disease

Zheng Z, Shi H, Jia J, Li D, Lin S, Vitamin D supplementation and mortality risk in chronic kidney disease: A meta-analysis of 20 observational studies. BMC Nephrol 2013; 14:199

Chronic Obstructive Pulmonary Disease

Zhu B, Zhu B, Xiao C, Zheng Z, Vitamin D deficiency is associated with the severity of COPD: A systemic review and meta-analysis. Int J Chron Obstruct Pulmon Dis 2015; 10:1907–16

Chronic Pancreatitis

Cai GH, Huang J, Zhao Y, Chen J, Wu HH, Dong YL, Smith HS, Li YQ, Wang W, Wu SX, Antioxidant therapy for pain relief in patients with chronic pancreatitis: A systematic review and meta-analysis. Pain Physician 2013; 16(6): 521–32

Cognitive Impairment

Etgen T, Sander D, Bickel H, Sander K, Forstl H, Vitamin D deficiency, cognitive impairment and dementia: A systematic review and meta-analysis. Dement Geriatr Cogn Disord 2012; 33(5): 297–305

Yurko-Mauro K, Alexander DD, Van Elswyk ME, Docosahexaenoic acid and adult memory: A systematic review and meta-analysis. PLoS One 2015; 10(3): e0120391

Zhang XW, Hou WS, Li M, Tang ZY, Omega-3 fatty acids and risk of cognitive decline in the elderly: A meta-analysis of randomized controlled trials. Aging Clin Exp Res 2016; 28(1): 165–6

Colon Cancer

Kim DH, Smith-Warner SA, Spiegelman D, Yaun SS, Colditz GA, Freudenheim JL, Giovannucci E, Goldbohm RA, Graham S, Harnack L, Jacobs EJ, Leitzmann M, Mannisto S, Miller AB, Potter JD, Rohan TE, Schatzkin A, Speizer FE, Stevens VL, Stolzenberg-Solomon R, Terry P, Toniolo P, Weijenberg MP, Willett WC, Wold A, Zeleniuch-Jacquotte A, Hunter DJ, Pooled analysis of 13 prospective cohort studies on folate intake and colon cancer. Cancer Causes Control 2012; 21(11): 1919–30

Colorectal Adenoma

Keum N, Lee DH, Greenwood DC, Zhang X, Giovannucci EL, Calcium intake and colorectal adenoma risk: Dose-response meta-analysis of prospective observational studies. Int J Cancer 2015; 136(7): 1680–87

Colorectal Cancer

Bonovas S, Fiorino G, Lytras T, Malesci A, Danese S, Calcium supplementation for the prevention of colorectal adenomas: A systematic review and meta-analysis of randomized controlled trials. World J Gastroenterol 2016; 22(18): 4594–603

Chen GC, Pang Z, Liu QF, Magnesium intake and risk of colorectal cancer: A meta-analysis of prospective studies. Eur J Clin Nutr 2012; 66(11): 1182–86

Ko HJ, Youn CH, Kim HM, Cho YJ, Lee GH, Lee WK, Dietary magnesium intake and risk of cancer: A meta-analysis of epidemiologic studies. Nutr Cancer 2014; 66(6): 915–23

Larsson SC, Orsini N, Wolk A, Vitamin B6 and risk of colorectal cancer: A meta-analysis of prospective studies. JAMA 2010; 303(11): 1077–83

Liu Y, Yu QY, Zhu ZL, Tang PY, Li K, Vitamin B2 intake and the risk of colorectal cancer: A meta-analysis of observational studies. Asian Pac J Cancer Prev 2015; 16(3): 909–13

Mohr SB, Gorham ED, Garland CF, Grant WB, Garland FC, Cuomo RE, Could vitamin D sufficiently improve the survival of colorectal cancer patients? J Steriod Biochem Mol Biol 2015; 148:245–52

Ou Y, Jiang B, Wang X, Ma W, Guo J, Selenium and colorectal adenomas risk: A meta-analysis. Nutr Cancer 2012; 64(8): 1153–59

Sun NH, Huang XZ, Wang SB, Li Y, Wang LY, Wang HC, Zhang CW, Zhang C, Liu HP, Wang ZN, A dose-response meta-analysis reveals an association between vitamin B12 and colorectal cancer risk. Public Health Nutr 2016; 19(8): 1446–56

Coronary Artery Disease
Wen YT, Dai JH, Gao Q, Effects of omega-3 fatty acid on major cardiovascular events and mortality in patients with coronary heart disease: A meta-analysis of randomized controlled trials. Nutr Metab Cardiovasc Dis 2014; 24(5): 470–75

Xin YI, Zhou Y, Jiang D, Li X, Guo Y, Jiang X, Efficacy of folic acid supplementation on endothelial function and plasma homocysteine concentration in coronary artery disease: A meta-analysis of randomized controlled trials. Exp Ther Med 2014; 7(5): 1100–10

Depression
Petridou ET, Kousoulis AA, Michelakos T, Papathoma P, Dessypris N, Papadopoulos FC, Stefanadis C, Folate and B12 serum levels in association with depression in the aged: A systematic review and meta-analysis. Aging Ment Health 2016; 20(9): 965–73

Spedding S, Vitamin D and depression: A systematic review and meta-analysis comparing studies with and without biological flaws. Nutrients 2014; 6(4): 1501–18

Stokes CS, Grunhage F, Baus C, Volmer DA, Wagenpfeil S, Riemenschneider M, Lammert F, Vitamin D supplementation reduces depressive symptoms in patients with chronic liver disease. Clin Nutr 2016; 35(4): 950–57

Yang JR, Han D, Qiao ZX, Tian X, Qi D, Qiu XH, Combined application of eicosapentaenoic acid docosahexaenoic acid on depression in women: A meta-analysis of double-blind randomized controlled trials. Neurpsychiatr Dis Treat 2015; 11:2055–61

Diabetes

Chen C, Yu X, Shao S, Effects of omega-3 fatty acid supplementation on glucose control and lipid levels in type 2 diabetes: A meta-analysis. PLoS One 2015; 10(10): e0139565

Feng R, Li Y, Li G, Li Z, Zhang Y, Li Q, Sun C, Lower serum 25(OH) D concentrations in type 1 diabetes: A meta-analysis. Diabetes Res Clin Pract 2015; 108(3): e71–75

Jayawardena R, Ranasinghe P, Galappatthy P, Malkanthi R, Constantine G, Katulanda P, Effects of zinc supplementation on diabetes mellitus: A systematic review and meta-analysis. Diabetol Metab Syndr 2012; 4(1): 13

Liu C, Lu M, Xia X, Wang J, Wan Y, He L, Li M, Correlation of serum vitamin D level with type 1 diabetes mellitus in children: A meta-analysis. Nutr Hosp 2015; 32(4): 1591–94

Lv WS, Zhao WJ, Gong SL, Fang DD, Wang B, Fu ZJ, Yan SL, Wang YG, Serum 25-hydroxyvitamin D levels and peripheral neuropathy in patients with type 2 diabetes: A systematic review and meta-analysis. J Endocrinol Invest 2015; 38(5): 513–18

San Mauro-Marin I, Ruiz-Leon AM, Camina-Martin MA, Garicano-Vilar E, Collado-Yurrita L, Mateo-Silleras B, Redondo Del Rio MP, Chromium supplementation in patients with type 2 diabetes and high risk of type 2 diabetes: A meta-analysis of randomized controlled trials. Nutr Hosp 2016; 33(1): 27

Song Y, Wang L, Pittas AG, Del Gobbo LC, Zhang C, Manson JE, Hu FB, Blood 25-hydroxy vitamin D levels and incident type 2 diabetes:

A meta-analysis of prospective studies. Diabetes Care 2013; 36(5): 1422–28

Suksomboon N, Poolsup N, Yuwanakorn A, Systematic review and meta-analysis of the efficacy and safety of chromium supplementation in diabetes. J Clin Pharm Ther 2014; 39(3): 292–306

Xu T, Chen GC, Zhai L, Ke KF, Nonlinear reduction in risk for type 2 diabetes by magnesium intake: An updated meta-analysis of prospective cohort studies. Biomed Environ Sci 2015; 28(7): 527–34

Zheng JS, Huang T, Yang J, Fu YQ, Li D, Marine N-3 polyunsaturated fatty acids are inversely associated with the risk of type 2 diabetes in Asians: A systematic review and meta-analysis. PLoS One 2012; 7(9): e445525

Dry Eyes

Liu A, Ji J, Omega-3 essential fatty acids therapy for dry eye syndrome: A meta-analysis of randomized controlled studies. Med Sci Monit 2014; 20:1583–89

Eczema

Kim G, Bae JH, Vitamin D and atopic dermatitis: A systematic review and meta-analysis. Nutrition 2016; 32(9): 913–20

Endometrial Cancer

Bandera EV, Gifkins DM, Moore DF, McCullough ML, Kushi LH, Antioxidant vitamins and the risk of endometrial cancer: A dose-response meta-analysis. Cancer Causes Control 2009; 20(5): 699–711

Esophageal Cancer

Bo Y, Lu Y, Zhao Y, Zhao E, Yuan L, Lu W, Cui L, Lu Q, Association between dietary vitamin C intake and risk of esophageal cancer: A dose-response meta-analysis. Int J Cancer 2016; 138(8): 1843–50

Exercise-Induced Bronchoconstriction

Hemila H, Vitamin C may alleviate exercise-induced bronchoconstriction: A meta-analysis. BMJ Open 2013; 3(6): e002416

Fatty Liver Disease

Parker HM, Johnson NA, Burdon CA, Cohn JS, O'Connor HT, George J, Omega-3 supplementation and non-alcoholic fatty liver disease: A systematic review and meta-analysis. J Hepatol 2012; 56(4): 944–51

Sato K, Gosho M, Yamamoto T, Kobayashi Y, Ishii N, Ohashi T, Nakade Y, Ito K, Fukuzawa Y, Yoneda M, Vitamin E has a beneficial effect on non-alcoholic fatty liver disease: A meta-analysis of randomized controlled trials. Nutrition 2015; 31(7–8): 923–30

Wang X, Li W, Zhang Y, Yang Y, Qin G, Association between vitamin D and non-alcoholic fatty liver disease/non-alcoholic steatohepatitis: Results from a meta-analysis. Int J Clin Exp Med 2015; 8(10): 17221–34

Fibromyalgia

Hsiao MY, Hung CY, Chang KV, Han DS, Wang TG, Is serum hypovitaminosis D associated with chronic widespread pain including fibromyalgia? A meta-analysis of observational studies. Pain Physician 2015; 18(5): E877–87

Gastrointestinal Cancers

Gong HY, He JG, Li BS, Meta-analysis of the association between selenium and gastric cancer risk. Oncotarget 2016; 7(13): 15600–5

Kong P, Cai Q, Geng Q, Wang J, Lan Y, Zhan Y, Xu D, Vitamin intake reduces the risk of gastric cancer: Meta-analysis of randomized and observational studies. PLoS One 2014; 9(12): e116060

Li P, Xu J, Shi Y, Ye Y, Chen K, Yang J, Wu Y, Association between zinc intake and risk of digestive tract cancers: A systematic review and meta-analysis. Clin Nutr 2014; 33(3): 415–20

Tio M, Andrici J, Cox MR, Eslick GD, Folate intake and the risk of upper gastrointestinal cancers: A systematic review and meta-analysis. J Gastroenterol Hepatol 2014; 29(2): 250–58

Gestational Diabetes

Askari G, Iraj B, Salehi-Abargouei A, Fallah AA, Jafari T, The association between serum selenium and gestational diabetes mellitus: A systematic review and meta-analysis. J Trace Elem Med Biol 2015; 29:195–201

Lu M, Xu Y, Association between vitamin D status and the risk of gestational diabetes mellitus: A meta-analysis. Arch Gynecol Obstet 2016; Jan 29: Epub ahead of print

Lu M, Xu Y, Lv L, Zhang M, Association between vitamin D status and the risk of gestational diabetes mellitus: A meta-analysis. Arch Gynecol Obstet 2016; 293(5): 959–66

Zhang MX, Pan GT, Guo JF, Li BY, Qin LQ, Zhang ZL, Vitamin D deficiency increases the risk of gestational diabetes mellitus: A meta-analysis of observational studies. Nutrients 2015; 7(10): 8366–75

Glaucoma

Lv W, Zhong X, Xu, L, Han W, Association between dietary vitamin A intake and the risk of glioma: Evidence from a meta-analysis. Nutrients 2015; 7(11): 8897–8904

Xu F, Zhang L, Li M, Plasma homocysteine, serum folic acid, serum vitamin B12, serum vitamin B6, MTHFR and risk of pseudoexfoliation glaucoma: A meta-analysis. Graefes Arch Clin Exp Ophthalomol 2012; 250(7): 1067–74

Glioma

Zhou S, Wang X, Tan Y, Qiu L, Fang H, Li W, Association between vitamin C intake and glioma risk: Evidence from a meta-analysis. Neuroepidemiology 2015; 44(1): 39–44

Gout

Juraschek SP, Miller ER 3rd, Gelber AC, Effect of oral vitamin C supplementation on serum uric acid: A meta-analysis of randomized controlled studies. Arthritis Care Res (Hoboken) 2011; 63(9): 1295–306

Graves' Disease

Xu MY, Cao B, Yin J, Wang DF, Chen KL, Lu QB, Vitamin D and Graves' disease: A meta-analysis update. Nutrition 2015; 7:3813–27

Heart Disease

Del Gobbo LCD, Imamura F, Wu JH, de Oliveira Otto MC, Chiuve SE, Mozaffarian D, Circulating and dietary magnesium and risk of cardiovascular disease: A systematic review and meta-analysis of prospective studies. Am J Clin Nutr 2013; 98(1): 160–73

Djousse L, Akinkuolie AO, Wu JH, Ding EL, Gaziano JM, Fish consumption, omega-3 fatty acids and risk of heart failure: A meta-analysis. Clin Nutr 2012; 31(6): 846–53

Jain A, Mehta R, Al-Ani M, Hill JA, Winchester DE, Determining the role of thiamine Deficiency in systolic heart failure: A meta-analysis and systematic review. J Card Fail 2015; 21(12): 1000–1007

Heart Failure

Loffredo L, Perri L, Di Castelnuovo A, Iacoviello L, De Gaetano G, Violi F, Supplementation with vitamin E alone is associated with reduced myocardial infarction: A meta-analysis. Nutr Metab Cardiovasc Dis 2015; 25(4): 354–63

Hemodialysis

Chi H, Lin X, Huang H, Zheng X, Li T, Zou Y, Omega-3 fatty acid supplementation on lipid profiles in dialysis patients: Meta-analysis. Arch Med Res 2014; 45(6): 469–77

Deved V, Poyah P, James MT, Tonelli M, Manns BJ, Walsh M, Hemmelgarn BR, Alberta Kidney Disease Network, Ascorbic acid for anemia management in hemodialysis patients: A systematic review and meta-analysis. Am J Kidney Dis 2009; 54(6): 1089–97

Sarathy H, Pramanik V, Kahn J, Abramowitz MK, Meier K, Kishore P, Melamed ML, The effects of short-term vitamin D supplementation on glucose metabolism in dialysis patients: A systematic review and meta-analysis. Int Urol Nephrol 2015; 47(3): 537–49

Hepatitis C

Villar LM, Del Campo JA, Ranchal I, Lampe E, Romero-Gomez M, Association between vitamin D and hepatitis C virus infections: A meta-analysis. World J Gastroenterol 2013; 19(35): 5917–24

Hypercholesterolemia

McRae MP, Vitamin C supplementation lowers serum low-density lipoprotein cholesterol and triglycerides: A meta-analysis of 13 randomized controlled trials. J Chiropr Med 2008; 7(2): 48–58

Hypertension

Binia A, Jaeger J, Hu Y, Singh Z, Zimmermann D, Daily potassium intake and sodium-to-potassium ratio in the reduction of blood pressure: A meta-analysis of randomized controlled trials. J Hypertens 2015; 33(8): 1509–20

Burgaz A, Orsini N, Larsson SC, Wolk A, Blood 25-hydroxyvitamin D concentration and hypertension: A meta-analysis. J Hypertens 2011; 29(4): 636–45

Kass L, Weekes J, Carpenter L, Effect of magnesium supplementation on blood pressure: A meta-analysis. Eur J Clin Nutr 2012; 66(4): 411–18

Ke L, Mason RS, Kariuki M, Mpofu E, Brock KE, Vitamin D status and hypertension: A review. Integr Blood Press Control 2015; 8:13–35

McRae MP, High-dose folic acid supplementation effects on endothelial function and blood pressure of hypertensive patients: A meta-analysis of randomized controlled trials. J Chiropr Med 2009; 8(1): 15–24

Miller PE, Van Elswyk M, Alexander DD, Long-chain omega-3 fatty acids eicosapentaenoic acid and docosahexaenoic acid and blood pressure: A meta-analysis of randomized controlled trials. Am J Hypertens 2014; 27(7): 885–96

Van Bommel E, Cleophas T, Potassium treatment for hypertension in patients with high salt intake: A meta-analysis. Int J Clin Pharmacol Ther 2012; 50(7): 478–82

Inflammatory Bowel Disease

Del Pinto R, Pietropaoli D, Chandar AK, Ferri C, Cominelli F, Association between inflammatory bowel disease and vitamin D deficiency: A systematic review and meta-analysis. Inflamm Bowel Dis 2015; 21(11): 2708–17

Furuya-Kanamori L, Wangdi K, Yakob L, McKenzie SJ, Doi SA, Clark J, Paterson DL, Riley TV, Clements AC, 25-Hydroxyvitamin D concentrations and Clostridium difficile infection: A meta-analysis. JPEN J Parenter Enteral Nutr 2015: 0148607115623457

Raftery T, Martineau AR, Greiller CL, Ghosh S, McNamara D, Bennett K, Meddings J, O'Sullivan M, Effects of vitamin D supplementation on intestinal permeability, cathelicidin and disease markers in Crohn's disease: Results from a randomized double-blind placebo-controlled study. United European Gastroenterology Journal 2015; 3(3): 294–302

Sadeqhian M, Saneei P, Siassi F, Esmaillzadeh A, Vitamin D status in relation to Crohn's disease: Meta-analysis of observational studies. Nutrition 2016; 32(5): 505–14

Kashin-Beck Disease

Zou K, Liu G, Wu T, Du L, Selenium for preventing Kashin-Beck osteoarthropathy in children: A meta-analysis. Osteoarthritis Cartilage 2009; 17(2): 144–51

Liver Cancer

Gao M, Sun K, Guo M, Gao H, Liu K, Yang C, Li S, Liu N, Fish consumption and n-3 polyunsaturated fatty acids, and risk of hepatocellular carcinoma: Systematic review and meta-analysis. Cancer Causes Control 2015; 26(3): 367–76

Lung Cancer

Chen G, Wang J, Hong X, Chai Z, Li Q, Dietary vitamin E intake could reduce the risk of lung cancer: Evidence from a meta-analysis. Int J Clin Exp Med 2015; 8(4): 6631–37

Chen GC, Zhang ZL, Wan Z, Wang L, Weber P, Eggersdorfer M, Qin LQ, Zhang W, Circulating 25-hydroxyvitamin D and risk of lung cancer: A dose-response meta-analysis. Cancer Causes Control 2015; 26(12): 1719–28

Dai WM, Yang B, Chu XY, Wang YQ, Zhao M, Chen L, Zhang GQ, Association between folate intake, serum folate and the risk of lung cancer: A systematic review and meta-analysis. Chin Med J (Engl) 2013; 126(10): 1957–64

Luo J, Shen L, Zheng D, Association between vitamin C intake and lung cancer: A dose-response meta-analysis. Sci Rep 2014; 4:6161

Zhang L, Wang S, Che X, Li X, Vitamin D and lung cancer risk: A comprehensive review and meta-analysis. Cell Physiol Biochem 2015; 36(1): 299–305

Zhu YJ, Bo YC, Liu XX, Qiu CG, Association of dietary vitamin E intake with risk of lung cancer: A dose-response meta-analysis. Asia Pac J Clin Nutr 2017; 26(2): 271–77

Lupus Erythematosus

Sahebari M, Nabavi N, Salehi M, Correlation between serum 25(OH)D values and lupus disease activity: An original article and a systemic review with meta-analysis focusing on serum vitamin D confounders. Lupus 2014; 23(11): 1164–77

Macular Degeneration

Huang P, Wang F, Sah BK, Jiang J, Ni Z, Wang J, Sun X, Homocysteine and the risk of age-related macular degeneration: A systematic review and meta-analysis. Sci Rep 2015; 5:10585

Melanoma

Caini S, Boniol M, Tosti G, Magi S, Medri M, Stanganelli I, Palli D, Assedi M, Marmol VD, Gandini S, Vitamin D and melanoma and non-melanoma skin cancer risk and prognosis: A comprehensive review and meta-analysis. Eur J Cancer 2014; 50(15): 2649–58

Zhang YP, Chu RX, Liu H, Vitamin A intake and risk of melanoma: A meta-analysis. PLoS One 2014; 9(7): e102527

Metabolic Syndrome

Capdor J, Foster M, Petocz P, Samman S, Zinc and glycemic control: A meta-analysis of randomized placebo controlled supplementation trials in humans. J Trace Elem Med Biol 2013; 27(2): 137–42

Dibaba DT, Xun P, Fly AD, Yokota K, He K, Dietary magnesium intake and risk of metabolic syndrome: A meta-analysis. Diabet Med 2014; 31(11): 1301–9

Ju SY, Choi WS, Ock SM, Kim CM, Kim DH, Dietary magnesium intake and metabolic syndrome in the adult population: Dose-response meta-analysis and meta-regression. Nutrients 2014; 6(12): 6005–19

Migraine

Chiu HY, Yeh TH, Huang YC, Chen PY, Effects of intravenous and oral magnesium on reducing migraine: A meta-analysis of randomized controlled trials. Pain Physician 2016; 19(1): E97–E112

Multiple Sclerosis

Duan S, Lv Z, Fan X, Wang L, Han F, Wang H, Bi S, Vitamin D status and the risk of multiple sclerosis: A systematic review and meta-analysis. Neurosci Lett 2014; 570:108–13

Zhu Y, He ZY, Liu HN, Meta-analysis of the relationship between homocysteine, vitamin B12, folate and multiple sclerosis. J Clin Neurosci 2011; 18(7): 933–38

Neural Tube Defects

Peake JN, Copp AJ, Shawe J, Knowledge and periconceptional use of folic acid for the prevention of neural tube defects in ethnic communities in the United Kingdom: Systematic and meta-analysis. Birth Defects Res A Clin Mol Teratol 2013; 97(7): 444–51

Obesity

Manousopoulou A, Al-Daghri NM, Garbis SD, Chrousos GP, Vitamin D and cardiovascular risk among adults with obesity: A systematic review and meta-analysis. Eur J Clin Invest 2015; 45(10): 1113–26

Onakpoya I, Posadzki P, Ernst E, Chromium supplementation in overweight and obesity: A systematic review and meta-analysis of randomized clinical trials. Obes Rev 2013; 14(6): 496–507

Yao Y, Zhu L, He L, Duan Y, Liang W, Nie Z, Jin Y, Wu X, Fang Y, A meta-analysis of the relationship between vitamin D deficiency and obesity. Int J Clin Exp Med 2015; 8(9): 14977–84

Oral Cleft

Badovinac RL, Werler MM, Williams PL, Kelsey KT, Hayes C, Folic acid-containing supplement consumption during pregnancy and risk or oral clefts: A meta-analysis. Birth Defects Res A Clin Mol Teratol 2007; 79(1): 8–15

Orthostatic Hypotension

Ometto F, Stubbs B, Annweiler C, Duval GT, Jang W, Kim HT, McCarroll K, Cunningham C, Soysal P, Isik AT, Luchini C, Solmi M, Sergi G, Manzato E, Veronese N, Hypovitaminosis D and orthostatic hypotension: A systematic review and meta-analysis. J Hypertens 2016; 34(6): 1036–43

Osteoporosis

Silk LN, Greene DA, Baker MK, The effect of calcium or calcium and vitamin D supplementation on bone mineral density in healthy males: A systematic review and meta-analysis. Int J Sport Nutr Exerc Metab 2015; 25(5): 510–24

Zheng J, Mao X, Ling J, He Q, Quan J, Low serum levels of zinc, copper and iron as risk factors for osteoporosis: A meta-analysis. Biol Trace Elem Res 2014; 160(1): 15–23

Pancreatic Cancer

Fan H, Kou J, Han D, Li P, Zhang D, Wu Q, He Q, Association between vitamin C intake and the risk of pancreatic cancer: A meta-analysis of observational studies. Sci Rep 2015; 5:13973

Lin HL, An QZ, Wang QZ, Liu CX, Folate intake and pancreatic cancer risk: An overall and dose-response meta-analysis. Public Health Nutr 2013; 127(7): 607–13

Peng L, Liu X, Lu Q, Tang T, Yang Z, Vitamin E intake and pancreatic cancer risk: A meta-analysis of observational studies. Med Sci Monit 2015; 21:1249–55

Parkinson's Disease

Etminan M, Gill SS, Samii A, Intake of vitamin E, vitamin C and carotenoids and the risk of Parkinson's disease: A meta-analysis. Lancet Neurol 2005; 4(6): 362–65

Lv Z, Qi H, Wang L, Fan X, Han F, Wang H, Bi S, Vitamin D status and Parkinson's disease: A systemic review and meta-analysis. Neurol Sci 2014; 35(11): 1723–30

Schottker B, Ball D, Gellert C, Brenner H, Serum 25-hydroxyvitamin D levels and overall mortality: A systematic review and meta-analysis of prospective cohort studies. Ageing Res Rev 2013; 12(2): 708–18

Shen L, Ji HF, Associations between vitamin D status, supplementation, outdoor work and risk of Parkinson's disease: A meta-analysis assessment. Nutrition 2015; 7(6): 4817–27

Pediatric Cancer

Revuelta Iniesta R, Rush R, Paciarotti I, Rhatigan EB, Brougham FH, McKenzie JM, Wilson DC, Systematic review and meta-analysis:

Prevalence and possible causes of vitamin D deficiency and insufficiency in pediatric cancer patients. Clin Nutr 2016; 35(1): 95–108

Preeclampsia
An LB, Li WT, Xie TN, Peng X, Li B, Xie SH, Xu J, Zhou XH, Guo SN, Calcium supplementation reducing the risk of hypertensive disorders of pregnancy and related problems: A meta-analysis of multicentre randomized controlled trials. Int J Nurs Pract 2015; 21 Suppl 2:19–31

Ma Y, Shen X, Zhang D, The relationship between serum zinc level and preeclampsia: A meta-analysis. Nutrients 2015; 7(9): 7806–20

Patrelli TS, Dall'asta A, Gizzo S, Pedrazzi G, Piantelli G, Jasonni VM, Modena AB, Calcium supplementation and prevention of preeclampsia: A meta-analysis. J Matern Fetal Neonatl Med 2012; 25(12): 2570–74

Xu M, Guo D, Gu H, Zhang L, Lv S, Selenium and preeclampsia: A systematic review and meta-analysis. Biol Trace Elem Res 2016; 171(2): 283–92

Premature Mortality
Jiang S, Pan Z, Li H, Li F, Song Y, Qiu Y, Meta-analysis: Low-dose intake of vitamin E combined with other vitamins or minerals may decrease all-cause mortality. J Nutr Sci Vitaminol (Tokyo) 2014; 60(3): 194–205

Kim Y, Je Y, Vitamin D intake, blood 25(OH) D levels, and breast cancer risk or mortality; a meta-analysis. Br J Cancer 2014; 110(11): 2772–84

Zhang YP, Wan YD, Sun TW, Kan QC, Wang LX, Association between vitamin D deficiency and mortality in critically ill adult patients: A meta-analysis of cohort studies. Crit Care 2014; 18(6): 684

Preterm Birth
Zhou SS, Tao YH, Huang K, Zhu BB, Tao FB, Vitamin D and risk of preterm birth: Up-to-date meta-analysis of randomized controlled trials and observational studies. J Obstet Gynaecol Res 2017; 43(2): 247–56

Prostate Cancer
Bai XY, Qu X, Jiang X, Xu Z, Yang Y, Su Q, Wang M, Wu H, Association between dietary vitamin C intake and risk of prostate cancer: A meta-analysis involving 103,658 subjects. J Cancer 2015; 6(9): 913–21

Cui R, Liu ZQ, Xu Q, Blood alpha-tocopherol, gamma-tocopherol levels and risk of prostate cancer: A meta-analysis of prospective studies. PLoS One 2014; 9(3): e93044

Hurst R, Hooper L, Norat T, Lau R, Aune D, Greenwood DC, Vieira R, Collings R, Harvey LJ, Sterne JA, Beynon R, Savovic J, Fairweather-Tait SJ, Selenium and prostate cancer: Systematic review and meta-analysis. Am J Clin Nutr 2012; 96(1): 111–22

Renal Cell Cancer

Jia L, Jia Q, Shang Y, Dong X, Li L, Vitamin C intake and risk of renal cell carcinoma: A meta-analysis. Sci Rep 2015; 5:17921

Lin G, Ning L, Gu D, Li S, Yu Z, Long Q, Hou LN, Tan WL, Examining the association of circulating 25-hydroxyvitamin D with kidney cancer risk: A meta-analysis. Int J Clin Exp Med 2015; 8(11): 20499–507

Mao B, Li Y, Zhang Z, Chen C, Chen Y, Ding C, Lei L, Li J, Jiang M, Wang D, Wang G, One-carbon metabolic factors and risk of renal cell cancer: A meta-analysis. PLoS One 2015; 10(10): e0141762

Shen C, Huang Y, Yi S, Fang Z, Li L, Association of vitamin E intake with reduced risk of kidney cancer: A meta-analysis of observational studies. Med Sci Monit 2015; 21:3420–26

Respiratory Infections

Charan J, Goyal JP, Saxena D, Yadav P, Vitamin D for prevention of respiratory tract infections: A systematic review and meta-analysis. J Pharmacol Pharmacother 2013; 3(4): 300–3

Mao S, Zhang A, Huang S, Meta-analysis of Zn, Cu and Fe in the hair of Chinese children with recurrent respiratory tract infection. Scan J Clin Lab Invest 2014; 74(7): 561–67

Rheumatoid Arthritis

Lee YH, Bae SC, Song GG, Omega-3 polyunsaturated fatty acids and the treatment of rheumatoid arthritis: A meta-analysis. Arch Med Res 2012; 43(5): 356–62

Lin J, Liu J, Davies ML, Chen W, Serum vitamin D level and rheumatoid arthritis disease activity review and meta-analysis. PLoS One 2016; 11(1): e0146351

Xin L, Yang X, Cai G, Fan D, Xia Q, Liu L, Hu Y, Ding N, Xu S, Wang L, Li X, Zou Y, Pan F, Serum levels of copper and zinc in patients with rheumatoid arthritis: A meta-analysis. Biol Trace Elem Res 2015; 168(1): 1–10

Yu N, Han F, Lin X, Tang C, Ye J, Cai X, The association between serum selenium levels with rheumatoid arthritis. Biol Trace Elem Res 2016; 172(1): 46–52

Schizophrenia

Chen AT, Chibnall JT, Nasrallah HA, A meta-analysis of placebo-controlled trials of omega-3 fatty acid augmentation in schizophrenia: Possible stage-specific effects. Ann Clin Psychiatry 2015; 27(4): 289–96

Firth J, Stubbs S, Sarris J, Rosenbaum S, Teasdale S, Berk M, Yung AR, The effects of vitamin and mineral supplementation on symptoms of schizophrenia: A systemic review and meta-analysis. Psychol Med 2017; 16:1–13

Sepsis

Alhazzani W, Jacobi J, Sindi A, Hartog C, Reinhart K, Kokkoris S, Gerlach H, Andrews P, Drabek T, Manzanares W, Cook DJ, Jaeschke RZ, The effect of selenium therapy on mortality in patients with sepsis syndrome: A systematic review and meta-analysis of randomized controlled trials. Crit Care Med 2013; 41(6): 1555–64

de Haan K, Groeneveld AB, de Geus HR, Egal M, Struijs A, Vitamin D deficiency as a risk factor for infection, sepsis and mortality in the critically ill: Systematic review and meta-analysis. Crit Care 2014; 18(6): 660

Upala S, Sanguankeo A, Permpalung N, Significant association between vitamin D deficiency and sepsis: A systematic review and meta-analysis. BMJ Anesthesiology 2015; 15:84

Sleep Apnea

Upala S, Sanguankeo A, Association between 25-hydroxyvitamin D and obstructive sleep apnea: A systematic review and meta-analysis. J Clin Sleep Med 2015; 11(11): 1347

Spina Bifida

Atta CA, Fiest KM, Frolkis AD, Jette N, Pringsheim T, St Germaine-Smith C, Rajapakse T, Kaplan GG, Metcalfe A, Global birth prevalence of spina bifida by folic acid fortification status: A systematic review and meta-analysis. Am J Public Health 2016; 106(1): e24–34

Stroke

Adebamowo SN, Spiegelman D, Willett WC, Rexrode KM, Association between intakes of magnesium, potassium and calcium and risk of stroke: 2 cohorts of US women and updated meta-analysis. Am J Clin Nutr 2015; 101(6): 1269–77

Chen GC, Lu DB, Pang Z, Liu QF, Vitamin C intake, circulating vitamin C and risk of stroke: A meta-analysis of prospective studies. J Am Heart Assoc 2013; 2(6): e000329

Dong H, Pi F, Ding Z, Chen W, Pang S, Dong W, Zhang Q, Efficacy of supplementation with B vitamins for stroke prevention: A network meta-analysis of randomized controlled trials. PLoS One 2015; 10(9): e137533

Larsson SC, Orsini N, Wolk A, Long-chain omega-3 polyunsaturated fatty acids and risk of stroke: A meta-analysis. Eur J Epidemiol 2012; 27(12): 895–901

Park JH, Saposnik G, Ovbiagele B, Markovic D, Towfighi A, Effect of B-vitamins on stroke risk among individuals with vascular disease who are not on antiplatelets: A meta-analysis. Int J Stroke 2016; 11(2): 206–11

Tian DY, Tian J, Shi CH, Song B, Wu J, Ji Y, Wang RH, Mao CY, Sun SL, Xu YM, Calcium intake and the risk of stroke: An up-dated meta-analysis of prospective studies. Asia Pac J Clin Nutr 2015; 24(2): 245–52

Tuberculosis

Zeng J, Wu G, Yang W, Gu X, Liang W, Yao Y, Song Y, A serum vitamin D level < 25 nmol/l pose high tuberculosis risk: A meta-analysis. PLoS One 2015; 10(5): e126014

Venous Thrombosis

Zhou K, Zhao R, Geng Z, Jiang L, Cao Y, Xu D, Liu Y, Huang L, Zhou J, Association between B-group vitamins and venous thrombosis: Review and meta-analysis of epidemiological studies. J Thromb Thrombolysis 2012; 34(4): 459–67

Vitiligo

Upala S, Sanguankeo A, Low 25-hydroxyvitamin D levels are associated with vitiligo: A systematic review and meta-analysis. Photodermatol Photoimmunol Photomed 2016; April 14: 10.1111/phpp.12241

Zeng Q, Yin J, Fan F, Chen J, Zuo C, Xiang Y, Tan L, Huang J, Xiao R, Decreased copper and zinc in sera of Chinese vitiligo patients: A meta-analysis. J Dermatol 2014; 41(3): 245–51

GLOSSARY

Adaptive immunity—The immune response mediated by lymphocytes is called adaptive immunity. B cells and T cells are the two major types of lymphocytes. B cells produce antibodies against pathogens, and T cells bind directly to pathogens.

Antioxidant—A molecule that inhibits the oxidation of other molecules is called an antioxidant. Antioxidants, such as vitamin C or vitamin E, can block the oxidation of biomolecules, such as lipids, proteins, or DNA in the body.

Apoptosis—The death of a cell that occurs in a programmed manner and leads to the elimination of the cell without affecting neighboring cells is called apoptosis. It is also called "programmed cell death."

Autoimmunity—The immune response that attacks the host's own healthy cells and tissues, mistaking them as foreign, is called autoimmunity. This aberrant immune response can lead to autoimmune diseases.

Autophagy—A cellular process by which unwanted debris in a cell is cleaned out is called autophagy. Autophagy plays important roles in the body's ability to getting rid of toxins and repair damage. However, cancer cells may utilize autophagy, also called "self-eating," to avoid destruction by the immune system.

Cofactor—A nonprotein molecule or metallic ion that supports enzymes in carrying out specific biochemical reactions is called a cofactor or an enzyme cofactor. A cofactor is like a facilitator.

DNA methylation—Cells control gene expression by adding methyl groups to a specific region of DNA in the chromosome. DNA methylation often turns off a target gene. Insufficient DNA methylation is a hallmark of cancerous cells.

Endothelial dysfunction—Normal functions of the endothelium in a blood vessel include acting as a barrier to control the traffic of substances into or out of the blood vessel, blood coagulation, and immune function. An imbalance between vasodilating and vasoconstricting molecules produced in the endothelium can lead to endothelial dysfunction, which can be caused by hypertension, diabetes, or high blood cholesterol.

Epigenetics—The study of how genes interact with environmental factors—such as diet, stress, or chemical pollutants—without the involvement of changes to the DNA sequence is called epigenetics.

Free radical—A molecule that contains one or more unpaired electrons is called a free radical. Free radicals are highly reactive molecules that can damage lipids, proteins, or DNA in a cell.

Gene polymorphism—The existence of multiple variants of a single gene in a given population is called gene polymorphism. Some variants of gene polymorphism are silent, while others may elevate the risk of diseases.

Inflammatory cytokine—Cell signing proteins that help cell-to-cell communication in immune responses as well as the movement of immune cells toward inflammatory sites are called inflammatory cytokines.

Innate immunity—Our first line of defense against pathogens—including the skin, respiratory and gastrointestinal tract, and macrophages residing in these regions—is called innate immunity. It acts as a physical and chemical barrier to defend against invaders.

Lipid peroxidation—Free radicals, such as hydroxyl radicals, "steal" electrons from the lipids in cell membranes, causing the oxidation of lipid molecules and subsequent destruction of cell membranes, which is called lipid peroxidation.

Meta-analysis—A statistical method that combines and analyzes data obtained from several selected studies to draw a single conclusion is called meta-analysis. Meta-analysis shows greater statistical power than that of any individual study.

One-carbon metabolism—*One-carbon* means "one methyl group." One-carbon metabolism is a biochemical pathway in which vitamin B6, vitamin 9 (folate), and vitamin B12 participate in enzymatic reactions by which one-carbon (methyl group) is transferred from one molecule to another molecule in a cell. One-carbon metabolism is crucial for the synthesis of certain amino acids, as well as the synthesis and repair of DNA.

Osteoblast—A cell that promotes bone formation in the bone tissues is called an osteoblast.

Osteoclast—A cell that promotes bone removal from the bone tissues is called an osteoclast.

Oxidation-reduction reaction—A chemical reaction in which a molecule loses electrons or is oxidized and another molecule gains electrons or is reduced is called an oxidation-reduction reaction, also known as "redox reaction."

Oxidative damage—Excessive amounts of free radicals cause deleterious and destructive effects on biomolecules, such as lipids, proteins, or DNA in a cell. That is called oxidative damage.

Oxidative stress—The condition when the amount of free radicals produced exceeds the antioxidant capacity in the body is called oxidative stress, which can lead to oxidative damage to biomolecules, such as lipids, proteins, or DNA in a cell.

Transcription factor—Transcription factors are proteins that help transcribe genetic information from DNA to messenger RNA by binding to specific DNA sequence in the cell nucleus.

ABBREVIATIONS

ADP—Adenosine diphosphate

ATP—Adenosine triphosphate

BDNF—Brain-derived neurotropic factor

BMI—Body mass index

DHA—Docosahexaenoic acid

DNA—Deoxyribonucleic acid

DXA—Dual-energy X-ray absorptiometry

EPA—Eicosapentaenoic acid

ER and **PR** (positive breast cancer)—Estrogen receptor and progesterone receptor (positive breast cancer)

ESR—Electron spin resonance

FAD—Flavin adenine dinucleotide

FDA—Federal Drug Administration

FLG—Filaggrin

FMN—Flavin mononucleotide

FVC—Forced vital capacity

HDL—High-density lipoprotein

HIV—Human immunodeficiency virus

HIV-RNA—Human immunodeficiency virus–ribonucleic acid

HLA—Human leukocyte antigen

HLA-RB1—Human leukocyte antigen—retinoblastoma1

HPV—Human papillomavirus

ICA—Internal carotid artery

IV—Intravenous

LASIK—Laser-assisted in situ keratomileusis

LDL—Low-density lipoprotein

MRI—Magnetic resonance imaging

NAD—Nicotinamide adenine dinucleotide

NADP—Nicotinamide adenine dinucleotide phosphate

NIH—National Institutes of Health

NNK—Nicotine-derived nitrosamine ketone

NSAID—Nonsteroidal anti-inflammatory drug

PDGF—Platelet-derived growth factor

PLP—Pyridoxal-5`-phosphate

PMP—Pyridoxamine-5`-phosphate

TPP—Thiamine pyrophosphate

USDA—United States Department of Agriculture

WHO—World Health Organization

INDEX

Page numbers followed by *t* refer to tables.